PANDEMIC DISEASE IN THE MEDIEVAL WORLD

THE MEDIEVAL GLOBE

The Medieval Globe provides an interdisciplinary forum for scholars of all world areas by focusing on convergence, movement, and interdependence. Contributions to a global understanding of the medieval period (broadly defined) need not encompass the globe in any territorial sense. Rather, *TMG* advances a new theory and praxis of medieval studies by bringing into view phenomena that have been rendered practically or conceptually invisible by anachronistic boundaries, categories, and expectations. *TMG* also broadens discussion of the ways that medieval processes inform the global present and shape visions of the future.

Volume 1

PANDEMIC DISEASE IN THE MEDIEVAL WORLD

RETHINKING THE BLACK DEATH

Edited by MONICA H. GREEN

ARC MEDIEVAL PRESS

Copyeditor
Shannon Cunningham

Editorial Assistant
Ann Hubert

Page design and typesetting
Martine Maguire-Weltecke

Printed and bound in the United States of America

Library of Congress Cataloging in Publication Data
A catalog record for this book is available from the Library of Congress

ISBN 978-1-942401-00-1
e-ISBN 978-1-942401-01-8

www.arc-humanities.org

CONTENTS

LIST OF ILLUSTRATIONS

Figures

Plates

Graphs

Maps

Tables

PREFACE

THE BLACK DEATH AND EBOLA: ON THE VALUE OF COMPARISON

MONICA H. GREEN

> It was as if the voice of existence in the world had called out for oblivion and restriction, and the world had responded to its call.
>
> Ibn Khaldun, d. 1406

THE ESSAYS THAT make up *Pandemic Disease in the Medieval World: Rethinking the Black Death* grew out of dialogue first begun in 2009. The volume itself began to come together in the spring of 2013 and was sent to press a year later. Little did we know that by the time the volume would appear in November 2014, the world's relationship to epidemic infectious disease would have taken such an abrupt turn. At the time of this writing, the 2014 West African Ebola epidemic has already caused over twenty-one thousand cases and taken over eight thousand lives.[1] Declared a Public Health Emergency of International Concern on August 8, 2014 by the World Health Organization (WHO), the Ebola outbreak prompted a United Nations (UN) Security Council meeting several weeks later. At that session on September 18, the resulting UN resolution called the outbreak a "threat to international peace and security," garnering the highest level of support in the history of the organization. The West African Ebola outbreak has disrupted the economies and trade relations of countries in West Africa and beyond. It has decimated the already strained healthcare personnel of the three most affected countries. It has left hundreds of children orphaned and disrupted the education and welfare of many thousands more. For the families whose loved ones make up those statistics, no relativizing of numbers can offer solace. From the perspective of the devastated countries of Guinea, Sierra Leone, and Liberia, the Tunisian historian Ibn Khaldun's bleak assessment of the world after the Black Death could just as well have been written today.

1 I will refer to this as the 2014 outbreak, even though evidence suggests it began in late 2013 and, at the time of writing, gives every sign of continuing well into 2015.

Plague is not Ebola Virus Disease. Many of the easy parallels that were drawn in the popular press in mid-2014 between the unfolding Ebola outbreak and the medieval Black Death were exaggerated or careless. In several respects, Ebola is better compared to other diseases. The current Ebola epidemic has brought back memories of the 2002–2003 SARS epidemic, whose intercontinental spread was also abetted by airline travel; or the ongoing HIV/AIDS pandemic, which has been surrounded by intense debates about drug development and ethical provision of treatment. In its mode of transmission via human bodily fluids, Ebola is similar to cholera, though this virus is fragile in the extreme compared to the hardy bacterium, which thrives in open brackish water. In its current form—a virus passing directly from one human to another—Ebola more closely resembles smallpox, which made its zoonotic leap into humans several thousand years ago. Nevertheless, with comparable case fatality rates and rapid progress from infection to death, plague and Ebola elicit a terror few other infectious diseases have produced. With this re-issue of our essays in book form, it will be good to set the Black Death—or really, the Second Plague Pandemic in all its immensity—into a larger context. And in that task, comparisons with the current Ebola outbreak are indeed useful, both for better understanding our collective past and for anticipating our common future.

If a Tree Falls? Invisible Pandemics

In August through October of 2014, dire predictions of Ebola's exponential growth were being made on the basis of mathematical modeling. One particularly alarming model, released 23 September, predicted that the epidemic might reach 1.4 million cases by January 2015, in Sierra Leone and Liberia alone (Meltzer et al. 2014). Similarly, predictions of exported cases—fueled by the documented transfer of the disease to Nigeria late in July, followed by a similar case that reached the United States in September—raised fears of outbreaks not simply elsewhere in Africa, but in large population centers in Asia and Latin America, which might not have the public health infrastructure to identify and contain new cases. The West African Ebola epidemic has not, as of this writing, become a pandemic. But it certainly had the potential to become one. And that is the more important point.

All pandemics start as local outbreaks. In the case of the West African Ebola epidemic, it is now understood to have started as early as December 2013 in a rural area of Guinea (Baize et al. 2014; Saéz et al. 2014/2015). It was not until March 2014 that the outbreak was officially acknowledged, and then only because the alarum had been raised by local doctors and the international medical charity, Médecins Sans Frontières (Doctors Without Borders), which already had a presence in Guinea to treat HIV/AIDS and malaria. In the early, "silent" phase of transmission—when deaths were mounting but no diagnosis had been made to link them to Ebola—the disease was able to establish itself in three countries.

A major objective of the present volume is to make the radical claim that the Second Plague Pandemic likely had "silent" phases, too. As awful as we have always thought the Black Death to be, the essays in this volume argue that it was likely even worse, because its full geographical or chronological extent had never before been conceptualized. As Robert Hymes recounts in his essay here, many historians of China have long doubted whether plague was even present in medieval China. That debate is sure to continue, but it now has to take seriously the implications of the phylogenetics of *Yersinia pestis*, which point strongly not simply to *Y. pestis*'s origins in regions that now fall within China's western borders, but also to a sudden evolutionary divergence of the organism around the thirteenth century. Just as historians of late antiquity have only recently realized how profound a role plague may have played in weakening the Roman Empire (see particularly Mitchell 2014), so with the Black Death we now have reason to suspect that it, too, had periods not simply when it was moving through wild animal communities with little or no human involvement, but also periods when it produced human outbreaks that we have failed to recognize as indications of epidemic disease. As we fully acknowledge here, to date we have no explanation for how plague might have moved across central Eurasia in the thirteenth and early fourteenth centuries.[2] And its postulated presence in sub-Saharan Africa still demands full investigation.[3] But as both Ann Carmichael and Nükhet Varlık show in this volume, careful gathering and sifting of local historical data can produce evidence suggestive of plague's stealthy focalization in new ecological niches.

2 Despite the rapid growth of Mongol studies in the past two decades (Biran 2013), the few scholars who have engaged with the question of plague simply repeat findings from McNeill 1976 or draw on western sources; an exception is Schamiloglu (1993). Aside from Buell (2012) (who denies that there were any significant outbreaks of human plague in Mongol China) and Hymes (in this volume, who asserts that there were several, pushing their presence back to the thirteenth century), there has as yet been no engagement with the genetics research on *Y. pestis* by historians of Central Asia.

3 After these essays originally went to press, I discovered that Gérard Chouin, now at the College of William and Mary, has taken his earlier suggestions about the possibility of a Black Death impact in late medieval West Africa and expanded them into a full research project. See Chouin 2013.

Relatively speaking, the 2014 Ebola outbreak did not long escape notice. But what if something like the Ebola outbreak had started a hundred years earlier, before cell phones and satellites and the Internet? We don't know how old Ebola Virus Disease is, and have no way of knowing right now whether it has caused any large-scale human outbreaks prior to its official biomedical discovery in 1976. We do not have to imagine, however, the possibility of silent epidemics, or even pandemics. We already know, from the reconstructed history of the early decades of HIV/AIDS, how a local disease can become a pandemic—invisibly. HIV/AIDS did not begin in 1981, when the first study by the Centers for Disease Control described five cases of unexplained *Pneumocystis carinii* pneumonia in Los Angeles. Rather, it began in Cameroon around 1920 and spread soon thereafter to Leopoldville in the Belgian Congo (now Kinshasa in the Democratic Republic of the Congo) and beyond (Faria et al. 2014). By the time the first published clinical descriptions appeared in 1981, the virus had already spread to all five inhabited continents and at least a million people were already infected.

Animal and Human Origins

Both plague and the 2014 Ebola outbreak reflect our recent understanding that many infectious diseases are of zoonotic origin.[4] In some cases, those viruses or microbial pathogens have been long accustomed to their animal hosts and cause only minimal disease. Once transferred into humans, however, these viruses or microbes become merciless killers. Ebola and plague are zoonotics in different senses, of course. Like HIV/AIDS,[5] the current West African Ebola outbreak seems to have arisen from one animal-to-human transfer of the virus, and then took off in a series of continued human-to-human transfers because of shared practices of caretaking in the home or preparations for burial (Gire et al. 2014). Plague, in contrast, can only maintain short bursts of human-to-human transfer and then only under two conditions: either in the form of septicemic plague, when certain medical interventions—such as lancing of buboes (see the

---

4 Morse and colleagues (2012) estimate that roughly 80% of viruses, 50% of bacteria, 40% of fungi, 70% of protozoa, and 95% of helminths that infect human beings are of zoonotic origin.

5 I am referring here, of course, only to HIV-1, Group M, which has been responsible for the global pandemic and which, according to current understanding, passed to humans via a single transmission from a *Pan troglodytes troglodytes* chimpanzee. On the Ebola virus, see Baize et al. 2014 and Gire et al. 2014.

image on p. 230 of this volume)—can transmit the disease from patient to caretaker; or, as a more common mode, in the form of pneumonic plague, when the plague bacterium is transferred in aerosolized form from a person with infiltrated lungs to others not yet infected. Needing crowded (and often cold) conditions, pneumonic plague outbreaks burn out quickly. However, if we think of plague not as a single organism but as an ecological package—the rodent-arthropod-bacterium nexus—then situations that bring that package into close, commensal relationships with human populations can create sustained human disease at the population level. For both diseases, therefore, the potential to tap into human networks of communication is what allows them to turn from small outbreaks into widely disseminated diseases.

A study that appeared in September 2014 suggested that Ebola was likely already present in the animal populations of at least twenty-two African countries (Pigott et al. 2014). Although not yet definitively proven as the main transmitters of the Ebola virus, bats are the likeliest suspect (Saéz et al. 2014/2015); as flying animals, their ability to transmit the disease across wide regions is distinctive. That Ebola was already a disease "underfoot" across wide swaths of Central Africa was, of course, already known, a fact underscored by the second outbreak in the Democratic Republic of the Congo in 2014, which caused sixty-six cases, including forty-nine deaths (WHO 2014). However, unnoticed by Pigott and colleagues, and by all other accounts of the Ebola outbreak in West Africa in the summer and fall of 2014, was the fact that studies going back to the late 1970s already documented that individuals in Liberia and Sierra Leone carried antibodies to Ebola in their blood. It would seem, therefore, that Ebola was already widely disseminated in animal populations in sub-Saharan Africa (including West Africa) prior to 2013, and it is possible for similar outbreaks to occur so long as animals infected with the virus are consumed for food.[6]

Even before extensive genetics studies were done of the Ebola virus circulating in West Africa, it was noted that the 2014 disease outbreak

6 Van der Waals et al. (1986) and Knobloch et al. (1982), neither of which were cited by Schoepp et al. (2014), which found nearly comparable levels of seroprevalence of Ebola antibodies. Cf. Becquart et al. (2010) for a similar study of Gabon based on samples taken in 2006–08. Importantly, scientists have noted for more than a decade that major die-offs were occurring from Ebola in primate populations in West Central Africa; see Muyembe-Tamfum et al. 2012. Saéz et al. (2014/2015), however, found no evidence of such die-offs in primate or other non-bat populations in the area of Guinea where the 2014 outbreak is thought to have begun.

was different from all previous ones, moving faster and into larger populations. But this is not because the *virus* was significantly different from those strains that had already caused several dozen outbreaks across Central Africa since 1976; rather, the 2014 outbreak was different because *Africa* was different. In seeking to understand what sparked the initial zoonotic transfer, questions have been raised as to whether new agricultural practices or other interventions have disrupted ecosystems in West Africa, making certain kinds of human-animal contact more likely (Wallace et al. 2014). More significantly, it has been noted that Africa in 2014 was different from Africa in 1976 in that there was greater socioeconomic diversity and new kinds of interconnectivity (Osterholm 2014). Whereas earlier outbreaks had occurred mostly in isolated rural regions, where there were few cars or other connections to major population centers, the 2014 outbreak was characterized by its quick linkage to large urban areas, which in turn facilitated further spread both near and far.

Plague, too, is now "underfoot" in many regions of the world. How it came to be so was not (so far as we know) because of transmission by bats, but because the micro-environments which *Yersinia pestis* demands—the rodent-arthropod-bacterium nexus—managed to hook into human networks supporting the material exchange of goods (grain, textiles, furs). That has happened at least three times in history, and (to judge from the surviving genetic evidence) likely more.[7] To what extent the three known plague pandemics—the Justinianic (so-called because it seemed to begin in 541 CE, during the reign of the Roman emperor Justinian), the Second Pandemic (commencing with the Black Death), and the Third Pandemic (commencing in the mid-nineteenth century)—were all magnified in their intensity by changing climate conditions has not yet been pinned down, though evidence is mounting for a major climatic element in the first two cataclysms (Sarris 2012; Campbell 2013; Brooke 2014). But for both the Justinianic Plague and the Black Death, the climate element did not *cause* the pandemics. Rather, it seems to have served as an *amplifier* of conditions that were already in the making. Even if the dust-veil event of 536 CE, which was followed by several years of cold weather and darkened skies, can be called the precipitator of the plague epidemics that broke out around the Mediterranean, that still does not explain how *Yersinia pestis* had *already* managed to wend its way from the Qinghai-Tibet Plateau into nearby territories like the kingdom of Aksum (encompassing parts of

---

7 See below, pp. 40–41, on the so-called "Angola" strain of *Yersinia pestis*, and also pp. 14, 39, 43n21, 199n12, 200n16, and 208n30, on the still unexplained dissemination of the so-called MEDIEVALIS strain across much of Eurasia.

modern Yemen, Ethiopia, and neighboring states at the mouth of the Red Sea), which was one of the main trading hubs linking Indian Ocean trade with that of the Mediterranean basin in the fifth and sixth centuries (Gebre Selassie 2011; Seland 2014). Even if the extreme weather that Campbell (2013) has now documented for the 1340s precipitated the sudden explosion of plague into new European and Mediterranean environments, and (if we can extrapolate) facilitated the focalization and persistence of plague in the European Alps as the chill of the Little Ice Age took hold, as Carmichael suggests in this volume, Hymes (also this volume) suggests we still must look at the extreme warfare, more than one hundred years earlier in an entirely different part of the Eurasian continent, to see what forces nudged *Yersinia pestis* out of its marmot burrows. And as Harrison (2012) has documented for plague and several other epidemic diseases that terrorized the world in the past five hundred years, human networks of trade have continued to play their role.

Whether climate change has played a role in the two dozen Ebola outbreaks known to have occurred since 1976 is not at all clear. Nevertheless, in assessing the pandemic potential of both diseases, we have to look to common *human* practices that facilitate disease transmission and the ways that local practices can connect to global networks. Seemingly innocent practices of human provision—eating bats or chimpanzees and hunting marmots, whether for food or for furs—have created conditions ripe for disease transfer. But those individual circumstances of disease transfer only develop pandemic potential when they are linked to wider networks of human exchange.

Comparing Crises

The time is not yet ripe for a historical post-mortem on all we have seen in terms of political posturing, economic collapse, or human bravery and compassion in the past few months of the 2014 West African Ebola epidemic. Nor was *Pandemic Disease in the Medieval World: Rethinking the Black Death* conceived specifically for comparative purposes, since it is not a general summary of the later medieval plague pandemic. The reader will find here no definitive estimates of total mortality or rehearsals of social catastrophe narrated by Boccaccio and his contemporaries. We do not offer an account of the history of quarantine nor, indeed, do we have much to say about the history of medical remedies for plague. Rather, we present this as an opportunity to think through, in a new way, what it really means for infectious disease to emerge or re-emerge—to move quickly and widely through human populations which are never (whatever we like to think to the contrary) wholly divorced from their ecological landscapes.

There is an important trend now in historical studies: not only to move analysis beyond the limits of the nation-state and even the human organism, but also to move it into deeper time scales. Although some diseases (like malaria and various kinds of parasites) have likely been with humans for many millennia (e.g., Webb forthcoming), increasing congregations of human populations into urban settlements have amplified the impact of infectious diseases in a shorter timescale, perhaps some 4,000 to 6,000 years, in both the Old World and the New. No definitive shift separates us from that history of increasing urbanization and the networking of human communities through long-distance trade. Granted, the revolution in scientific understanding of infectious diseases brought about by the great late nineteenth-century revelations of germ theory did put us on a whole new footing with respect to *understanding* infectious disease. But only one infectious disease has since been thoroughly eradicated (smallpox). Malaria and tuberculosis are still high on the list of the world's killers; plague, as we have noted, is embedded in the landscapes of four continents, still regularly producing outbreaks in Madagascar, Peru, Vietnam, Central Africa, and China; cholera still rears its head in any number of places, most recently in Haiti and Ghana. And for all of these diseases, antibiotic resistance is weakening the arsenal of defenses we have. Ebola's "small" numbers or (currently) limited geography should not, therefore, in any way be dismissed. Rather, we should think of this as a real-time lesson in how local diseases become global.

Recent comparisons of Ebola and plague have often been accompanied by an implicit shudder of horror: "How *medieval*." Yes, the practice of quarantine—so discredited when it was invoked by the Liberian government in August 2014 in its own capital of Monrovia, and implicitly by many other nations as they closed their borders to travellers from West Africa and cut off air transport—is medieval in its origins, even if practices of segregation and exclusion of suspected infectious persons are much older (Grmek 1980). Yes, the sight of bodies being piled in streets calls to mind the chilling stories of the Black Death's devastation. When Centers for Disease Control director Thomas Frieden described the situation in West Africa in October 2014 as "something out of Dante," he can be forgiven for apparently eliding the description of hell in the *Inferno* (which was written more than a quarter century before the arrival of the Black Death in Europe) with the hellish scenes Dante's Italian kindred would describe several decades later.[8] But this derogatory deployment of

8 Sun et al. 2014: "Frieden had seen plenty of death over the years, but this was far worse than he expected, a plague on a medieval scale. 'A scene out of Dante,' he called it."

"the medieval" does not get us very far. Universities are "medieval," too, as are public health regulations, autopsies, and the licensing of medical practitioners. The presence of a highly sophisticated biomedical infrastructure in the later twentieth century did not stop the HIV/AIDS pandemic from exploding, and it has not (yet) stopped the current Ebola outbreak. The journal that gave birth to these essays, *The Medieval Globe*, was founded to ask what it means for the Middle Ages to stop being "Other" and to become knowable. With climate change, among other factors, pushing the homeostasis of our own world out of balance, the past—which is the only knowable guide we have to the future—merits revisiting.

* * *

My thanks to Robert and Saul Hymes for their very helpful suggestions. Once again, let me take this opportunity to thank Carol Symes, founding executive editor of *The Medieval Globe*, for taking a leap of faith in agreeing to let this volume inaugurate the journal. Thanks as well to Simon Forde and all the production staff at Arc-Medieval Press.

Phoenix, Arizona
13 January 2015

Bibliography

Baize, Sylvain, Delphine Pannetier, Lisa Oestereich, Toni Rieger, et al. 2014. "Emergence of Zaire Ebola Virus Disease in Guinea," *New England Journal of Medicine* 371: 1418–25 (October 9) [preliminary report published online on April 16; final report published online on September 19]

Becquart, Pierre, Nadia Wauquier, Tanel Mahlakõiv, Dieudonné Nkoghe, et al. 2010. "High Prevalence of Both Humoral and Cellular Immunity to *Zaire ebolavirus* among Rural Populations in Gabon," *PLoS ONE* 5, no. 2: e0009126

Biran, Michal. 2013. "The Mongol Empire: The State of the Research," *History Compass* 11, no. 11: 1021–33

Brooke, John. 2014. *Climate Change and the Course of Global History: A Rough Journey* (Cambridge: Cambridge University Press)

Buell, Paul D. 2012. "Qubilai and the Rats," *Sudhoffs Archiv* 96, no. 2: 127–44

Campbell, Bruce M. S. 2013. "The Great Transition: Climate, Disease and Society in the 13th and 14th Centuries," The Ellen McArthur Lectures, University of Cambridge <http://www.econsoc.hist.cam.ac.uk/podcast-campbell.html> [accessed January 9, 2014]

Chouin, Gérard. 2013. "Fossés, enceintes et peste noire en Afrique de l'Ouest forestière (500–1500 AD): réflexions sous canopée," *Afrique: Archéologie & Arts* 9: 43–66

Faria, Nuno R., Andrew Rambaut, Marc A. Suchard, Guy Baele, et al. 2014. "The Early Spread and Epidemic Ignition of HIV-1 in Human Populations," *Science* 3 (October): 56–61

Gebre Selassie, Yohannes. 2011. "Plague as a Possible Factor for the Decline and Collapse of the Aksumite Empire: A New Interpretation," *ITYOPIS — Northeast African Journal of Social Sciences and Humanities* 1: 36–61

Gire, Stephen K., Augustine Goba, Kristian G. Andersen, Rachel S. G. Sealfon, et al. 2014. "Genomic Surveillance Elucidates Ebola Virus Origin and Transmission during the 2014 Outbreak," *Science* <doi: 10.1126/science.1259657> (August 28)

Grmek, Mirko Dražen. 1980. "Le concept d'infection dans l'antiquité et au moyen âge, les anciennes measures sociales contra les maladies contagieuses et la foundation de la première quarantine à Dubrovnik (1377)," in *Radovi sa Međunarodnog simpozija u povodu šestote obljetnice dubrovačke karantene: Dubrovnik, 29. i 30. rujna 1977*, Rad Jugoslavenske akademije znanosti i umjetnosti, 384: Razred za medicinske znanosti, 16, 9–55, Zagreb: Jugoslavenska akademija znanosti i umjetnosti

Harrison, Mark. 2012. *Contagion: How Commerce Has Spread Disease* (New Haven: Yale University Press)

Ibn Khaldun, Abū Zayd. 1375–79/1967. *The Muqaddimah: An Introduction to History*, trans. Franz Rosenthal (Princeton, NJ: Princeton University Press) <http://www.scribd.com/doc/8205879/Muqaddamah-Ibn-Khaldun> [accessed January 14, 2013]

Knobloch, J., E. J. Albiez, and H. Schmitz. 1982. "A Serological Survey on Viral Haemorrhagic Fevers in Liberia," *Annales de l'Institut Pasteur/Virologie* 133, no. 2: 125–28

McNeill, William H. 1976. *Plagues and Peoples* (New York: Anchor)

Meltzer, Martin I., Charisma Y. Atkins, Scott Santibanez, Barbara Knust, et al. 2014. "Estimating the Future Number of Cases in the Ebola Epidemic — Liberia and Sierra Leone, 2014–2015," *Morbidity and Mortality Weekly Report* 63, no. 3: 1–14 (September 26)

Mitchell, Stephen. 2014. *A History of the Later Roman Empire, AD 284–641*, 2nd ed. (New York: Wiley-Blackwell)

Morse, S. S., J. A. K. Mazet, M. Woolhouse, C. R. Parrish, et al. 2012. "Prediction and Prevention of the Next Pandemic Zoonosis," *Lancet* 380: 1956–65

Muyembe-Tamfum, J. J., S. Mulangu, Justin Masumu, J. M. Kayembe, et al. 2012. "Ebola Virus Outbreaks in Africa: Past and Present," *Onderstepoort Journal of Veterinary Research* 79, no. 2: art. 451 <http://dx.doi. org/10.4102/ojvr.v79i2.451>

Osterholm, Michael. 2014. "What We Need to Fight Ebola," *Washington Post*, August 1, 2014 <http://www.washingtonpost.com/opinions/what-we-need-to-fight-ebola/2014/08/01/41f4dbb8-182d-11e4-9349-84d4a85be981_story.html> [accessed August 1, 2014]

Pigott, David M., Nick Golding, Adrian Mylne, Zhi Huang, et al. 2014. "Mapping the Zoonotic Niche of Ebola Virus Disease in Africa," *eLIFE* 3: e04395 (September 8)

Saéz, Almudena Marí, Sabrina Weiss, Kathrin Nowak, Vincent Lapeyre, et al. 2014/2015. "Investigating the Zoonotic Origin of the West African Ebola Epidemic," *EMBO Molecular Medicine* (published online December 30)

Sarris, Peter. 2012. "Unlucky For Some? David Keys' *Catastrophe* Thirteen Years On," paper presented at Amherst College, April 14 , 2012 (cited with permission)

Schamiloglu, Uli. 1993. "Preliminary Remarks on the Role of Disease in the History of the Golden Horde," *Central Asian Survey* 12: 447–57

Schoepp, Randal J., Cynthia A. Rossi, Sheik H. Khan, Augustine Goba, et al. 2014. "Undiagnosed Acute Viral Febrile Illnesses, Sierra Leone," *Emerging Infectious Diseases* 20, no. 7 (July): 1176–82

Seland, Eivind Heldas. 2014. "Early Christianity in East Africa and Red Sea/Indian Ocean Commerce," *African Archaeological Review* 31, no. 4: 637–47 (published online November 18)

Sun, Lena H., Brady Dennis, Lenny Bernstein, Joel Achenbach. 2014. "Out of Control: How the World's Health Organizations Failed to Stop the Ebola Disaster," *Washington Post* (October 4) <http://www.washingtonpost.com/sf/national/2014/10/04/how-ebola-sped-out-of-control/> [accessed October 10, 2014]

Van der Waals, F.W., K. L. Pomeroy, J. Goudsmit, D. M. Asher, et al. 1986. "Hemorrhagic Fever Virus Infections in an Isolated Rainforest Area of Central Liberia: Limitations of the Indirect Immunofluorescence Slide Test for Antibody Screening in Africa," *Tropical and Geographical Medicine* 38, no. 3: 209–14

Wallace, Robert G., Marius Gilbert, Rodrick Wallace, Claudia Pittiglio, et al. 2014. "Did Ebola Emerge in West Africa by a Policy-Driven Phase Change in Agroecology?," *Environment and Planning A* 46: <doi:10.1068/a4712com>

Webb, James L. A., Jr. Forthcoming. "Early Malarial Infections and the First Epidemiological Transition," in *From Colonisation to Globalisation: Species Move-*

ments in Human History, ed. Michael Petraglia and Nicole Boivin (Cambridge: Cambridge University Press)

WHO (World Health Organization). 2014. "Ebola Response Roadmap Situation Report" (October 31)

WHO Ebola Response Team. 2014. "Ebola Virus Disease in West Africa — The First 9 Months of the Epidemic and Forward Projections," *New England Journal of Medicine* (September 23) <doi: 10.1056/NEJMoa1411100>

Monica H. Green (Monica.Green@asu.edu) is a historian of medieval European medicine and global health. In 2009 and 2012, she ran a National Endowment for the Humanities Summer Seminar in London on "Health and Disease in the Middle Ages," which had as its central goal the exploration of ways that the scientific and humanistic disciplines could engage in productive dialogue about the history of disease and health-seeking behaviors. During this same period, she has also argued for the development of a new field, "Global History of Health," which explores the evolution of the major pathogens that have afflicted the human species since its origin up to the present day, and the ways that human cultural changes have facilitated or hindered those pathogens' trajectories. In addition to many works on the cultural history of medieval medicine, she is the author of "The Value of Historical Perspective," in *The Ashgate Research Companion to the Globalization of Health*, ed. Ted Schrecker (Aldershot: Ashgate, 2012), pp. 7–37; and "The Globalisations of Disease," which will be published in 2015.

Abstract The 2014 West African Ebola epidemic shocked a world that had grown insensitive to the threat of major epidemic infectious disease outbreaks. Looking for analogies, popular media that year often invoked the Black Death as a comparison. In this preface to the book edition of *Pandemic Disease in the Medieval World: Rethinking the Black Death*, it is argued that while most of the extreme comparisons of the Black Death and Ebola were unhelpful, the largest pandemic in human history can be used comparatively to think through certain frameworks of global health and emerging disease analysis. All pandemics start as local outbreaks. Studying the processes by which local outbreaks (often invisible in their early phases) grow into disease events of major historical import focuses our attention on the contingent historical circumstances that can move microorganisms through vast human networks of contact and exchange.

Keywords pandemics, global health, 2014 West African Ebola epidemic, Second Plague Pandemic, HIV/AIDS, zoonoses

INTRODUCING *THE MEDIEVAL GLOBE*

CAROL SYMES

WHEN A CERTAIN Genoese mariner sailed southward to find the elusive Indies, he was guided by two favorite books. We know one as *The Travels of Marco Polo*: the product of a collaboration between that Venetian merchant-adventurer and his cellmate in a Genoese prison, a purveyor of popular romances named Rustichello of Pisa. This book was composed around 1298, in a literary creole designated today as "Franco-Italian," but it was soon circulating widely in many different languages and editions. (There is no "original" text; the copy owned and annotated by that famous mariner was a later Latin translation.[1]) The other book, attributed to one Johan (or John) de Mandeville, was published around the middle of the fourteenth century, in the French dialect then prevalent in England. It, too, survives in numerous variants, none of which is the "original" text. In its own time, the former work was often titled *Le devisement du monde* (The Description of the World), *Le livre des merveilles* (The Book of Marvels), or *Il milione* (The Million). The latter work was also known as *Le livre des merveilles*.

Along with their titles, these influential texts share some other salient characteristics: authorial and linguistic indeterminacy, a tangled history of transmission and reception, the tendency to imprint ancient imaginaries on a mesh of contemporary fantasy and observation. What were these books supposed to be about? How were they understood by generations of readers? To what extent do they constitute evidence for contemporary worldviews? Such questions are open to debate. In essence, these books are not travel narratives or practical manuals: they are *mises-en-abyme*. The mysterious conditions of their making underscore the challenges of knowing anything about the world they purport to describe—the difficulty, even, of talking about that world in terms that mirror its own conceptual categories. ("Franco-Italian," "the French dialect of England," the literary work as a fixed entity: all of these are anachronisms.) Yet like so many readers before me, I have drawn inspiration from one of these books.

---

1 It is now in the library of the Institución Colombina in Sevilla (Spain). For an excellent introduction to this multi-layered text, see Gaunt (2013). See also Kinoshita (2013), whose new annotated translation of the text is forthcoming. On the reasons for the southerly course charted by Columbus, see Wey Gómez (2008).

> On this topic, I've many times recalled something I heard when I was young, about how a brave man once left our parts in order to explore the world. So he passed through India and the islands beyond India (where there are more than five thousand islands) and went so far by sea and by land—so far around the world for so many seasons—that he found an island where he heard his own language spoken, and even heard the oxen being called in the very same words as in his own country, so that he was much amazed. Because he did not know how that could ever be. But I say that he had gone so far by land and by sea that he had gone around the whole earth, that he had come right back around to his own borders. And if he had only gone a bit further on, he would have found his own lands and his own knowledge. But he went all the way back the way he had come and so lost much of his effort, just as he himself said, a great while after, when he finally returned.[2]

This story captures the alienation experienced by anyone who ventures beyond the bounds of homely knowledge. It warns that my own neighborhood will come to seem so strange, in a global context, that I won't recognize it. But it also holds out hope that I'll achieve, in time, a broader vision.

The Medieval Globe is dedicated to exploring varieties of connectivity, communication, and exchange during a period central to human history: the millennium or so prior to 1500. It is an interdisciplinary journal for all scholars studying any aspect of this era, including those who work in parts of the medieval world that may seem well trodden and familiar (in my case, Western Europe). A global approach to medieval studies need not encompass the globe in any territorial sense. Rather, *The Medieval Globe* seeks to advance a new theory and praxis of medieval studies by encouraging the investigation of phenomena that have been rendered practically or conceptually invisible by modern categories and expectations: move-

---

2 "Et pur ceo m'ad il souvenuz mointefoiz d'une chose qe jeo oÿ compter quant jeo fuy jeovenes, comment un vaillant homme s'em party jadis de noz parties pur aler ceercher le mounde. Si passa Ynde et les isles outre Ynde ou il y a plus de V^{m} isles, et tant ala par mer et par terre et tant envirouna le mounde par mointes saisouns q'il troeva un isle ou il oÿ parler soun langage et toucher les boefs en disant tieles paroles come l'em fait en son pays don't il s'enmerveilla moult. Qar il ne savoit coment ceo poait estre. Mes jeo dy q'il avoit tant irré par terre et par mer q'il avoit environé toute la terre, qu'il estoit revenuz envyronant jusqes a ses marches, et s'il vousist avoir passé avant q'il eust troevé et son pays et sa connaissance. Mes il retorna ariere par illecques ou il estoit venuz, si perdy assez de ses peines si come il mesmes le disoit un grand piece après q'il fust revenuz" (Mandeville [*c.* 1357]/2000: 337, my translation). On the manuscript history and variants of this text, see the editorial introduction of Christiane Deluz (Mandeville [*c.* 1357]/2000: 28–84).

ments, networks, interactions, affinities, borrowings, ways of knowing, forms of agency, systems of belief. This enterprise has the potential to expand our understanding of long-term global developments while simultaneously transforming the ways that we approach this particular age.

Although "the medieval globe" might seem to be a contradiction in terms, its components have an old and complicated relationship. The "discovery" of a "new world" unsettled Europeans' understanding of their place in world history at a time when the expansion of the mighty Ottoman empire, and intensified contact with the civilizations of South and East Asia, were also posing new threats and opportunities. Meanwhile, notions of territorial sovereignty in Europe itself were being based on powerful historical fictions that some states had a warrant to colonize others. Although the terms "medieval" and "Middle Ages" were not coined until the early nineteenth century (Stein 1995), the complex associations that eventually crystallized in these terms were already forming in the very early sixteenth (Dagenais and Greer 2000; Summit and Wallace 2006; Davis 2008). On the one hand, this medieval past became a source of legitimacy and identity, an object of reverence and nostalgia; on the other, it was construed as a "feudal age" of cruelty and ignorance. Non-European cultures were accordingly described as "medieval" in order to subordinate and denigrate them (Wolf 1982; Davis and Altschul 2009). The current use of "medieval" as a synonym for "primitive" or "inhuman" continues this trend (e.g., Holsinger 2007); at the same time, the Middle Ages continues to be the cradle of the West's vaunted superiority, the font of romantic mythologies and "natural" rights (Geary 2002; Symes 2011a; Geary and Klaniczy 2013).

In many ways, then, the concept of "the Middle Ages" made possible "the modern world-system" heralded by Wallerstein (1974); "the medieval" and "the global" defined each other. If they now appear to denote mutually exclusive realms of inquiry, that is because triumphal narratives of modernity require them to remain separate (Abu-Lughod 1989; Gaonkar 2000; Bennett 2006; Goody 2006; Sassen 2008; Symes 2011b). Nationalist origin stories and universal teleologies do not work when events and their outcomes are viewed as the products of chancy, contingent forces (Smail et al. 2011). Only in the past two decades, for example, have Europe's component regions—and "Europe" itself—been recognized as colonized and postcolonial spaces (e.g., Bartlett 1994; Cohen 2000; Fernández-Armesto and Muldoon 2008; Murray 2009). Yet there is still tremendous resistance to critical approaches that would threaten claims of political autonomy or territory staked in medieval precedent. New paradigms that would debunk the presumption of an essential binary between "East" and "West" (or "Muslim" and "Christian," for example) also generate resistance, and are consequently all the more important (see, e.g., Lieberman 1999; McCormick 2001; Grabar 2006; Komaroff 2006; Lieberman 2007–09; Sizgorich 2009; Flood 2009; Foltz 2010; Mallette 2010; Beihammer 2011).

For all of these reasons, the problem of how we conceptualize and study a global Middle Ages is not going to be easy to solve. How can we even discuss this era meaningfully, given the value-laden vocabulary we must use? What should we call the communities and regions of encounter that formed and reformed throughout this period when they do not map onto discrete territories or modern nation-states? What names might we give to peoples or religions that better reflect indigenous identities and beliefs? How do we deal with the fact of asynchronous developments within and between societies as diverse as Heian Japan, classical Angkor, the Delhi Sultanate, Song China, Carolingian Europe, the Emergent Mississippian Culture of North America, and the Aztecs of the Postclassical Period? Yet the difficulty of the task is part of the reason for undertaking it. No human endeavor can be divorced from global phenomena, and it is imperative that we learn how the interconnected pasts of medieval societies shaped the complex world we have inherited from them.

In pursuit of this goal, *The Medieval Globe* (*TMG*) will promote scholarship in three related areas of study: the means by which peoples, things, and ideas came into contact with one another; the deep roots of global developments; and the ways that perceptions of "the medieval" have been (and are) created around the world. *TMG* is also committed to supporting innovative, collaborative work in a variety of genres: full-length articles, scholarly dialogues, multi-authored discussions of critical problems, review essays, editions or translations of source materials, and other formats. The common denominator among articles accepted for publication will be their authors' willingness to explore points of convergence or movement (potential or actual), to address topics of broad scholarly interest, or to pioneer portable methodologies.

The need for such a forum is clear. Many programs and research centers traditionally devoted to the European Middle Ages are being reconfigured to enable the study of co-eval cultures across the world; these include my own Program for Medieval Studies at the University of Illinois, the launching pad for *TMG*. Students entering the many specialized fields and disciplines embraced by this globalized medieval studies will need to be trained accordingly (Heng 2009) and will also need appropriate outlets for their work. Scholars of other eras, dissatisfied with the modernist (Western) perspectives that have dominated global studies to date, will also find a home in this emerging community. *TMG* envisions a new place for "the medieval" in global studies, but it also insists that all ages have been fundamental to the formation of our world (Shryock and Smail 2011; Smail and Shryock 2013). Its role is to mediate, to make the *medium ævum* truly an "age between".

This inaugural double issue of *The Medieval Globe* is a special showcase for these aspirations. Its editor, Monica H. Green, has assembled a team of experts from many diverse disciplines to address a global, medieval phenomenon that is still affecting human beings and ecosystems around the world. She has also nurtured communication among these contributors and ensured that their work engages the broadest possible audience. The essays gathered here, individually and collectively, bring state-of-the-art scientific and humanistic methods to bear on both new and old bodies of evidence. They greatly advance our understanding of the medieval Black Death, and they also reveal how much our current knowledge of this pandemic—its causes, effects, and more recent manifestations—has been limited by assumptions that have not yet yielded to those methods. As important and far-reaching as this issue is, it is not intended to be definitive; rather, it provides a series of firm footholds for future scholarship and lays out an ambitious agenda for collaborative research. I cannot think of a better introduction to *The Medieval Globe.*

Acknowledgments

I am grateful to members of *The Medieval Globe*'s editorial board for their comments on an earlier draft of this essay, whose shortcomings remain my own. I am also grateful to the many students and colleagues at the University of Illinois and at Harvard University, who helped me to grapple with the implications of this initiative. Special thanks are due to Megan McLaughlin, Elizabeth Oyler, D. Fairchild Ruggles, and Eleanora Stoppino; and (above all) to Charles D. Wright, director of the Program in Medieval Studies at Illinois, whose leadership made it possible to dream of compassing the medieval globe. I also thank our College of Liberal Arts and Sciences for providing the funding for an editorial assistant and thus enabling graduate student involvement in the production of this journal.

The next issue of *TMG* (2.1, forthcoming in 2015) will feature articles fostered by our conference on "The Medieval Globe: Communication, Connectivity, Exchange," held in April of 2012: the source of inspiration for this journal. I warmly acknowledge those who participated in that inspiring encounter: Jonathan Conant, Kathleen Davis, Margot Fassler, Geraldine Heng, Sharon Kinoshita, Linda Komaroff, Elizabeth Lambourn, Carla Nappi, Michael Puett, Christian Raffensperger, and Nicolás Wey Goméz. Finally, I thank guest editor Monica Green for approaching me with the idea for this special issue in the spring of 2013, and for skillfully bringing it to fruition.

Bibliography

Abu-Lughod, Janet L. 1989. *Before European Hegemony: The World System, A.D. 1250–1350* (Oxford: Oxford University Press)

Bartlett, Robert. 1994. *The Making of Europe: Conquest, Colonization, and Cultural Change, 950–1350* (Princeton, NJ: Princeton University Press)

Beihammer, Alexander D. 2011. "Defection across the Border of Islam and Christianity: Apostasy and Cross-Cultural Interaction in Byzantine-Seljuk Relations," *Speculum* 86: 597–651

Bennett, Judith M. 2006. *History Matters: Patriarchy and the Challenge of Feminism* (Philadelphia: University of Pennsylvania Press)

Cohen, Jeffrey Jerome (ed.). 2000. *The Postcolonial Middle Ages* (New York: St. Martin's Press)

Dagenais, John, and Margaret Greer. 2000. "Decolonizing the Middle Ages," in *Decolonizing the Middle Ages*, ed. by John Dagenais and Margaret Greer, special issue, *Journal of Medieval and Early Modern Studies* 30: 431–48

Davis, Kathleen. 2008. *Periodization and Sovereignty: How Ideas of Feudalism and Secularization Govern the Politics of Time* (Philadelphia: University of Pennsylvania Press)

Davis, Kathleen, and Nadia Altschul (eds.). 2009. *Medievalisms in the Postcolonial World: The Idea of "The Middle Ages" outside Europe* (Baltimore: Johns Hopkins University Press)

Fernández-Armesto, Felipe, and James Muldoon (eds.). 2008. *Internal Colonization in Medieval Europe* (Farnham: Ashgate Variorum)

Flood, Finbarr Barry. 2009. *Objects of Translation: Material Culture and Medieval "Hindu-Muslim" Encounters* (Princeton, NJ: Princeton University Press)

Foltz, Richard. 2010. *Religions of the Silk Road: Premodern Patterns of Globalization*, 2nd ed. (New York: Palgrave Macmillan)

Gaonkar, Dilip Parameshwar. 2000. *Alternative Modernities* (Durham, NC: Duke University Press)

Gaunt, Simon. 2013. *Marco Polo's "Le devisement du monde": Narrative Voice, Language and Diversity* (Cambridge: D.S. Brewer)

Geary, Patrick J. 2002. *The Myth of Nations: The Medieval Origins of Europe* (Princeton, NJ: Princeton University Press)

Geary, Patrick J., and Gábor Klaniczay (eds.). 2013. *Manufacturing Middle Ages: The Entangled History of Medievalism in Nineteenth-Century Europe* (Leiden: Brill)

Goody, Jack. 2006. *The Theft of History* (Cambridge: Cambridge University Press)

Grabar, Oleg. 2006. "The Shared Culture of Objects," in *Islamic Visual Culture, 1100–1800: Constructing the Study of Islmaic Art II*, 51–67 (Aldershot: Ashgate Variorum)

Heng, Geraldine. 2009. "The Global Middle Ages: An Experiment in Collaborative Humanities, or Imagining the World, 500–1500 C.E.," *English Language Notes* 47: 205–16

Holsinger, Bruce. 2007. *Neomedievalism, Neoconservatism, and the War on Terror* (Chicago: Prickly Paradigm Press)

Kinoshita, Sharon. 2013. "Reorientations: The Worlding of Marco Polo," in *Cosmopolitanism and the Middle Ages*, ed. John Ganim and Shayne Legassie, 39–57 (New York: Palgrave Macmillan)

Kinoshita, Sharon (trans.). Forthcoming. *Marco Polo and Rustichello of Pisa: The Description of the World* (Cambridge, MA: Hackett)

Komaroff, Linda (ed.). 2006. *Beyond the Legacy of Ghengis Khan* (Leiden: Brill)

Lieberman, Victor (ed.). 1999. *Beyond Binary Histories: Re-Imagining Eurasia to c. 1830* (Cambridge: Cambridge University Press)

Lieberman, Victor. 2007–09. *Strange Parallels: Southeast Asia in Global Context, c. 800–1830*, 2 vols. (Cambridge: Cambridge University Press)

Mallette, Karla. 2010. *European Modernity and the Arab Mediterranean: Toward a New Philology and a Counter-Orientalism* (Philadelphia: University of Pennsylvania Press)

Mandeville, John [Johan or Jean]. [*c*. 1357]/2000. *Le livre des merveilles du monde*, ed. Christiane Deluz (Paris: Centre national de la recherche scientifique Éditions)

McCormick, Michael. 2001. *Origins of the European Economy: Communications and Commerce, AD 300–900* (Cambridge: Cambridge University Press)

Murray, Alan V. (ed.). 2009. *The Clash of Cultures on the Medieval Baltic Frontier* (Farnham: Ashgate)

Sassen, Saskia. 2008. *Territory, Authority, Rights: From Medieval to Global Assemblages* (Princeton, NJ: Princeton University Press)

Shryock, Andrew, and Daniel Lord Smail. 2011. *Deep History: The Architecture of Past and Present* (Berkeley: University of California Press)

Sizgorich, Thomas. 2009. *Violence and Belief in Late Antiquity: Militant Devotion in Christianity and Islam* (Philadelphia: University of Pennsylvania Press)

Smail, Daniel Lord. 2011. "Genealogy, Ontogeny, and the Narrative Arc of Origins," *French Historical Studies* 34: 21–35

Smail, Daniel Lord, Clare Haru Crowston, Kristen B. Neuschel, and Carol Symes. 2011. "History and the Telescoping of Historical Time," *French Historical Studies* 34: 1–55

Smail, Daniel Lord, and Andrew Shryock. 2013. "History and the "Pre"," *American Historical Review* 118: 709–37

Stein, Robert M. 1995. "Medieval, Modern, Post-Modern: Medieval Studies in a Post-Modern Perspective" (paper presented at the conference "Cultural Frictions: Medieval Cultural Studies in Post-Modern Contexts," at Georgetown University) <http://www.medievalists.net/2010/01/23/medieval-modern-post-modern-medieval-studies-in-a-post-modern-perspective/> [accessed October 10, 2014]

Summit, Jennifer, and David Wallace. 2007. "Rethinking Periodization," in *Medieval/Renaissance: After Periodization*, ed. Jennifer Summit and David Wallace, special issue, *Journal of Medieval and Early Modern Studies* 37: 447–51

Symes, Carol. 2011a. "The Middle Ages between Nationalism and Colonialism," *French Historical Studies* 34: 37–46

Symes, Carol. 2011b. "When We Talk about Modernity," *American Historical Review* 116: 715–26

Wallerstein, Immanuel. 1974. *The Modern World-System: Capitalist Agriculture and the Origins of the European World Economy in the Sixteenth Century* (New York: Academic Press)
Wey Goméz, Nicolás. 2008. *The Tropics of Empire: Why Columbus Sailed South to the Indies* (Cambridge, MA: MIT Press)
Wolf, Eric. 1982. *Europe and the People without History* (Berkeley: University of California Press)

Carol Symes (symes@illinois.edu) is the founding executive editor of *The Medieval Globe.* She is the Lynn M. Martin Professorial Scholar at the University of Illinois, where she is an associate professor of history with joint appointments in medieval studies, global studies, and theatre. Her own research focuses on the history of documentary practices and communication technologies, the social and cultural history of Western Europe from *c.* 1000 to 1300, and the abiding influence of medievalism in the modern world.

Abstract The concept of "the medieval" has long been essential to global imperial ventures, national ideologies, and the discourse of modernity. And yet the projects enabled by this powerful construct have essentially hindered investigation of the world's interconnected territories during a millennium of movement and exchange. The mission of *The Medieval Globe* is to reclaim this "middle age" and to place it at the center of global studies.

Keywords Medieval, Middle Ages, medievalism, global studies, empire, postcolonial studies, colonization, nationalism, modernity, Columbus, Marco Polo, John Mandeville.

EDITOR'S INTRODUCTION TO *PANDEMIC DISEASE IN THE MEDIEVAL WORLD: RETHINKING THE BLACK DEATH*

MONICA H. GREEN

AFTER THE JUSTINIANIC Plague (*c.* 541–*c.* 750), which has been called the First Plague Pandemic, the Black Death or Second Plague Pandemic was likely the first semi-global phenomenon that fully merits the name—affecting "all people" (*pan* + *demos*).[1] Total (absolute) mortality would be higher from several nineteenth-century cholera outbreaks, the 1918–19 influenza pandemic, or the current HIV/AIDS pandemic. But when expressed as a percentage of the population, the mortality caused by the Black Death is the highest of any large-scale catastrophe known to humankind, save for the impact of smallpox and measles on indigenous peoples in first-contact events of the early modern period. The Black Death killed an estimated 40% to 60% of all people in Europe, the Middle East, and North Africa when it first struck there in the mid-fourteenth century. Its demographic effects are well known (particularly with respect to Western Europe), and there is a considerable body of historical scholarship on population losses and the economic and political changes that ensued. Such questions about its aftermath are important, of course; but so, too, are questions of why and how the pandemic happened in the first place and how it was sustained. For these questions, we currently have no definitive answers. Even its full geographic extent is still unknown: we are only now beginning to engage with scientific and documentary evidence

1 On the modern definition of "pandemic," see Morens, Folkers, and Fauci (2004), who identify wide geographic extension, disease movement, high attack rates and explosiveness, minimal population immunity, novelty, infectiousness, contagiousness, and severity as the most commonly used features in describing disease outbreaks as "pandemic". Of these, only contagiousness does not commonly apply to plague since it is normally spread by an arthropod vector, except that pneumonic plague (one of plague's most lethal forms) is directly contagious from person to person. In this essay, I use the term "the Black Death" as synonymous with the Second Plague Pandemic as a whole. Individual contributors to this special issue retain the original usage, applying the term to the first wave of plague that struck the Mediterranean and Western Europe in the mid-fourteenth century. On the issue of plague's chronology and periodization and the definition of "pandemic," see below.

for plague in East Asia, and we can only suspect (as we will see) whether the disease might have also reached other regions of Afroeurasia as well.

A catastrophe of this magnitude demands explanation. The present collection of essays starts from the premise that studies of the Black Death must embrace a new reality: the fact that the field of microbiology has, in the past two decades, leapt past the barriers of the late nineteenth-century biological laboratory and created new ways to explore the history of pathogenic organisms. Microbiology has effected a transformation in our understanding of the disease's history. It has reconstructed the phylogenetic (evolutionary) history of the plague organism, *Yersinia pestis*, from modern molecular samples, and it has developed techniques to retrieve and reconstruct genetic material of the pathogen from historical remains. The question "What was the pathogen?" has been decisively resolved. In 2011, over a decade of innovative research (and controversy) in the retrieval and analysis of ancient DNA (aDNA) fragments and other proteins culminated in the reconstruction of the full genome of *Yersinia pestis*, using the remains of persons buried in London's famed Black Death cemetery (East Smithfield), which can be precisely dated to the first outbreak of plague in London, in 1348–50 (Bos et al. 2011; see also DeWitte 2014, in this issue).[2] Even if we cannot yet rule out the possibility that there was more than one organism or other causative factor leading to the mass mortalities in this period, there is no longer any question that *Y. pestis* was a key player.

The essays in this first issue of *The Medieval Globe* take the new microbiological consensus on the Black Death as a given. Yet the assembled contributors do not contest a key point raised by so-called "plague deniers," who in the past several decades have raised doubts about the role of *Y. pestis* in the pandemic.[3] Their skepticism arose from the fact that the speed of the disease's spread, and the level of well-documented human mortality it caused during the fourteenth century, in no way match the patterns seen in the Third Plague Pandemic, which is normally dated from around 1894 to the 1930s and during which the foundation was laid for our modern bacteriological and epidemiological understandings of the pathogen and the disease it causes in animals and humans. There is good

---

2 A superb summary of the developments in microbiology as it relates to historical plagues can be found in Little (2011). The presence of *Y. pestis* in remains from the time of the Justinianic Plague has now been documented as well. See Green (2014, in this issue) for further details on the contributions of genetics to plague studies.

3 Benedictow (2010) summarizes these perspectives and, in the tenor of his own arguments, reveals how contentious the issue has become.

reason, now, to question the role that early twentieth-century epidemiology has played in our general constructions of plague's histories, because plague is not always or everywhere the same in its vectors or animal hosts (Royer 2014; see Varlık 2014 and Carmichael 2014, both in this issue). Nevertheless, rather than dismiss the skeptics' focus on the discrepancies between twentieth-century understandings of plague's epidemiology and our medieval evidence, this collection of essays is motivated by an acceptance of the discrepancies. We concede that there is currently no plausible, comprehensive theory that can explain in full detail how the non-motile, single-celled organism that modern science knows as *Yersinia pestis*—which may have originated as a new species as little as about 3000 to 4000 years ago (Cui et al. 2013)—could, in an age before steam-powered (let alone jet) travel, have been disseminated across so much of the Eurasian and North African landscape in just a few decades.

Admitting ignorance of the full epidemiological character and amplifying factors of the Second Pandemic does not, however, mean that we have no useful knowledge at all. This may still be *terra incognita*, but we are not without a compass. Genetic science confirms the very close identity of the strain of the *Y. pestis* bacillus found in fourteenth-century human remains and the organism as it is found disseminated now throughout most of the inhabited world (Bos et al. 2011; Cui et al. 2013).[4] The organism itself, therefore, serves as a tracer element, a living chain of evidence that can tie together vastly distant times and places. To borrow a phrase coined by the French historian Emmanuel Le Roy Ladurie (1973), back when the possibilities of modern genetics analysis could barely be fantasized: we have here a "microbial unification of [half] the world." That biological fact enables us to take an interpretative stance: given the same pathogen, more or less the same epidemiological parameters can be inferred in terms of necessary environmental conditions, modes of transmission, and symptomatologies in infected hosts. We may not yet know all the species of arthropod vectors or mammalian hosts we need to search out; we may not yet know all the climatic and other environmental factors that contributed to the propagation of *Y. pestis*. We certainly do not know

4 Ancient DNA (aDNA) retrieved from the period of the Justinianic Plague also fits into phylogenetic understandings that have already been postulated for the evolution of *Y. pestis* since its divergence from its most recent common ancestor; see Harbeck et al. 2013 and Wagner et al. 2014. On the dissemination of *Y. pestis* in the Third Pandemic, see Morelli et al. 2010. Plague foci currently exist in North and South America, Africa, and Eurasia. Although plague reached Australia in 1900, it does not seem to have established permanent foci there; see Curson and McCracken 1989.

all the human factors of trade in grains or textiles or other material goods and foodstuffs that created the microenvironments allowing *Y. pestis* to spread. But we do know that we need to search out those connections.

Accepting the precepts of an evolutionary perspective on the history of *Y. pestis* suggests that the field of historical plague studies as it relates to the Second Pandemic must be redefined in three dimensions: its geographic extent, its chronological extent, and the methodological registers we use to investigate it. The essays in this volume pursue, from various perspectives, all these agendas.

First, the **geography** of the Second Pandemic must be expanded. Black Death studies can no longer be defined as if the disease struck only Western and Central Europe, as is often depicted in maps, sourcebooks, and textbooks.[5] Analyses of the evolutionary history of *Y. pestis* from modern samples have suggested since 2004 that the geographic origins of the pathogen were likely on the Tibetan-Qinghai Plateau (Achtman et al. 2004).[6] *Y. pestis* had to move across as many animal species (arthropod vectors as well as mammalian hosts) as climatic zones in order to cause the massive mortality in human bodies that it did in the fourteenth century (and episodically thereafter). But again, the microbiology makes clear that it did move. Contributors to this volume cover geographic terrain from China to all sides of the Mediterranean and on to England. In my own essay, I suggest that even the Indian Ocean basin merits exploration as a route possibly as important as the Silk Roads; at least, that is a possibility worth exploring given that genetics research ties sub-Saharan Africa to our premodern plague narratives. The call for an expanded geography also includes calling for a veritable menagerie of possible hosts for the organism. *Y. pestis* always needs precise microenvironments to thrive and even more precise circumstances of transfer across species to create human plague. But limiting plague's narrative to one or two kinds of rats and fleas occludes too much: it defies the evidence that modern entomology and zoology have brought forward, which reminds us repeatedly that human plague is a relatively rare epiphenomenon in *Y. pestis*'s evolution. Although humans have regularly been involved in plague's long-distance spread, *Yersinia pestis* survives because it establishes itself in microenvironments that more or less replicate those of its origin. Marmots and gerbils (and guinea pigs and prairie dogs) are more important for that long-term survival than rats.

---

5 Even for Europe, such maps pose major interpretative problems (Mengel 2011).

6 A summary of debates on the geographic origin of *Y. pestis* can be found in Green (2014, in this issue); see also Hymes (2014, in this issue).

Second, the **chronology** of the Black Death must be expanded.[7] The term "Black Death" has often been used to denote just the first "wave" of plague that struck the Mediterranean and Western Europe between 1347 and 1353. Usage of the term in that narrow sense is still justified, especially when examining many kinds of synchronous sources at the period of the highest collective human mortality. However, beyond its Eurocentricity, the narrow time frame beginning in 1347—or 1346, if we include the outbreak in Kaffa, where besieging Mongols are famously said to have hurled infected bodies over the city walls—obscures two epidemiological facts that must be addressed: first, that plague came to Kaffa *from somewhere*; and second, that plague did not simply come to Western Eurasia, *it stayed*. How much earlier than 1346/7 we must look for the "origin" of the Black Death is not yet clear. In 2013, microbiologists Cui and colleagues proposed a polytomy, a sudden divergence or "Big Bang" of *Y. pestis* into four new lineages, likely caused because it was moving into new host species (Cui et al. 2013). They suggested a median date of *c.* 1268 with a 95% confidence interval of 1142–1339. As Robert Hymes suggests in his epilogue to this collection, "A Hypothesis on the East Asian Beginnings of the *Yersinia pestis* Polytomy," Cui and colleagues' proposed dating coincides intriguingly with events taking place in the first decades of the thirteenth century near the edge of the Tibetan-Qinghai Plateau—events that might possibly serve as the "disseminating factor" necessary to start the process of *Y. pestis*'s spread to other environments. The possible role of climatic change in catalyzing the thirteenth-century polytomy, or, indeed, in any other major outbreak of plague, has not yet been defined decisively, but evidence is increasingly suggesting that though small localized outbreaks of plague occur regularly wherever it has established enzootic foci, the commonality of more widespread outbreaks is due to climatic factors.[8]

---

7 This issue of chronological definition was addressed by Little (2011: 271): "the Black Death [is] a name that many historians restrict to the massive mortality throughout Europe between 1347 and 1353 but is better understood as a pandemic that began in Central Asia in the 1330s, subsequently spread through Europe and the Middle East starting in the late 1340s, and made frequent returns in those regions for over four centuries." And just as this issue argues for extending the Second Plague Pandemic forward into the nineteenth century, arguments are also being made to extend the Third Pandemic back into the eighteenth century; a beginning date of *c.* 1772 is implied by Benedict (1996) and taken as the foundation for research in Xu et al. (2014).

8 On the correlation of climate with widespread outbreaks, as established by modern observational science and predictions about what current climate change might do to plague dynamics in the future, see, e.g., Stenseth et al. 2006; Ben Ari et al. 2011; and Gage 2012. In-progress work by Bruce Campbell (2013) suggests that major climatic

As for the end date of the Second Pandemic, we clearly must look well beyond 1353. For Western Europe, we have long known that plague outbreaks continued to occur up through the early eighteenth century, but even such oft-cited dates as 1679 (for the last plague outbreak in England) and 1722 (for the Continent, following the last major outbreak in Marseille, 1720) may be illusory (Cummins, Kelly, and Ó Gráda 2013; Ermus 2014). If, moreover, we add in the Islamicate world, the 1722 end date for the Second Pandemic becomes meaningless. Outbreaks in North Africa, the Ottoman empire, and even Russia certainly continued well into the nineteenth century (Varlık 2014, in this issue; Mikhail 2012; Robarts 2010). Were all these outbreaks repeated importations from enzootic loci "elsewhere"? Or do they reflect local cases of plague persistence? Because we currently lack any aDNA from sites in Central Eurasia, we cannot settle these questions now. For example, a strain of *Y. pestis* recently documented in Libya comes from Branch 2 of the general phylogenetic tree, which diverged from Branch 1, the lineage involved in both the Black Death (as documented from London remains) and the global Third Pandemic; this divergence occurred some seven hundred to eight hundred years ago (Cui et al. 2013). Since strains from Branch 1 are also documented in other parts of North Africa, the Libyan case suggests that we may well be looking at the remnants of more than one pandemic leaving its traces in that region (Cabanel et al. 2013). There may, in other words, have been multiple amplifications of *Y. pestis* in the late medieval and early modern periods that have left living descendants to this day. Can we really say that the Second Plague Pandemic ever ended?

Third, it is now obligatory that plague studies be broadened into a **multidisciplinary mode**. There is no single discipline or investigative approach that can be privileged: microbiologists may study the evolution or particular genetic characteristics of the pathogen, but that single-celled organism only creates "plague" when it passes through various environments, different hosts as well as different ecosystems. Entomologists must study the arthropod vectors, zoologists must study the many different possible mammalian hosts for the disease, from the tiniest rodents up through carnivores and camels. Bioarcheologists are the guardians of all aspects of retrieval, classification, and analysis of material remains, not only of humans and their artifacts but also all the species that form

changes occurred throughout the northern hemisphere in the early 1340s, which may have been a particular precipitating factor for the events that pushed plague into the Black Sea and Mediterranean basins. On climate and the Justinianic Plague, see Green 2014, in this issue.

the chains through which *Y. pestis* passes. And finally, humanists—historians, but also linguists and art historians and others who painstakingly interpret the cultural products of human societies—are needed to reconstruct not only the ways in which humans contributed to the creation of conditions ripe for amplification of *Y. pestis* on pandemic scales, but also the many human responses to plague and catastrophic mortality, be they medical or religious, palliative or murderous.

The following essays attempt to lay out a forward path for studies of plague in this multidisciplinary and collaborative mode. In the opening essay, "Taking 'Pandemic' Seriously: Making the Black Death Global," I ask what the implications are for our histories of the Black Death when we take into account the major transformations in the biological sciences during the past fifteen years. I argue that approaching plague studies from the perspective of global health history allows the creation of frameworks of analysis that are both richly multidisciplinary and productive of new research agendas. The field of global history writ large is already known for embracing broad expanses of both time and place, literally covering the globe but also (in its mode as Deep History) going back to the time of human origins—and, in some cases, beyond. Global history is also generally quite interdisciplinary, recognizing that narratives at those levels of scale cannot rely solely on written documentation. But with different sources and methods come different research goals. What the microbiologist or historical epidemiologist wants to explain is different from what the historian of religious persecution or public health seeks to document. A major obstacle to fruitful dialogue between the humanistic and scientific approaches has been historians' aversion to agendas that smacked of "retrospective diagnosis": the imposition of modern categories of scientific disease classification on evidence from the past; this aversion has been especially strong among recent generations of historians of medicine. My essay suggests that using the categories of modern science to reconstruct plague's histories—adopting an outsider's (*etic*) perspective on the material history of plague—is actually essential to reconstructing the history of participants' *experiences* of those material conditions and the resulting experiences of sudden death, economic devastation, and social chaos (an *emic* perspective). Both are valid, and both are necessary to a historical enterprise that unites the efforts of scientists and humanists alike.

As has been noted, the common practices of long-distance trade or animal husbandry that facilitated the spread of *Y. pestis* to lands far distant from the Tibetan-Qinghai Plateau are yet to be discovered. But spread it did, and it is certain that human activities, unwitting though they may have been, were responsible. Epidemiologically, we would now "blame" the grain distributor or the trader in furs or the second-hand clothes dealer for creating mobile microenvironments that facilitated the spread of *Y. pestis*. But these causes would not have been apparent to medieval actors, and it has long been known that, in their terror, people in the fourteenth century looked in many directions to answer the question "Why?" In Christian Europe, reproachful eyes often turned toward resident Jewish communities.[9] In "The Black Death and its Consequences for the Jewish Community in Tàrrega: Lessons from History and Archeology," Anna Colet, Josep Xavier Muntané i Santiveri, Jordi Ruíz Ventura, Oriol Saula, M. Eulàlia Subirà de Galdàcano, and Clara Jáuregui unite an *emic* approach to the perspectives of historical human actors with the *etic* approach implicit in archeology's reconstruction of material culture. Beginning in 2007, excavations were undertaken on the Maset hill in a suburb of the Catalonian town of Tàrrega: a site subsequently identified as that of the town's medieval Jewish cemetery. Analysis of the human remains found in several communal graves (a burial practice rare among medieval Jews) shows that many had suffered a violent death. Linking this material evidence to written documentation of attacks against the Jewish community of Tàrrega in July 1348, Colet and her colleagues find astonishing parallels between two very different kinds of evidence. Arriving in the port of Barcelona, the plague had spread inland to Cervera and then to Tàrrega. And immediately on the heels of the plague spread waves of hate, according to official records kept by the Crown of Aragon, which reports that twenty Jews were killed in Barcelona, eighteen in Cervera, and three hundred in Tàrrega. This contemporary record of mass murder in Tàrrega, one of the earliest to be associated with the plague's arrival on the European mainland in the spring of 1348, is now confirmed by the archaeological evidence published here. This evidence corroborates not only violent deaths and the postmortem desecration of some bodies, but also the careful attempts, probably by the community's surviving Jews, to give the deceased a ritually appropriate burial.

Archeology takes us in a very different direction in Sharon DeWitte's contribution, "The Anthropology of Plague: Insights from Bioarcheological Analyses of Epidemic Cemeteries." Bioarcheology is a relatively recent designation for archeological work that encompasses paleopathology (the determination of disease or nutritional deficits from human remains) and combines it with fuller contextual analysis to create a rich understanding

---

9 It has long been recognized that minority Jewish communities were not targeted in the Islamic regions of the medieval world (Dols 1974). On the varied attempts to explain the contagion, see Stearns 2011.

of how whole communities lived (and died). As recently as a decade ago, it was believed that plague was one of the diseases that bioarcheology could not reconstruct. The "osteological paradox" holds that bone only reacts slowly to most stressors. Whereas violent trauma (as in the case of the Tàrrega victims) will immediately create lesions in bone, disease or nutritional deficits take time to work their destructive effects. Hence, anything that kills quickly (like plague, which can strike a human down in anywhere from two to ten days) does not have time to damage the bone in any discernible way. Now, of course, bioarcheology is at the forefront of historical plague studies, not simply because *Y. pestis* aDNA can be extracted from teeth excavated by archeologists, but because new innovative techniques of epidemiological analysis at the population level allows us to assess the health state of victims, and also the cultural attitudes and responses toward mass mortality as evidenced in burial practices themselves. Excavations of mass gravesites in London have been particularly revelatory because the sites can be precisely dated and contextualized from supporting documentary information. DeWitte's summary of current research (much of it her own) also allows us to see some of the directions in which multidisciplinary work on plague and other epidemic diseases will take us in the future.

In his essay, "Plague Depopulation and Irrigation Decay in Medieval Egypt," Stuart Borsch examines plague depopulation's very direct effect on the economic infrastructure of Egypt in the late medieval period. Several essays in this volume focus on the ecologies that facilitate plague maintenance, amplification, or transmission. Borsch, in contrast, reminds us that plague can create a new ecology for humans. By eliminating human actors whose agricultural practices had regulated the environment, plague literally transformed the landscape of Egypt. Irrigation systems and the social and technological institutions that had built them up over many millennia fell into ruin because major population losses, caused by recurrent outbreaks of plague, severely circumscribed the amount of labor available to maintain this elaborate infrastructure, designed to control and exploit the flooding of the Nile River. By 1468, Egyptian officials themselves could not explain why their predictions for the annual flood had failed for the first time since records began to be kept, in the third millennium BCE. The magnitude of mortality from plague, which seems to have been far more extreme than can be documented for other disease pandemics, is likely the key factor in Egypt's drastic economic decline.

In her essay "Plague Persistence in Western Europe: A Hypothesis," Ann G. Carmichael explores an issue hinted at in Borsch's account of recurrent plague in Egypt. Although we do not know the precise mechanisms of its spread, there is little reason at this point to doubt medieval reports that the "great mortality" in Western Europe and North Africa came via ships, arriving first in the seaports of the Mediterranean and then at other ports on the Atlantic and North Sea coasts. But our modern knowledge of *Y. pestis*—drawn from studies of sylvatic (or "maintenance") foci of the organism in North and South America, Africa, and Asia—shows that *Y. pestis* can be readily established in rodent communities within a few years of its introduction to a new geographic area. Often, those new foci are established at high elevations.[10] Carmichael raises the question of whether the Alps became one such area where local foci were established in Europe, causing recurrent plague outbreaks in the early modern period. That is, documented waves of the plague in later centuries came, not through reintroductions of the organism via long-distance trade networks linked to Central Asia (though that may also have happened), but from Northern Europe's own sylvatic foci in local mountainous areas. Beginning her narrative with a handful of deaths in small mountain villages in 1567, Carmichael moves both forward and backward in time, ending with the second wave of the epidemic in Western Europe, that of 1359–63. *As was noted at the time*, this epidemic moved down from upland communities into metropolitan centers such as Milan, not from coastal cities into the interior; this was the mortality so famously recorded and bemoaned by the poet Francesco Petrarca (d. 1374), who had already lost his beloved Laura to the Black Death in 1348, and who was now to lose his son and a good friend in this new epidemic. In order to lay out this hypothesis (itself a wonderful example of how the new science of plague can stimulate new research questions for historians), Carmichael is impelled to raise questions about what animal species may have served as local hosts for *Y. pestis*. The fact that the European Alps, like the Tibetan-Qinghai Plateau, had a resident species of marmot is, she suggests, likely one part of the answer to how plague came to persist in late medieval and early modern Western Europe.

Like Borsch and Carmichael, Nükhet Varlık shows how command of what she calls "local knowledge" can, when set into larger frameworks of epidemiological and scientific analysis, yield results that enlighten not only contemporaries' experiences of plague in one part of the world, but our larger understanding of plague's causes and effects. In her essay "New Science and Old Sources: Why the Ottoman Experience of Plague Matters,"

10 This phenomenon has been noted for individual localities but has not been studied systematically, so far as I have been able to determine. See, for example, Eisen et al. 2010; Neerinckx et al. 2010; MacMillan et al. 2011; Eisen et al. 2012; Andrianaivoarimanana et al. 2013; and Schneider et al. 2014.

Varlık begins by noting that Eurocentric narratives of plague history have rendered invisible the geographic and temporal extent of plague—and, thus, human experiences of the disease—in other areas of the Eurasian world. While the Second Pandemic may have started at approximately the same time in Western Europe and in the lands that would later form the Ottoman empire, outbreaks of plague continued in Ottoman territories well into the nineteenth century, far beyond the chronological parameters that have been established with reference to European cases alone. Like Carmichael, Varlık explores the historical importance of determining whether plague established urban or rural foci, allowing *Y. pestis* to perpetuate itself independently of newly imported infections. And like Green and Carmichael, Varlık stresses the importance of adopting more complex models of plague-transmission, models which pay special attention to interspecies dynamics. Importantly, Varlık also gives us a lesson in seeing science itself as dynamic. Although the contributors to this special issue regularly rely on scientific claims about *Y. pestis*'s evolution or ecology or physiological effects, we recognize that this body of knowledge is ever changing. Just as the universalist claims of science must be made locally specific in the hands of the well-trained historian, so too must the scientific understandings of the past be recognized as the products of culturally specific moments. Varlık suggests the need to re-examine the ways that some basic tenets of plague science were formulated in the early twentieth century. "These imagined divisions of epidemiological experience," she says, "have resulted in separate histories of plague in Europe and the Middle East/Islamic world" (Varlık 2014, in this issue, p. 205).

Recognizing that plague remained a repeated threat in many communities into the nineteenth century—and remains a threat today for those human populations living around established plague foci—Fabian Crespo and Matthew B. Lawrenz bring the perspectives of biological anthropology and microbiology to bear in their essay "Heterogeneous Immunological Landscapes and Medieval Plague: An Invitation to a New Dialogue between Historians and Immunologists." Modern scientific understanding of mammalian immune systems has been transformed in the past four decades, in part because the HIV/AIDS pandemic made such knowledge desperately urgent. Certain misunderstandings of immunity have been widespread in discussions about historical plague, among them the misleading idea that whole populations can suddenly and permanently "acquire" immunity to certain pathogens if a part of that population survives an epidemic event. Crespo and Lawrenz are concerned, rather, to lay the foundation for experimental investigation of whether any immunological characteristics (innate and acquired) *already* present in Western Europe's diverse gene pool and ecology may have acted differentially in facilitating the survival of some exposed individuals rather than others. Just as DeWitte finds evidence for differential survival based on an individual's prior exposure to compromised nutrition or other stressors, Crespo and Lawrenz wish to explore from an immunological perspective the basic question of differential survival that is the foundation of all epidemiological investigation. Crespo and Lawrenz's articulation of these questions shows how fruitful dialogue between the many historicist disciplines can be. As they note, "historians must step in and help scientists put all these biological differences into context."

Our next essay, "The Black Death and the Future of the Plague," written by Michelle Ziegler, a microbiologist and specialist in disaster preparedness, considers the reasons why this most "medieval" of diseases remains of urgent concern today. As noted above, much of our modern understanding of plague's human epidemiology comes from studies made during the Third Plague Pandemic in the late nineteenth and early twentieth centuries: right at the time when germ theory was establishing a new paradigm for understandings of disease. Current scientific concerns are related not simply to fears of biological warfare (already attempted earlier in twentieth century) but also to threats of disease re-emergence and antibiotic resistance, threats that have only become fully apparent since the 1990s. The complete reconstruction of the genome of *Y. pestis* from fourteenth-century samples shows that the organism as it existed then is not radically different from the organism that exists in numerous strains throughout the world in the present day. In other words, in terms of the pathogenicity or virulence of the organism (and, probably, human susceptibility to it), the Black Death could happen all over again today, given the proper conditions. That raw fact is what propels millions of dollars of new research on *Y. pestis*. The medieval Black Death, therefore, is far more than a mere historical curiosity; it is, in all its complexity, the source of vital data that can help us to establish scenarios for pandemic disease now and in the future.

Late in the process of assembling this collection, we had the good fortune to be put in touch with Robert Hymes, a historian of China whose epilogue now rounds out our narrative. While Ziegler brings the Black Death's narratives into the twenty-first century, Hymes takes us back to its beginning—or, at least, the beginning as currently hypothesized by genetics science. Hymes offers a tentative rereading of Chinese historical sources from the thirteenth century, more than a century before plague arrived in the Mediterranean basin. Historiography on China has long been reluctant to see plague as a factor in East Asian history, where references to epidemics are abundant but descriptions of what could be interpreted specifically as "plague" are exiguous: even the recent publication of major genetics studies asserting an Asian origin of *Y. pestis* did not shake the fundamental skepticism of those who maintain that human plague was not a major factor in China's medieval history (Buell 2012). Hymes, however, takes the sudden divergence of *Y. pestis* postulated by genetics in 2013 (the polytomy mentioned above, estimated to have occurred between the twelfth and early fourteenth centuries) as an invitation to begin assembling several pieces of a scattered puzzle: the sequence of Mongol raids against towns on the northern border of the Tibet-Qinghai plateau starting in the 1210s; the reports that the Mongols themselves were experiencing unaccustomed illness on these campaigns; reports of epidemics in major cities, and so forth. He calls for a new reading of the Chinese sources from the period, one more sensitive to the claims that they themselves are making: including the claim that contemporaries were witnessing an *epidemic* that appears to have been *new* in its manifestations. Although Hymes's study is, like Carmichael's, presented as a hypothesis, the interpretative power of both essays comes from taking the historical sources as seriously as the science. Such meticulous scholarship has the potential to recreate, at a level of detail never before imaginable, the paths that different strains of *Y. pestis* might have taken as they reshaped the populations and landscapes of Eurasia.

Finally, in the interests of making new historical documentation available—and to allow students to see for themselves how historians craft understandings of the past—we offer a "featured source": "Diagnosis of a 'Plague' Image: A Digital Cautionary Tale." This essay returns us to London, the site of the Black Death cemetery at East Smithfield whence the *Yersinia pestis* genome was retrieved in 2011. Much of the work that geneticists have done in the past fifteen years has been premised on dramatic advances in computerization, which allow manipulation of many terabytes of genetic data simultaneously. For the humanities, computerization, and specifically the Internet, has made possible the wide dissemination of texts and images. That such new freedom should generate errors, too, is to be expected. The surprise lies in what we found while correcting the error of a "misdiagnosed" image of "plague" using appropriate humanistic analysis of its manuscript context and situated meaning: we were soberingly reminded that plague was not the only disease that troubled people in the middle of the fourteenth century. Although science plays no role in this analysis, I and my coauthors—historian of medicine Kathleen Walker-Meikle and canon law specialist Wolfgang P. Müller—happily acknowledge our debt to scientists who for many decades have been modeling the benefits of collaborative work.

This volume, the inaugural issue of *The Medieval Globe*, is put forward in the belief that dialogue between historical records and modern science, between quantifiable assessment of material remains and the intangibles of humanistic method, is not an exercise in presentism but an opportunity to take seriously the task of reconstructing the world that historical actors inhabited, right down to the microbes that killed them. In an earlier draft of her essay, Ann Carmichael quoted the environmental historian Richard C. Hoffman, who observed that we are dealing with events that "took place before we were in a position to see [them]" (Hoffman 1995: 59). We are in a position to see so much more now—from both *emic* and *etic* perspectives—and what we see is an enlarged, more dynamic, and more complex medieval globe.

Acknowledgments

I and all the contributors to this volume collectively owe thanks to several groups of people and institutions for making this work possible. Nine years ago at Arizona State University, I discovered in the Bioarcheology Program colleagues (most importantly, Jane Buikstra) whose professionalism and driving curiosity about disease experiences in the past have set the standard for the work I aspire to here. That enthusiasm was transferred for two wonderful summers to London, where the Wellcome Library hosted my National Endowment for the Humanities Summer Seminars; the participants there were the first to wrestle with the problem of opening up dialogue between the humanities and the historicist sciences on the huge question of plague's history. We owe a special debt of gratitude to Jelena Bekvalac and Rebecca Redfern of the Human Bioarchaeology Centre at the Museum of London for allowing us to examine their collections from the London Black Death Cemetery, and to Rachel E. Scott (now of DePaul University) who was our bioarcheological guide. In 2012, Michelle Ziegler created the Plague Working Group, an invaluable small community for discussing the latest work in the field. In 2013–14, the Institute for Advanced Study at Princeton provided me with an incomparable cohort of historians from across the chronological and geographic range, together with intellectual sustenance of every other kind; funding while at the Institute was provided by the National Endowment for the Humanities and the Willis F. Doney Membership Endowment.

The particular debt we owe collectively is to the World History Center of the University of Pittsburgh. By granting me an appointment as Visiting Scholar in 2013–14, the Center provided not simply another welcoming audience but also funds to subsidize conference travel critical to this project and, most importantly, to underwrite the open-access publication of this volume. None of these individuals or institutions bears responsibility for statements made in this or the following essays, though I hope all will recognize with pride their essential contributions. Any views, findings, conclusions, or recommendations expressed in this publication do not necessarily reflect those of the National Endowment for the Humanities.

Finally, we thank Carol Symes, founding editor of *The Medieval Globe*, for her belief that the Black Death could provide a valuable exploratory path between and beyond traditional geographic and disciplinary boundaries, and for investing extraordinary levels of patience and care in editing this issue.

Bibliography

Achtman, M., G. Morelli, P. Zhu, T. Wirth, et al. 2004. "Microevolution and History of the Plague Bacillus, *Yersinia pestis*," *Proceedings of the National Academy of Sciences* 101, no. 51: 17837–42

Andrianaivoarimanana, V., K. Kreppel, N. Elissa, J.-M. Duplantier, et al. 2013. "Understanding the Persistence of Plague Foci in Madagascar," *PLoS Neglected Tropical Diseases* 7, no. 11: e0002382

Ben Ari, T., S. Neerinckx, K. L. Gage, K. Kreppel, et al. 2011. "Plague and Climate: Scales Matter," *PLoS Pathogens* 7, no. 9: e1002160

Benedict, Carol. 1996. *Bubonic Plague in Nineteenth-Century China* (Stanford: Stanford University Press)

Benedictow, Ole. 2010. *What Disease was Plague? On the Controversy over the Microbiological Identity of Plague Epidemics of the Past* (Leiden: Brill)

Borsch, Stuart. 2014. "Plague Depopulation and Irrigation Decay in Medieval Egypt," *The Medieval Globe* 1: 125–156

Bos, K. I., V. J. Schuenemann, G. B. Golding, H. A. Burbano, et al. 2011. "A Draft Genome of *Yersinia pestis* from Victims of the Black Death," *Nature* 478, no. 7370: 506–10

Buell, Paul D. 2012. "Qubilai and the Rats," *Sudhoffs Archiv* 96: 127–44

Cabanel, N., A. Leclercq, V. Chenal-Francisque, B. Annajar, et al. 2013. "Plague Outbreak in Libya, 2009, Unrelated to Plague in Algeria," *Emerging Infectious Diseases* 19, no. 2: 230–36

Campbell, Bruce M. S. 2013. "The Great Transition: Climate, Disease and Society in the 13th and 14th Centuries," The Ellen McArthur Lectures, University of Cambridge <http://www.econsoc.hist.cam.ac.uk/podcast-campbell.html> [accessed January 9, 2014]

Carmichael, Ann G. 2014. "Plague Persistence in Western Europe: A Hypothesis," *The Medieval Globe* 1: 157–191

Colet, Anna, Josep Xavier Muntané i Santiveri, Jordi Ruíz Ventura, Oriol Saula, et al. 2014. "The Black Death and its Consequences for the Jewish Community in Tàrrega: Lessons from History and Archeology," *The Medieval Globe* 1: 63–96

Crespo, Fabian, and Matthew B. Lawrenz. 2014. "Heterogeneous Immunological Landscape and Medieval Plague: An Invitation to a New Dialogue between Historians and Immunologists," *The Medieval Globe* 1: 229–258

Cui, Y., C. Yu, Y. Yan, D. Li, et al. 2013. "Historical Variations in Mutation Rate in an Epidemic Pathogen, *Yersinia pestis*," *Proceedings of the National Academy of Science* 110, no. 2: 577–82

Cummins, Neil, Morgan Kelly, and Cormac Ó Gráda. 2013. "Living Standards and Plague in London, 1560–1665," *Social Science Research Network* <http://ssrn.com/abstract=2289094> [accessed September 10, 2014]

Curson, P. H., and K. McCracken. 1989. *Plague in Sydney: The Anatomy of an Epidemic* (Kensington: New South Wales University Press)

DeWitte, Sharon N. 2014. "The Anthropology of Plague: Insights from Bioarcheological Analyses of Epidemic Cemeteries," *The Medieval Globe* 1: 97–123

Dols, Michael. 1974. "The Comparative Communal Responses to the Black Death in Muslim and Christian Societies," *Viator* 5: 269–87

Eisen, R. J., K. S. Griffith, J. N. Borchert, K. MacMillan, et al. 2010. "Assessing Human Risk of Exposure to Plague Bacteria in Northwestern Uganda Based on Remotely Sensed Predictors," *American Journal of Tropical Medicine and Hygiene* 82, no. 5: 904–11

Eisen, R. J., J. N. Borchert, J. T. Mpanga, L. A. Atiku, et al. 2012. "Flea Diversity as an Element for Persistence of Plague Bacteria in an East African Plague Focus," *PLoS ONE* 7, no. 4: e3559

Ermus, Cindy. 2014. "Pestilence and Politics: A Global History of the Marseille Plague" (PhD dissertation, Florida State University)

Gage, K. L. 2012. "Factors Affecting the Spread and Maintenance of Plague," in *Advances in Yersinia Research*, ed. Alzira Maria Paiva de Almeida and Nilma Cintra Leal, special issue, *Advances in Experimental Medicine and Biology* 954, no. 1: 79–94

Green, Monica H. 2014. "Taking 'Pandemic' Seriously: Making the Black Death Global," *The Medieval Globe* 1: 27–61

Harbeck, M., L. Seifert, S. Hänsch, D. M. Wagner, et al. 2013. "*Yersinia pestis* DNA from Skeletal Remains from the 6th Century AD Reveals Insights into Justinianic Plague," *PLoS Pathogens* 9, no. 5: e1003349

Hoffman, R. C. 1995. "Environmental Change and the Culture of Common Carp in Medieval Europe," *Guelf Ichthyology Review* 3, no. 1: 57–85

Hymes, Robert. 2014. "A Hypothesis on the East Asian Beginnings of the *Yersinia pestis* Polytomy," *The Medieval Globe* 1: 285–308

Le Roy Ladurie, Emmanuel. 1973. "Un concept: l'unification microbienne du monde (XVIe–XVIIe siècles)," *Schweizerische Zeitschrift für Geschichte* 23, no. 4: 627–96 (An abbreviated English translation is also available: Emmanuel Le Roy Ladurie. 1981. "A Concept: The Unification of the Globe by Disease," trans. Sian Reynolds and Ben Reynolds, in *The Mind and Method of the Historian*, 28–83 (London: Harvester))

Little, Lester K. 2011. "Plague Historians in Lab Coats," *Past and Present* 213: 267–90

MacMillan, K., R. E. Enscore, A. Ogen-Odoi, J. N. Borchert, et al. 2011. "Landscape and Residential Variables Associated with Plague-Endemic Villages in the West Nile Region of Uganda," *American Journal of Tropical Medicine and Hygiene* 84, no. 3: 435–42

Mengel, David. 2011. "A Plague on Bohemia? Mapping the Black Death," *Past and Present* 211: 3–34

Mikhail, Alan. 2012. "Plague and Environment in Late Ottoman Egypt," in *Water on Sand: Environmental Histories of the Middle East and North Africa*, ed. Alan Mikhail, 111–32 (Oxford: Oxford University Press)

Morelli, G., Y. Song, C. J. Mazzoni, M. Eppinger, et al. 2010. "*Yersinia pestis* Genome Sequencing Identifies Patterns of Global Phylogenetic Diversity," *Nature Genetics* 42, no. 12: 1140–45

Morens, D. M., G. K. Folkers, and A. S. Fauci. 2009. "What Is a Pandemic?," *Journal of Infectious Diseases* 200, no. 7: 1018–21

Neerinckx, S., A. Townsend Peterson, H. Gulinck, J. Deckers, et al. 2010. "Predicting Potential Risk Areas of Human Plague for the Western Usambara Mountains, Lushoto District, Tanzania," *American Journal of Tropical Medicine and Hygiene* 82, no. 3: 492–500

Robarts, Andrew. 2010. "A Plague on Both Houses? Population Movements and the Spread of Disease across the Ottoman-Russian Black Sea Frontier, 1768–1830s" (PhD dissertation, Georgetown University)

Royer, Katherine. 2014. "The Blind Men and the Elephant: Imperial Medicine, Medieval Historians, and the Role of Rats in the Historiography of Plague," in *Medicine and Colonialism: Historical Perspectives in India and South Africa*, ed. Poonam Bala, 99–110 (London: Pickering & Chatto)

Schneider, M. C., P. Najera, S. Aldighieri, D. I. Galan, et al. 2014. "Where Does Human Plague Still Persist in Latin America?," *PLoS Neglected Tropical Diseases* 8, no. 2: e2680

Stearns, Justin K. 2011. *Infectious Ideas: Contagion in Premodern Islamic and Christian Thought in the Western Mediterranean* (Baltimore: Johns Hopkins University Press)

Stenseth, N. Chr., N. I. Samia, H. Viljugrein, K. L. Kausrud, et al. 2006. "Plague Dynamics are Driven by Climate Variation," *Proceedings of the National Academy of Sciences* 103, no. 35: 13110–15

Varlık, Nükhet. 2014. "New Science and Old Sources: Why the Ottoman Experience of Plague Matters," *The Medieval Globe* 1: 193–227

Wagner, D. M., J. Klunk, M. Harbeck, A. Devault, et al. 2014. "*Yersinia pestis* and the Plague of Justinian, 541–543 AD: A Genomic Analysis," *Lancet Infectious Diseases* 14, no. 4: 319–26

Xu, L., L. Chr. Stige, K. L. Kausrud, T. Ben Ari, et al. 2014. "Wet Climate and Transportation Routes Accelerate Spread of Human Plague," *Proceedings of the Royal Society B: Biological Sciences* 281, no. 1780: 20133159

Ziegler, Michelle. 2014. "The Black Death and the Future of the Plague," *The Medieval Globe* 1: 259–284

Monica H. Green (Monica.Green@asu.edu) is a historian of medieval European medicine and global health. In 2009 and 2012, she ran a National Endowment for the Humanities Summer Seminar in London on "Health and Disease in the Middle Ages," which had as its central goal the exploration of ways that the scientific and humanistic disciplines could engage in productive dialogue about the history of disease and health-seeking behaviors. During this same period, she has also argued for the development of a new field, "Global History of Health," which explores the evolution of the major pathogens that have afflicted the human species since its origin up to the present day, and the ways that human cultural changes have facilitated or hindered those pathogens' trajectories. In addition to many works on the cultural history of medieval medicine, she is the author of "The Value of Historical Perspective," in *The Ashgate Research Companion to the Globalization of Health*, ed. Ted Schrecker (Aldershot: Ashgate, 2012), pp. 17–37; and "The Globalisations of Disease," which will be published in 2015.

Abstract Extraction of the genetic material of the causative organism of plague, *Yersinia pestis*, from the remains of persons who died during the Black Death has confirmed that pathogen's role in one of the largest pandemics of human history. This then opens up historical research to investigations based on modern science, which has studied *Yersinia pestis* from a variety of perspectives, most importantly its evolutionary history and its complex ecology of transmission. The contributors to this special issue argue for the benefits of a multidisciplinary and collaborative approach to the many remaining mysteries associated with the plague's geographical extent, rapid transmission, deadly outcomes, and persistence.

Keywords *Yersinia pestis*, Second Plague Pandemic, Afroeurasia, anti-Jewish violence, bioarcheology, biological anthropology, microbiology, historical method.

TAKING "PANDEMIC" SERIOUSLY: MAKING THE BLACK DEATH GLOBAL

MONICA H. GREEN

IN 2009, WHEN the most recent major monograph was published on life in an Italian city of the mid-fourteenth century, its author deferred judgment on whether the disease that struck Italy in 1348—"an infinite mortality the likes of which ha[ve] never been seen on earth"—was in fact plague as defined by modern science (Wray 2009: 1). The authors contributing to this, the inaugural issue of *The Medieval Globe*, no longer feel that such caution is necessary. Since 1998, several international teams of microbiologists have tested and contested the possibilities for establishing the presence of plague's causative organism, *Yersinia pestis*, in the physical remains of Europeans who died at various moments in premodern history when major epidemics were raging. The reason that there is scientific consensus now, when there was not before, is a function of two developments, both of them having to do with trajectories in genetics research in the past thirty years that have come together quite recently.

On the one hand, researchers have been exploring methods to capture and analyze "ancient" DNA (aDNA), by which they mean any genetic material from older remains. Because *Y. pestis* would be circulating throughout the bloodstream by the time it kills a person, and because the hard enamel of intact teeth could potentially preserve small amounts of blood found within the dental pulp, teeth became the focal point of attempts to retrieve *Y. pestis* from human remains. But the challenges of developing viable methods of extraction and analysis were significant. DNA, like

In addition to the individuals and institutions thanked in the Editor's Introduction to this volume, I would here like to acknowledge my debt to the participants at a conference held in Oxford, "Proto-Globalisation in the Indian Ocean World," in November 2013, and to Patrick Manning, Mark Horton, and Neil Kodesh for their guidance on incorporating Africa into this narrative. Funding for this project was provided by fellowships from the Institute for Advanced Study at Princeton (with funds from the National Endowment for the Humanities and the Willis F. Doney Membership Endowment) and the World History Center of the University of Pittsburgh (which has also subsidized open-access publication of this volume). Any views, findings, conclusions, or recommendations expressed in this publication do not necessarily reflect those of the National Endowment for the Humanities.

every other part of the body, begins to decay immediately after death, so degradation of the genetic material was the first of the challenges encountered by researchers. For example, the full genome of *Yersinia pestis* is about 5.6 million base pairs long. The fragments that researchers have had to deal with are rarely even fifty to seventy-five base pairs long. Add to this issue the problems of the material's possible contamination (which could occur when collecting it in the field, or in the lab, or at any point in between), and it is quite understandable, looking back on them now, why the "aDNA debates" of the late 1990s and 2000s were so intense. Already in 2004, however, another diagnostic mechanism—a protein assay that tested for an antigen produced uniquely by *Yersinia pestis*—was shown to be useful in determining the presence of *Y. pestis* not simply in modern diagnostics and epidemiological surveys, but also in historical samples. Meanwhile, studies reporting success in extracting *Y. pestis* aDNA kept appearing, each with more confidence, and by 2011 it was announced that the complete genome of *Y. pestis*, assembled from fourteenth-century remains, had been sequenced (Bos et al. 2011; Little 2011).

At the same time as this aDNA work was being pursued, highly sophisticated studies were being done of modern samples of *Y. pestis*, which is now a globally distributed pathogen. Scientific studies of *Y. pestis* have been going on since the late nineteenth century, but have increased in pace and intensity in recent years, both because *Y. pestis* is a useful model for studying pathogen virulence, and also because there are heightened concerns of bioterrorism and disease re-emergence (Ziegler 2014, in this issue). One main objective of phylogenetic studies of *Y. pestis*'s modern genome (which was first fully sequenced in 2001) has been to reconstruct the organism's evolutionary history. The principle is simple: by categorizing like genetic variations with like, the modern samples can be grouped into clusters, from which phylogenetic relationships can then be inferred. In other words, different modern strains are placed at different end points of a family tree, with inferred branches connecting back down to a common root. Doing this on the basis of long sections of the genome (or now, more commonly, using multiple samples of the whole genome itself) allows for analysis of the organism's phylogeny down to the level of individual base-pair changes (what are called single nucleotide polymorphisms, or SNPs).

The most critical development comes from the fact that both of these lines of research have now converged. Fusing the phylogenetic work and the aDNA work shows that the fourteenth-century genome does in fact fit onto a branch of the phylogenetic tree that had already been postulated (Cui et al. 2013; see **Plate 1 below**). In other words, the organism found in historical human remains is not simply *Y. pestis*, but a kind of *Y. pestis* not too far distant in its genetic structure (and in its potential virulence) from the organism known in the world today. Is it possible that other pathogens were involved in causing the extreme mortality levels of the fourteenth century, in addition to *Y. pestis*? Yes, or at least we cannot rule out that possibility now. Is it possible that other strains of the organism might be found that complicate the narrative I have sketched above? Absolutely. Is it possible that science will keep doing what it always does, making new discoveries? We should hope so.[1] But the microbiological science, whose rigorous methods are becoming standardized and are proving equally fruitful in exploring the histories of other pathogens and organisms, is building up a mounting body of evidence.[2] This confirms that we know enough about the history of *Y. pestis* as a biological organism to structure research programs around certain shared assumptions about its character and behavior. This is not "fringe" science. It is leading-edge work and it demands the serious attention of historians and all others investigating plague in history.

But the skeptic will ask: So what if we can say definitively that people died of *Y. pestis* infections in disease outbreaks of the past? How does that change the work of historians or those working in other historicist disciplines? It is the purpose of this special issue of *The Medieval Globe* to argue that the new microbiology matters not simply because it solves the question "What was the disease?," but because in solving that question (as I believe it does) it opens up entirely new questions, ones we did not previously know we needed to ask. First and foremost, it grounds plague history in the eastern part of the Eurasian landmass. As will be explained in more detail below, study after study is narrowing in on the Tibetan Plateau and Qinghai as the likely place where *Yersinia pestis* diverged from the rela-

1 I have omitted from this assessment a survey of climate science that may eventually implicate major geological or other events in the disturbed ecosystems that initiated the premodern pandemics. Although there is now compelling evidence for coincidental events (e.g., the dust-veil event of *c.* 535 as background to the Justinianic Plague, and a volcanic explosion *c.* 1257 as well as major climatic events in the 1340s that may have contributed to the Black Death), no evidence has yet been brought forth that would link such events directly to the biological evolution of *Y. pestis*. Such evidence may soon be forthcoming, however, since it is clear that alterations in the weather (like excessive rain) contribute to flea production and hence to the possibility of the spread of *Y. pestis*.

2 On continuing efforts to make aDNA research as methodologically rigorous as work on modern genetic materials, see Seifert et al. 2013, and papers presented at the 2013 aDNA conference at the Royal Society in London.

tively harmless soil pathogen *Y. pseudotuberculosis* and became one of the most highly lethal organisms in the world. Plague's history is now firmly on the map in a way it has never been before, and that (as well as other considerations) demands that we rethink almost everything that has been said to date about the disease. As historian Lester Little noted, referring to the significance of the Tübingen-McMaster study of 2011 that reconstructed the Black Death genome from a London cemetery (Bos et al. 2011):

> They are calling for work on the contexts of particular epidemics, including such factors as climate, presence and characteristics of vectors, interactions with concurrent diseases, living conditions, and means of communication and travel. If nothing else, this finding is an open invitation to historians, among others, to re-enter the fray. (Little 2011: 289–90)

That "fray" is already quite active, with various participants coming from different disciplinary backgrounds and, with some cause, bringing with them a wariness of differing approaches. At the conference "Human Evolution, Migration and History Revealed by Genetics, Immunity and Infection," which was held in London in 2011, the organizers (two biologists and a physician) expressed concern that relying on what was already known to historians offered too limiting a view of the history of pathogens and human evolution.

> [W]e have, often, an equally fragmentary account of the historical timeline to which we seek to tether the twists and turns of the biological story. The warning is that we should resist the temptation to link relationships casually through *cherry picking those milestones in human history that are best recorded*. While it is tempting to look for the correlates in evolutionary selection of the Black Death, the fall of the Roman Empire or the colonization of South America, how many equally or more dramatic bottlenecks have been imposed in the past millennia by pathogens, climate change or natural disasters for which we lack a good historical record (or any awareness at all)? (Altmann et al. 2012: 765–66, my emphasis).

Altmann and colleagues then go on to suggest that *Yersinia pestis* should be excepted from this caution on the grounds that it is of relatively recent origin and genetically monomorphic (not showing significant levels of genetic diversity). Yet from the historian's perspective—we who study humans and only secondarily the pathogen—plague's history is still stunningly lacunous. Yes, there is no question that a major plague outbreak happened between 1347 and 1353 in the Mediterranean basin and Western Europe. Whether we estimate its highest mortality rates at 30%, 40%, or 60% (as have variously been proposed), its effects were catastrophic. But while we may have good—in some cases, excellent—records to document human fatalities from plague in those areas, the new plague science tells us that there is much about this disease of which we still lack awareness, including most of the factors that caused it to become, for many centuries, a defining feature not only in the landscape of Western Europe, North Africa, and the Middle East, but also in Russia, India, and East and Central Africa: all the latter being places where it still remains in enzootic foci. As will be noted below, most of the new plague science is also relevant to studies of the First Plague Pandemic, the Justinianic Plague which raged, at least in the Mediterranean basin, from *c.* 541 to *c.* 750 (Little 2007; Mitchell 2014).

This essay, then, argues that it is no longer helpful for historians to take a posture of scientific agnosticism when it comes to the history of plague. I will focus here mainly on the Second Pandemic, sketching out two areas where we have yet to search fully for plague's historical effects: its range across different host species and its geographical extent outside of the Tibetan Plateau and Qinghai region. The revised zoology reminds us to take into account not only the incidental animal species that immediately spread *Y. pestis* to humans in epidemic outbreaks, but also the many other species involved in the long-distance spread of the disease. Taking the genetics science seriously also demands that we revise our geography of plague's history. This new geography is not limited to the Mediterranean and the lands surrounding it. It extends from the Tibetan highlands and Western China overland into Western Eurasia but also, I will suggest, southward, into the Indian Ocean basin and nearly all points connected to it.[3]

An Elephant of a Disease: Widening the Zoological Lens

The Indian tale of the six blind men and the elephant is a useful metaphor for thinking about plague. Believing that the elephant was like a fan (by touching only its ear) or like a tree trunk (by feeling only its thick legs), individual blind men could not perceive the huge and complex beast in its entirety. In thinking about plague, we too need to keep in play all the elements that allowed a single-celled, non-motile bacterium to become a (semi-)global pandemic. There is plenty of scientific literature to explain

3 On the possibility that plague spread east and southeast from the Tibetan-Qinghai Plateau in the medieval period, see Hymes 2014, in this issue. To date, I know of no evidence—genetic, skeletal, or documentary—that suggests that plague reached either Madagascar or Australia prior to the Third Pandemic radiation at the end of the nineteenth century.

the mechanisms connecting pathogen, natural hosts, accidental (or intermediate) hosts, environmental and climatic factors, and human elements. On some issues there is widespread consensus; on others, research is only beginning. Here, I wish to focus on the need for more historical study of the animal hosts that may be involved in plague transmission. We need to look at more than the elephant's tail.

The Tibetan-Qinghai Plateau, whose average elevation is several thousand meters above sea level, is as far removed in its climatic and ecological environment from most of the areas hardest hit by plague in the fourteenth century as it is in geographic distance. *Y. pestis* had to move across many animal species (arthropod vectors as well as mammalian hosts) as well as climatic zones in order to cause the massive human mortality that it did in the fourteenth century (and episodically thereafter). Tracing *Y. pestis* across many animal species will be a necessary part of retracing its geographical spread. That includes re-examining the role of one particular species, *Homo sapiens*, who is likely responsible for plague's most extensive dissemination. But we'll get to that species later.

As Michelle Ziegler explains (2014, in this issue), the trifold litany of plague modes usually cited in historical accounts—bubonic, pneumonic, and septicemic—needs to be broadened now to include the gastrointestinal. As Ziegler notes, these different presentations of plague are better thought of by their method of transmission: insect bite and abrasion or cutting (bubonic and septicemic), inhalation (pneumonic), and ingestion (gastrointestinal), respectively. These are not different diseases, of course. They are all caused by *Y. pestis*. They differ only in the path by which the organism enters the body and the speed with which it reaches the bloodstream, and, in clinical terms, by the symptoms induced when different immune responses are triggered, depending on what tissues the organism first encounters (Pechous et al. 2013). It is important to begin with this distinction, because while any or all of these modes of transmission may be operative in a given outbreak, each can have its own characteristic microenvironment.

Most historical work has focused on bubonic plague, and the rat-flea mode of transmission that was documented early in the Third Pandemic at the turn of the twentieth century. But rats are not the only carriers of plague: they are not even efficient ones in terms of the organism's evolutionary survival.[4] There are several hundred animal species that can be

---

4 A new line of research has raised the question of whether human lice might also be a factor in plague's spread (e.g, Ayyadurai et al. 2010). If so, this would radically increase the importance of studying practices of clothing exchange and resale,

infected with plague.[5] For studying human outbreaks, interest has focused on "commensals," those species that "share our tables," living around human settlements, eating our foodscraps. But the new geography of plague tells us they we need to look at much wider biological systems to understand how *Y. pestis* moved many thousands of miles across varying ecological environments to reach large human population settlements. Beyond commensal rodents, we need to look at wild rodents, lagomorphs (hares, rabbits, etc.), and ruminants (cattle, goats, sheep, camels, deer), as well as the carnivore species that prey on them.

For their 2013 study of historical variations in the mutation rates of *Y. pestis*, Cui and colleagues drew on 133 complete genome sequences of the organism, which had been collected from nineteen different mammalian genera infected with *Y. pestis*, as well as from a variety of fleas, ticks, and lice that prey on them (Cui et al. 2013, supplemental data: 10). Eleven of the mammalia were rodent species, one was a type of lagomorph, and then there were other various grazing animals (sheep, bharals) and carnivores (badgers, weasels, canids, and foxes). There were also humans. But the list of susceptible animals is far larger than that. A surveillance study in India carried out between 1989 and 2007 found that *Tatera indica cuvieri* (Hardwicke), the Indian gerbil, made up the highest percentage of plague-infected rodents (41.9%), followed by *Rattus rattus rufescens* Gray and *Rattus rattus wroughtoni* Hinton, and finally the lesser bandicoot rat or Indian "Mole-Rat" (Biswas et al. 2011). These several species have different relations to human populations, the rats being "peri-domestic," while the gerbils are wild. But all of them shared two species of flea, showing how transmission could occur across rodent populations and move from rural enzootic foci into proximity with humans.

Similar field surveillance of plague transmission in rodent communities has been going on for over a century and has shown repeatedly that multiple species are involved (e.g., Davis 1953). Especially important is research showing the importance of looking beyond rodents. Camels have been known to be plague carriers for over a century, but they seem to infect humans for the most part when sick animals are slaughtered and eaten, thus producing gastrointestinal plague. Such a case has been doc-

---

and their implications for transmission of disease among humans, without the intervention of a flea vector. (See Veracx et al. 2012 for the connections between human head and body lice.)

5 Anisimov, Lindler, and Pier (2004) note that over two hundred species of wild rodents and over eighty different flea species are known to be involved in plague transmission.

umented as recently as 2009 (Federov 1960; Christie, Chen, and Elberg 1980; cf. Ziegler 2014, in this issue). How commonly camels were involved in plague transmission in the past has yet to be explored. But we can see the possible scenarios. Small rodents called jirds (in the genus *Meriones*) are known to live around the tents of nomads and have been documented as being infected but plague-resistant, most recently in Algeria. This raises the specter that even isolated nomadic herders or traders might have helped transmit plague across wide expanses not otherwise thought hospitable to *Y. pestis* transmission (Bitam et al. 2010; see also Varlık 2014, in this issue). Various species of *Meriones* are found from Northern Africa to Mongolia, in a variety of different climatic environments. Jirds can be commensal as well as sylvan, making possible plague transmission from enzootic foci to human communities. Since camels were domesticated as early as the fourteenth or fifteenth century BCE and served as the major beast of burden for overland trade in the Middle East from about the second century of the Common Era (Bulliet 1975), they should surely be factored into our calculus of how *Y. pestis* moved as far as it did.

I am not proposing a grand new monocausal thesis here. Few of these species, by themselves, make sense as plague-transmitters across the wide terrains of Afro-Eurasia,[6] and the climate science needed to help understand faunal dispersals (independent of human herding or trade) is only beginning to emerge. But it is important to stress that historical research, likely combining the efforts of historians working with documentary sources and bioarcheologists working with biological remains (and climatologists as well), will be necessary to assess whether some of these possibilities are more plausible than others. The phylogenies of commensal animals are now being studied as bioproxies for human histories: that is, tracking the histories of animals that have moved at great distances along with humans can serve to document human movements even when all other traces have vanished (Jones et al. 2013). But as the case of plague makes plain, the movements of such commensals are important in their own right, since these species can serve to recreate fairly homogenous microenvironments in many different parts of the world.[7] Introduce even a limited number of *Yersinia pestis*-bearing fleas into such populations, and you may well have the ingredients for epizootics that spill over into human populations.

6 A conference on precisely this issue was held in Leipzig in 2010 (Franz, Riha, and Schubert 2010).

7 Anthropogenic replication of microenvironments has likewise been key to the global spread of other vector-borne diseases, like malaria and dengue fever. See Green (forthcoming) for an overview.

Reaching Africa: *Yersinia pestis* in Evolutionary Time and Place

As noted above, one of the key developments in genetics has been the construction of robust phylogenetic trees that postulate the evolutionary relationships among various strains of *Y. pestis*, as documented from aDNA and modern samples. Evolution, of course, is a historical phenomenon par excellence, involving that most essential object of the historian's quest: change over time. Earlier calculations of *Y. pestis*'s history, working from the assumption that there was a biomolecular clock that "ticked" at a regular rate, postulated that *Y. pestis* diverged from the most recent common ancestor it shares with *Yersinia pseudotuberculosis* anywhere from 1,056 years before the present (50% confidence limit) to 20,436 years (95% confidence limit) (Achtman et al. 1999).[8] The complete sequencing of the fourteenth-century genome—which at last put a time-date stamp on one point of the organism's premodern evolutionary tree—allowed a recalibration of that molecular clock. A new history of *Y. pestis* was proposed, which estimated its emergence as having taken place as recently as about 3335 years before the present, with 95% confidence intervals still within the range of recorded human history (4394 BCE to 510 CE) (Cui et al. 2013).

The calculation of time using molecular evidence is still a highly contested area of paleogenetics (Ho and Larson 2006; Larson 2013). The phrase "about 3335 years [ago]" has no calendrical authority, but is rather just a computational cipher. In fact, the notion of a fixed "molecular clock" is now seeming like a red herring: genetic change likely occurs for various reasons and at various rates, and is therefore historically variable.[9] Still, the phylogenetic tree of *Y. pestis* (as it has been refined over the course of the past decade and a half) does offer important chronological infor-

8 These biomolecular clock rates were initially calibrated in the 1980s on the basis of changes observed under laboratory conditions in *Enterococcus coli* and *Staphylococcus enterica* type *typhimurium*. The lower limit cited here, 1056 years before the present, would, if true, obviously put *Y. pestis* out of the running as the causative agent of the Justinianic Plague. But the authors, assuming that the First Plague Pandemic was caused by *Y. pestis*, simply adjusted the clock back: "Justinian's plague was 1,500 years ago, and, therefore, *Y. pestis* is at least 1,500 years old" (Achtman et al. 1999: 14047). A revised calculation was offered in Achtman et al. 2004, and again in Cui et al. 2013, which I discuss below.

9 See, for example, Wagner et al. 2014, which offers a second fixed point in time for *Y. pestis*'s historical genome and suggests that "[w]hatever the cause of this rate variation, these data suggest that previous molecular-clock-derived estimates of the timescale of *Y. pestis* evolution, including the date of its divergence from *Y. pseudotuberculosis*, might be erroneous."

mation in that it suggests a *sequence* of chronological change: "this" happened before "that." And once we tie that relative chronological information to fixed geographic space, the real value of the new work in genetics for the historian becomes apparent: the fact that approximate place in time can be connected to specific place in space.

The question of plague's geographic origins has long troubled historians. Oddly, the lines of argument have gone in different directions: for the Justinianic Plague, the standard argument had been to assume an African origin;[10] for the Black Death, its genesis has been placed more or less vaguely in "the East." Given a confused historical record and the current distribution of *Y. pestis* across most of Asia and Africa (World Health Organization 2008, Neerinckx et al. 2008), it is little wonder the question has long been unresolved. In 1976, McNeill, who placed the origins of *Y. pestis* "at some perhaps geologically ancient time," chose to remain on the fence: "There appears to be no basis for deciding which of these two natural reservoirs [Central Africa or northeastern India, i.e., the Himalayas] is the oldest" (McNeill 1976: 139).[11] For McNeill, the obscure geographic origins of *Y. pestis* could be shrugged off so long as it was seen to exist "time out of mind." Even the emerging evolutionary narrative in the 1990s left the question ambiguous because a widely used classification system, dating from the 1950s, collapsed African and Asian strains into a single subspecies grouping, the biovar "Antiqua" (Giuyoule et al. 1994; Achtman et al. 1999). Extensive work has now been done on the genetic diversity of *Yersinia pestis* as it is currently found throughout the world, allowing the pathogen's evolutionary history to come more clearly into view. That work does not prove in any absolute sense where *Y. pestis* originated as an organism. But as a hypothesis, it accords with the emerging evolutionary and historical understanding of the organism.

---

10 Horden 2005; Sarris 2007: 120–23; and Sallares 2007. McCormick (2007: 303–04), relying on Actman et al. 1999, defers judgment on the question. No written evidence has yet been gathered that can push plague's presence in sub-Saharan Africa back definitively before 1877; see Neerinckx et al. 2010.

11 For reasons that I will address in the last section of this essay, I consider all of this prior work "retrospective diagnosis" in the older sense, based exclusively on textual sources whose ability to properly document a specific microbiological pathogen is not robust. It is for this reason, too, that I will not engage here with the many maps that have been published in history textbooks and elsewhere, "plotting the course" of plague's spread with arrows and routes that have no foundation in documentary evidence, let alone material remains. On the many pitfalls in mapping as it relates to plague's histories, see Mengel 2011.

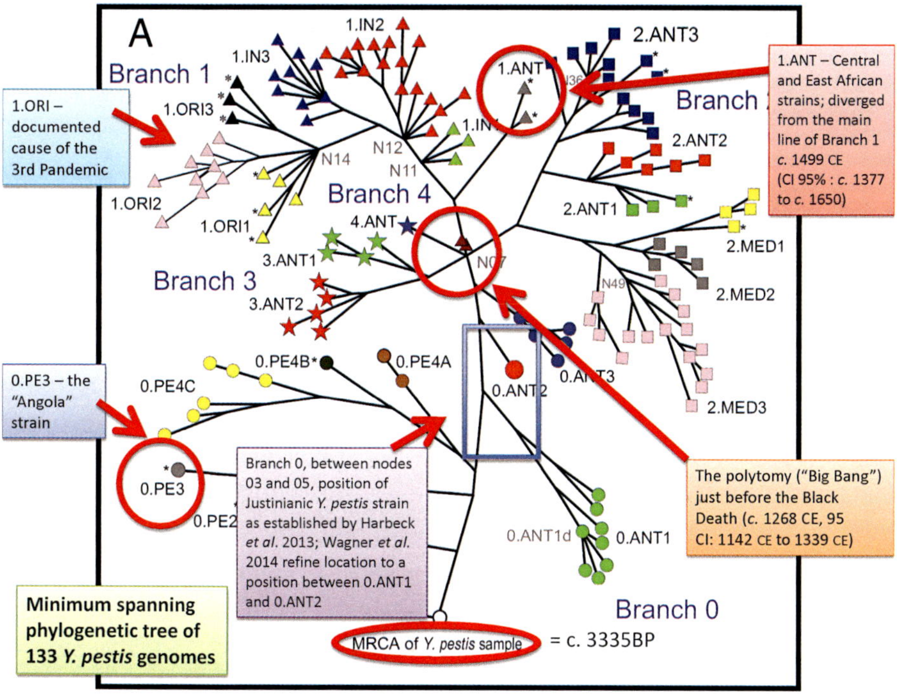

Plate 1. Phylogenetic Tree of *Yersinia Pestis. Adapted with permission from Cui et al. 2013.*

A basic principle of evolutionary theory is that the greatest subspecies diversification will be found in the area where the species has lived the longest. This is no constant, of course, since changed environmental conditions can drive any life form out of its original habitat. And strains go extinct, erasing from view certain lines of development. But as a rule of thumb, the association of geography with subspecies diversification generates valuable hypotheses. For *Y. pestis*, the current hypothesis—first proposed on genetics grounds in 2004 and elaborated further since then—is that the organism took its origin in the Tibetan-Qinghai Plateau, now a part of modern China.[12] If this is true, then all narratives of plague's history must be connected to that place of origin. And if it is true, it resolves definitively the Africa vs. Asia dilemma of plague's origin. This is one of the biggest game-changers in historical studies of plague since

12 The Chinese plague researcher Wu Lien-teh seems to have been the first to suggest, on epidemiological grounds, that *Yersinia pestis* had its origin within the boundaries of what we now call China (Wu 1924). The hypothesis was first advanced on genetic grounds by Achtman et al. 2004; see most recently Li et al. 2009, Morelli et al. 2010, Cui et al. 2013, and Yan et al. 2014.

the identification of the rat-flea nexus at the turn of the twentieth century. But the emerging evolutionary narrative has a second result, and that is to suggest that we should broaden our narratives of the Second Pandemic to include sub-Saharan African and, by implication, the Indian Ocean basin.

The phylogenetic tree shown in **Plate 1** comes from Cui and colleagues' 2013 study of historical variations in the mutation rate of *Y. pestis* and summarizes the entire history of the organism as it is understood from genetics. The historical significance of its five major branches (or lineages) and twenty-five subbranches (or phylogroups) is as follows.[13]

- Branch 0 (the main stem of tree) contains almost all pestoides isolates, which, with the exception of the oldest strain, 0.PE7, are found primarily in voles (groups 0.PE1, 0.PE2, 0.PE3, 0.PE4, 0.PE7).[14] It also includes the earlier strains of the ANT group (0.ANT1-3).
- Harbeck and colleagues (2013), working from human remains found in Bavaria, established that the strain that caused the Justinianic Plague seemed to lie on branch 0 between nodes 03 and 05. Wagner and colleagues (2014) have refined that conclusion to put the Justinianic strain specifically between nodes 04 and 05 (that is, between the current extant strains 0.ANT1 and 0.ANT2).
- Node 07 is the polytomy event ('Big Bang') that leads to branches 1-4. Cui et al. (2013) calculate a date for the polytomy at *c.* 1268 (95% CI: 1142, 1339).
- Branch 1 contains African Antiqua (1.ANT) and all of the Intermediate (1.IN) and Orientalis (1.ORI) strains. Strains on this branch caused both the Black Death and the Third Pandemic. 1.ANT is localized now in Central and East Africa.[15]

---

13 The trifold categories of biovars—"Antiqua," "Medievalis," and "Orientalis"—formulated in the 1950s according to the ability of different strains to reduce nitrate and to ferment glycerol, have been shown to be misleading and are now otiose (Achtman et al. 2004); these phenotypical categories have no meaningful relationship with the strains likely to have caused the three plague pandemics. The labels "ANT," "MED," and "ORI" are, nevertheless, still found on laboratory samples, relics of that older classification system.

14 In 2012, Riehm et al. proposed an additional strain, 0.PE8 (MNG 2972) found in Mongolia, and suggested the possibility of yet another strain, 0.PE9 found in Tajikistan, Uzbekistan. The species from which the samples were collected were not reported. Neither strain is shown on the diagram of Cui et al. (2013).

15 Seifert et al. (2013: 5, table 2) refer to one sample of 1.ANT as "NCTC_570 Bombay 267." Assuming this is not simply a labeling error, it would be the only known case of

- Branch 2 contains all of Medievalis (2.MED) and yet another "Antiqua" strain (2.ANT). These strains are currently found throughout much of Eurasia, including India (cf. Kingston et al. 2009) and as far west as Turkey and Libya (Cabanel et al. 2013).
- Branches 3 and 4 (3.ANT and 4.ANT) were first announced in 2013 by Cui and colleagues; to date, these have been found only in China and Mongolia, in marmots and in the genus *Meriones*, which includes many kinds of jirds as well as gerbils.

Three features of this evolutionary tree are significant for plague's standard premodern history: that is, the narrative centered on plague's arrival in the Mediterranean and Western Europe. At the center of the tree, at node 07, is the polytomy ("Big Bang") dated by Cui and colleagues to *c.* 1268 CE, with a 95% confidence interval ranging from 1142 CE to 1339 CE.[16] This period of rapid diversification of *Y. pestis* (possibly caused by the organism moving into new climatic environments and new hosts) immediately preceded the Black Death, whose genome (taken from the London Black Death cemetery) lies near the root of Branch 1 (the maroon-colored triangles). Below the great polytomy, on Branch 0, lies the strain involved in the Justinianic Plague, which seems to fall between nodes 04 and 05 (Harbeck et al. 2013; Wagner et al. 2014).

The phylogenetic tree produced by Cui and colleagues was constructed from information drawn from the complete genomes of 133 samples of *Y. pestis*. Two of these (the two maroon triangles near the base of Branch 1) are medieval samples from the London Black Death cemetery. All the others (131) are samples collected between the late nineteenth and early twenty-first century; and all of these, save seventeen, come from areas now within the political boundaries of China and Mongolia. The outliers come from Russia (2), other areas within the former Soviet Union including Georgia (3), Africa (3), India (1), the United States of America (2), Myanmar (1), Madagascar (3), Nepal (1) and Iran/Kurdistan (1). Here I wish to focus on the three samples from Africa.

---

the African strain 1.ANT being found outside of Africa. Amann (2007: 22) gives the provenance of NCTC_570 Bombay 267 as "G. Liston in 1920 / fatal bubonic plague, Bombay." W. Glen Liston (1872–1950) was a leading plague researcher in Bombay (Mumbai) and helped establish the role of the flea in transmitting plague from rats to humans. I have not been able to determine anything further about the provenance of this sample.

16 See Hymes (2014, in this issue) for the significance of this date.

Little genetics work has been done on sub-Saharan Africa on a scale comparable to what has been done in China and Mongolia, a lacuna in research that makes the following speculations tentative in the extreme.[17] Nevertheless, such *hints* as are now available from *Y. pestis* genetics work suggest that a premodern history of plague in sub-Saharan Africa might be worth exploring. The earliest of the three African samples is also the single most problematic part of the phylogenetic tree of *Y. pestis* as it is currently understood. This strain, called "Angola" (0.PE3), comes from a laboratory sample collected in or before 1984.[18] All provenance information has been lost, and it is not known whether it was collected from a human being, a rodent, or an arthropod vector. It is in every sense a conundrum, because no other samples from this region have yet entered into the genomics databases for *Y. pestis*. The "Angola" strain is distinctive in two respects. First, it is the most divergent of all the strains thus far studied. 548 SNPs separate it from the most recent common ancestor (MCRA) that *Yersinia pestis* shares with its closest related species, *Yersinia pseudotuberculosis*. All other strains, save two, of *Y. pestis* that were studied from complete genomes by Cui and colleagues have less than 300 SNPs that separate them from the MRCA (the mean is 248). "Angola" is the ultimate outlier. Second, "Angola" also lies very close to the base of the phylogenetic tree of *Y. pestis*. Just how old it is as a strain is unclear, but it clearly derives from some very ancient form of the organism. Only

---

17 Work coming out of the Institut Pasteur in Paris in the 1990s (e.g., Guiyoule et al. 1994) drew heavily on samples from Kenya and the (then Belgian) Congo. More recent genetics work, however, has focused mostly on Madagascar, where a radiation of one of the Third Pandemic strains predominates (Morelli et al. 2010). According to the World Health Organization, foci exist in the Democratic Republic of the Congo, Kenya, Lesotho, Libya, Mauritania, Mozambique, Namibia, Senegal, Tanzania, Uganda, and probably Egypt (World Health Organization 1999: 16 and 26–31). I return to the implications of this sampling and research bias at the end of the essay. See also Varlık 2014, in this issue.

18 Dos Santos Grácio and Grácio (2011: 1) claim (without offering citations) that the "first reference to the occurence [*sic*] of plague in Angola was made in 1921. . . . However, others believed plague was already there, and that a sylvatic cycle with a reservoir in wild rodents was already present in Austral Africa before the XV century European arrival." The complete genome of the Angola strain (NC_010159) was sequenced in 2010 and can be found online at <http://www.ncbi.nlm.nih.gov/nuccore/NC_010159.1> [accessed September 10, 2014]. Morelli et al. (2010) first broached the idea that the Angola strain might be an extant remnant of the strain that caused the Justinianic Plague. That notion has since been challenged by Harbeck et al. (2013) on the basis aDNA retrieved from a gravesite in Bavaria.

two phylogroups that have yet been sequenced are more basal, and these come from Eurasia.[19]

So, how long has "Angola" been in sub-Saharan Africa? There is simply no way to tell at this point. But here is where a multidisciplinary perspective would allow us to take the question seriously, even if we cannot yet answer it. We actually have a least one account from a Greek writer in the first century CE, Rufus of Ephesus, reporting on other writers who described a "pestilential fever" characterized by swollen glands in the neck, armpits, groin, and back of the legs. According to Rufus, this condition was reported in Libya, Egypt, and Syria—in other words, around the Mediterranean littoral—at least six centuries before the Justinianic Plague arrived at the port of Pelusium in 541 CE.[20] By itself, Rufus's report is insufficient for a clear determination of the presence of plague in North Africa around the beginning of the Common Era. And connecting the Mediterranean to sub-Saharan Africa is even more problematic for this period of time. But we can see why the historiographic tradition linking plague with Africa in ancient times cannot be dismissed out of hand.

The real surprise that comes from genetics, however, is the possibility that it might help us to reconstruct a medieval or early modern history of plague in sub-Saharan Africa. The other African phylogroup represented on Plate 1 is 1.ANT (gray triangles, top center), which breaks off from the main stem of Branch 1 just above (i.e., just after) the 1348 London genome. 1.ANT, also called "Africa Antiqua," is the group of strains of *Y. pestis* found now in East and Central Africa, from Kenya to Uganda and into the Democratic Republic of Congo. In 2010, Morelli and colleagues proposed an age for the origin of this branch somewhere between 628–6914 years ago. In 2013, Cui and colleagues recalibrated this biological clock, suggesting that the African clades had branched off from the main Black Death clade at a later time: *c.* 1499, with a 95% confidence interval of *c.* 1377 to *c.* 1650.

19 These are 0.PE7, which was sampled for the study of Cui et al. (2013) from the Mongolian five-toed jerboa (*Allactaga sibirica*) and a human patient, both in the Chinese province of Qinghai; and 0.PE2, which was sampled from voles in an area of the Former Soviet Union and Georgia.

20 Rufus's original work no longer survives; rather, the excerpt describing buboes is reported by the fourth-century CE writer Oribasius, in his *Collectionum*. See Sallares (2007: 251) for the Greek text and, for an English translation of the passage, Simpson (1905: 4); see also Simpson (1905: 281) for an image of a popliteal (behind the knee) bubo. My thanks to Heinrich von Staden for confirming the reading of the Greek and advising me on the identification of the authorities Rufus cites, none of whom (*pace* Sallares) can be dated before the first century BCE.

Again, as stressed above, the chronology established by genetics is more valuable in suggesting *relative* position in time than absolute position. It establishes a historical sequence: X happened before Y. 1.ANT is, in terms of its place on the *Yersinia pestis* phylogenetic tree, one of the most closely related "descendants" of the strain that killed the individuals in London whose remains were studied in reconstructing the first complete sample of the Black Death genome. Or, one could say that it is a "distant cousin" of the London strain, rather than a direct descendant. This distinction is important, since the phylogenetic tree does not show us all the dead ends, the extinct sub-branches that may have moved into new geographic terrains or new hosts but then failed to establish mechanisms of long-term survival. The Black Death genome from London is an incredibly lucky find: that rare one-in-a-zillion fossil that captures a strain of the organism as it existed seven hundred years ago, before it hit a "dead end" in the human beings it killed in fourteenth-century London. The modern specimens of 1.ANT, in contrast, have had seven hundred more years to evolve. And like the "Angola" strain, they show that 1.ANT has undergone considerable unique evolution: on a differently calibrated tree, one where physical distance more closely approximates genetic difference, 1.ANT is the furthest spanning subbranch of lineage 1, representing up to 100 SNPs from the 07 polytomy and 300–305 SNPs from the most recent common ancestor of *Y. pestis* (Cui et al. 2013: 579 and supplementary data 8, fig. S3, A). Moreover, a study of this East and Central African strain done back in 1994 found a considerable level of local genetic diversity, suggesting that it had been established in the area for a considerable period of time (Guiyoule et al. 1994).

According to current biological theory, when populations diverge from a common ancestor, genetic differences between them can arise for several reasons. One of those reasons may be adaptations necessary for survival in a new host species. There are no marmots (one of the main host genera for *Y. pestis* in Eastern Eurasia) in Africa, nor, aside from commensal rodents, does there seem to be any major overlap in the known host species of *Y. pestis* on the Eurasia and African continents. In other words, adaptation to new host species may well account for the stark divergence of 1.ANT from other strains on Branch 1, none of which are currently known in Africa save for the modern 1.ORI strains.

So, to summarize, genetics currently tells us three things about 1.ANT. First, it does not derive directly from the "Angola" strain. Hence, whenever "Angola" did arrive in Africa, it did not give rise to 1.ANT. The history of those two strains, and specifically the history of their arrival in Africa, can thus be separated. Second, 1.ANT is older than the strains disseminated worldwide (including to parts of sub-Saharan Africa) during the Third (modern) Pandemic, the 1.ORI strains. So the history of 1.ANT can be separated from the narratives of the Third Pandemic.[21] And third, 1.ANT, the strain of *Y. pestis* associated (so far as we currently know) only with Central and Eastern Africa, is most closely related to the Black Death strain now documented from the London Black Death cemetery.

So when did 1.ANT arrive on the African continent? And by what route? As will be discussed in the next section, the arrival of plague into the Mediterranean basin (and so into North Africa) in the ancient Greco-Roman period was almost certainly via the Red Sea, where trade would have connected the Mediterranean to the Indian Ocean. Whether plague moved further south into the African continent, beyond the Horn of Africa, during the ancient Greco-Roman period is as yet unclear. Clearly, trade was occurring across the Sahara and, up to a point, in the Nile Valley, but we do not yet have strong evidence either for the presence of commensal rodents or for developed urban communities that would have facilitated plague's spread south of the Sahara before the seventh century CE.

By the time of the later medieval plague, however, the situation in sub-Saharan Africa was different. Considerable trade occurred across the Sahara in exchanges of gold, slaves, salt, and probably also ivory (McDougall 1990; Guérin 2013). Mansa Musa's famous pilgrimage from Mali to Mecca in 1324 remains symbolic of those medieval trade networks, a trip whose timing should not go unnoted. For just a few decades later, we find abandonment of sites in sub-Saharan Africa that had previously been thriving metropolitan centers. The sudden late medieval abandonment of earthwork settlements at Jenne-Jeno and Akrokrowa, in what is present-day Ghana, has proved a puzzle to archeologists. In 1998, McIntosh mused on the possibility that plague may have been involved in Jenne-Jeno's abandonment (McIntosh 1998: 247–50), while Chouin and DeCorse (2010) were willing to speculate openly about it as the cause of widespread abandonment:

> Looking at world history during this period, it seems that only one event can possibly explain such a large-scale phenomenon: the occurrence of

21 The historical works of Myron Echenberg on plague in Senegal and South Africa (Echenberg 2001 and 2007) do not draw on the genetics works that was only then emerging. Nevertheless, subsequent genetic analysis suggests that the strains of plague that hit northern, northwestern, and southern Africa in the twentieth century were of the 1.ORI phylogroups, and hence distinctive of the Third Pandemic; see Bitam et al. 2010; Morelli et al. 2010. On the recent discovery of a MED strain (found on Branch 2 of the phylogenetic tree in Cui et al. 2013) in Algeria, see Cabanel et al. (2013).

> the Black Death or Great Plague. . . . In affecting societies living in forest areas of southern Ghana, the Plague would have had exactly the same effect as in other parts of the world: it would have destroyed a large portion of the population living in densely populated settlements, resulting in their abandonment—a well-documented phenomenon in many other contexts. (Chouin and DeCorse 2010: 143)

But in placing plague in sub-Saharan Africa, Chouin and DeCorse were over-interpreting the superficial and unsubstantiated claims of a non-academic book published nearly thirty years earlier (Cartwright and Biddiss 1972).[22] To date, there is neither bioarcheological research nor aDNA to tell us what happened to these societies which, it seems, left no written records. Hence, the question of plague's possible penetration across the Sahara to West Central Africa must remain for the moment an open question.

The situation for East Africa is different. Here, the likely point of entrance for the strain of *Yersinia pestis* that now dominates in Central and East Africa, 1.ANT, was the Indian Ocean coast, where from the seventh century on there is increasing evidence of a "a deeply networked trade and contact situation" (Boivin et al. 2013: 1; cf. Horton 2004). With two exceptions, Indian Ocean transit of *Y. pestis* to East Africa below the Horn has not previously been suggested for plague prior to the Third (modern) Pandemic.[23] Nevertheless, we have cause to raise the question of the timing of plague's arrival. For in Eastern Africa, we have a phenomenon similar to that in West Africa, at virtually the same time: at least four important trading centers suffered major decline. On the coast, Shanga (on the Lamu Archipelago off the coast of modern-day Kenya) and Tumbatu

22 In fact, Cartwright and Biddiss never said anything about sub-Saharan Africa per se, referring only generically to "Africa" (1972: 32 and 51). Their narrative typically just summarizes the impact of the Black Death on Europe.

23 Horton (1996/2012) notes the coincidental timing of the Black Death and the decline of these towns, but implies that the latter is due to the general collapse of the international economy at that time. Horton and Middleton (2000: 82) offer a passing suggestion that plague may have indeed reached East Africa. They cite Dols (1977) in support of their claim that plague spread "throughout the Middle East and the Indian Ocean world," but Dols in fact claimed that transmission through the Indian Ocean was unlikely (Dols 1977: 43–44). The other claim of Indian Ocean transport was made by the microbiologist Mark Achtman, who proposed in 2010 that *Y. pestis* might have been brought to East Africa by the Chinese explorer Zheng He (1371–1433) (Morelli et al. 2010). Achtman has since retracted that suggestion (Cui et al. 2013), not because of its historical or epidemiological improbability, but rather because he recalibrated his biological clock, pushing the divergence of 1.ANT from the main branch to a later era and thus making Zheng He's role less likely.

(on Tumbatu Island) were abandoned, while Kilwa on the island of Kilwa Kisiwani (modern-day Tanzania) became derelict. Inland, Great Zimbabwe (near present day Masvingo, Zimbabwe), known for its monumental mortarless structures, was abandoned. The dating of Great Zimbabwe's abandonment has been intensely debated; carbon-14 dating performed in the early 1990s showed that Great Zimbabwe's growth had stopped by the mid-fourteenth century, and the site was abandoned definitively by the sixteenth, at the latest (Huffman and Vogel 1991; Pikirayi 2001: 150–51). While there was not complete devastation of the East African coast in this period (e.g., Wynne-Jones 2013), the pattern of coastal areas and an upland region (Great Zimbabwe is on a plateau, over a thousand meters high) being simultaneously affected bears the distinctive stamp of plague (Carmichael 2014, in this issue). Moreover, the conditions for plague's spread were there: intense human trade in various commodities across the Indian Ocean and the arrival of Asian commensal rodents in East Africa.

Reaching Tibet: A New Geography of Plague

> And the coral *which is brought from our homeland* is sold more in this land than any other kind.[24]

Marco Polo (d. 1324) was a latecomer to the vast trade networks that brought Mediterranean coral all the way to Kashmir (where he made this observation) and to Tibet, where he noted that coral brought "great delight" there, too.[25] Polo's *Description of the World,* read from the perspective of what we know now about the global spread of pathogens, opens a window onto the material connections of the premodern world. Coral was one of the few precious yet easily transportable substances that the Mediterranean world could trade eastward in exchange for so many kinds of materials and goods coming from East and South Asia (Sibon 2012). Tracing its trade, as well as that of other substances like Tibetan musk, Indian pepper, or East African ivory, helps us reconstruct human exchanges otherwise lost to his-

24 Chapter 48, on Kashmir ("Thesimur"): "Et le coral qui se porte de nos contrees se vent moult en ceste contree plus que en autre" (Polo [and Rustichello of Pisa 1298–99]/2003: 7, emphasis added). My thanks to Barbie Campbell Cole for bringing this statement to my attention, and to Markus Cruse for providing me with the citation.

25 Chapter 115, on Tibet ("Tebet"): "En ceste prouvince s'espant le corail et est moult chier, car il le meitent au col de leurs fames et de leur ydres par moult grant joie" (Polo [and Rustichello of Pisa 1298–99]/2003: 71).

tory. By themselves, these luxury goods were probably innocuous in terms of disease transmission.[26] But add in the furs that may have carried fleas and their excrement far beyond where their animal hosts would have taken them while living (Ducène 2005); the beasts of burden laden with these goods, with their own fleas and ticks; the shipholds and storage containers full of locally traded grain, and the rodents they attracted; and a medieval taste for luxury textiles that drove international trade (but also could transport fleas and their excrement), and we have a web of connections that make up Le Roy Ladurie's "microbial unification of the world" (Le Roy Ladurie 1973). We cannot, of course, be casual in our use of globalizing frameworks. Specifics in time and space matter hugely. Genetics has some contributions to make, archeology and history even more. But together, they suggest that a whole world region should be added to our narratives of the Black Death, a region that would connect the Tibetan Plateau and Qinghai to sub-Saharan Africa: the Indian Ocean basin.

It is nothing new to connect the Black Death narrative with trade, of course; it has long been suggested that plague moved to Western Eurasia and thence the Mediterranean and North Africa "via the Silk Road." That is simply a statement of its trajectory, however, rather than an actual documented mode of transmission, since it is likely that (whether carried by rodents or humans or other species) *Y. pestis* followed the topography of mountain passes, rivers, and valleys that traversed Central Asia and served as the network of trade connections that we aggregate under the rubric "Silk Road" (Beckwith 2009). Overland routes make most sense, of course, as trajectories for plague's arrival in the Black Sea region, whence it spread into the Mediterranean. But an important question needs to be asked: did it go in other directions as well? Arguments have been made by Buell (2012), Sussman (2011), and Anandavalli (2007) that plague (or at least major human outbreaks) cannot be documented in medieval China or India. Hymes's contribution to this issue challenges these claims with respect to the Gansu corridor and areas of China further east. Moreover, as science reminds us, there can be plague without "plague." Even in the absence of human outbreaks, *Y. pestis* can subsist and thrive in mammalian communities normally beneath the notice of humans. A new genetics of plague—especially the fact that the African 1.ANT strain demands explanation—suggests that southern routes of plague in the late medieval period merit further consideration.

---

26 Or perhaps one should say "usually innocuous." A twelfth-century Latin account explains that musk (both real and fake) was often sold in the skin of the musk deer (Wölfel 1939: 79–80), so perhaps it posed the same problem as the transmission of furs.

First of all, it is likely that we have underestimated the role of a southern route, via the Indian Ocean, for the First Plague Pandemic itself. Contrary to assumptions made by historians of late antiquity, it would seem that plague manifested first at the Egyptian port city of Pelusium (in the same site as modern-day Tell el-Farama) not because it "came out of Africa" (i.e., Egypt), but because it came via traffic from the Red Sea (Little 2007).[27] The port of Clysma in the Red Sea has recently been proposed as the possible entrance gate of *Yersinia pestis* into the Mediterranean (Tsimias et al. 2009). This argument was based solely on considerations of ancient geography, but the need to plot a route for *Y. pestis* out of the Tibetan Highlands fits both the emerging genetics data and the newer research on trade in the Indian Ocean basin, which can now very easily account for an intensity of travel that (however slowly) might have moved plague out of its Central Asian home into the very different environments of the Indian Ocean and ultimately the Red Sea and the Mediterranean littorals.

Secondly, the field of Indian Ocean studies is one of the areas that has been transformed radically in the decades since the main lines of argument in plague historiography were laid down (Seland 2014; Beaujard 2005 and 2012). We have long known about the *Periplus of the Erythraean Sea*, a Greek report on Indian Ocean trade and navigation, written in the mid-first century CE by an Egyptian merchant. It notes, for example, the import of coral at the Skythian port of Barbarikon/Minnagar, which was at the mouth of the Indus, and the export of "Chinese pelts" (Seland 2010: 59). More recent discoveries include the existence on Socotra Island (off the coast of modern Yemen and Somalia) of a cave with ancient inscriptions. These have been determined to be by sailors who visited the island between the first century BCE and sixth century CE. Texts written in Indian Brahmi script, and South-Arabian, Ethiopian, Greek, Palmyrene, and Bactrian scripts and languages give evidence of the breadth of Indian Ocean trade up to and including the time of the Justinianic Plague (Strauch 2012). For the later Middle Ages, we have equally remarkable letters and other documents of Jewish traders from the Cairo Genizah that show an intense and thriving trade across the Indian Ocean (Goitein and Friedman 2008).

The Socotra and Genizah finds are unusual, however, as is the Greek *Periplus*. For the most part, we have neither identifiable individuals nor

---

27 The claim that rats carrying plague brought the disease from the Tanzanian coast up to the Red Sea in the sixth century was premature (Horden 2005: 153). Instead, as discussed below, the archeological evidence now suggests the arrival of rats in East Africa somewhat later.

any written records at all. However, as with Marco Polo's coral, tracking unique commodities in their travels allows us to glimpse how intense Indian Ocean traffic was. Take pepper and musk, for example. Black pepper was, throughout antiquity and the Middle Ages, produced primarily on the Malabar Coast of what is now southwest India. Pepper's history has long been told in terms of trade with the West, but it is apparent now that China was one of the main markets for pepper in the Middle Ages. In other words, pepper was going both directions from the Malabar Coast, connecting China with all points in the Indian Ocean (Prange 2011). Similar motives in the trade of musk connected Tibet with the Indian Ocean world and parts beyond. The Egyptian encyclopedist and historian al-Nuwayrī (677/1279–732/1332), for example, explained that Tibetan musk (deemed far superior to that that came from China or elsewhere) was brought down to the Arabian Sea via the Indus Valley, whence it was shipped to various other ports in the western Indian Ocean (Akasoy and Yoeli-Tlalim 2007: 221). In fact, a whole array of archeological evidence—pottery, beads, tableware, and so forth—is stark witness to the intensity and extent of trade, both short- and long-distance, throughout much of the Indian Ocean basin.

Where there is extensive human traffic across a geographical expanse, it stands to reason that we should also look for commensals that traveled with these traders: a scenario perfect for the establishment of *Y. pestis* in new terrain (and amply documented from modern studies of *Y. pestis*'s very rapid establishment in North and South America and Madagascar during the twentieth century). And in East Africa, such commensals are readily found. The Asian house shrew, *Suncus murinus*; the black rat (ship rat), *Rattus rattus*; and the house mouse, *Mus musculus*, are all documented as imports from Asia (Boivin et al. 2013). The bones of *Rattus rattus*, the black rat, have been found in archeological remains from Unguja Ukuu, Tumbatu (one of the abandoned sites mentioned above), and Shanga along the Swahili Coast of East Africa. *Rattus rattus* may have arrived there as early as the seventh century and seems to have been common in urban contexts in the fourteenth.[28]

Hence, we have two parts of the "elephant" of plague here: the mechanisms of trade across the Indian Ocean basin, and the presence of a "rodent infrastructure" in East Africa to support a vector-borne disease when and if it arrived. We currently have, however, no paleogenetic work from this part of Africa; and indeed, very little genetics work has been done at all on

28 Nina Mudida and Mark Horton, personal communication (February 10, 2013).

the modern *Y. pestis* organism as it currently exists throughout much of sub-Saharan Africa, and where it still causes the second largest number of human cases per year. Indeed, we do not even have clear evidence of a trail of human plague from the Tibetan highlands down to the Indian Ocean ports in the fourteenth or fifteenth centuries, a point used by Anandavalli (2007) and Sussman (2011), in their respective studies, to argue against the presence of plague in medieval India. Yet we should be reminded of the mantra of bioarcheologists: absence of evidence is not evidence of absence. In a 2006 report of the 1994 plague outbreak in Surat, plague is given a history in India that goes back three thousand years.

> The first known outbreak of plague occurred from 1500–600 BC as recorded in *Bhagvata Purana*. The plague was seen again in 1031 AD when the disease reached India from Central Asia following the invasion of Sultan Mahmoud. In 1403 AD, Sultan Ahmed's Army was supposed to have been destroyed by a plague epidemic in Malwa. (Dutt, Akhtar, and McVeigh 2006: 757–58)

No supporting documentation was offered. But other, less extreme claims of the antiquity of plague in India, in some cases pushing it back to the eleventh century, occur in plague literature of the nineteenth and twentieth centuries (e.g., Simpson 1905: 40).[29] For India, then, we are at the same stage of feeble retrospective diagnosis from a handful of opaque written sources as we were when studying the history of plague in Europe prior to 1998. The first "clinical" description that meets Anandavalli's criteria for plague is a 1689 report by a historian, Khafi Khan, writing in Arabic, who recounts how "the plague (*taun*) and pestilence (*waba*), which had been ravaging Dakhin (South India) for several years, had spread to Bijapur. He describes the visible marks of the plague: 'swellings as big as a grape or banana under the arms, behind the ears, and in the groin'" (Anandavalli 2007: 25).[30] For Sussman, the "first" clinical report is that of the Mughal emperor Jahangir (d. 1627), who reported in 1619 that

> At this time, again, it appeared from the reports of the loyal that the disease of the plague was prevalent in Agra, so that daily about 100 people,

29 The possibility of a hitherto unrecognized pandemic in the eleventh/twelfth century merits more examination. There is a story of "epidemics (*wabā'*) and the plague (*ṭā'ūn*)" in early eleventh-century Tunisia "which carried off the greater part of the population" (Talbi 1981: 221). Dols (1977: 33) reports an outbreak in the Hijaz, Yemen, and Egypt in the twelfth century.

30 For the latest assessment of the semantic weight carried by these Arabic terms, see Stearns 2011.

> more or less, were dying of it. Under the armpits, or in the groin, or below the throat, buboes formed, and they died. This is the third year that it has raged in the cold weather, and disappeared in the commencement of the hot season. (Jahangir, as quoted by Sussman 2011: 336)

Is it possible that it was only in the seventeenth century that *Yersinia pestis* first came down from the Tibetan highlands into India?[31] Sometimes absence of evidence really does signal absence of the phenomenon. But India's proximity to the Tibetan highlands, the well-documented networks of trade that connected much of south and southeast Asia throughout the ancient and medieval periods, and, now, the evidence of deep genetic links between the strains of *Y. pestis* found in East and Central Africa and those that came out of Central Eurasia in the fourteenth century: all of these factors raise new questions about India's history with plague.

Anandavalli and Sussman are right to be cautious of reading too much into the ambiguous evidence of the few written sources they had at their disposal. Plague is hardly the only disease that presents in epidemic form, and careful interpretation of such sources always demands the expertise of scholars skilled in the nuances of the original languages. But it has been the objective of this essay to argue that historical narratives can be crafted from other sources, too. Transmission of plague through India (whether via the Indus Valley or the Ganges) begins to look plausible if we take seriously the emerging narrative derived from genetics, and posit an arrival of plague in late medieval East Africa.[32] Indeed, the fourteenth and fifteenth centuries were periods of intense upheaval in many areas of Asia, and it may be worthwhile to consider the possibility that a major social disruptor such as plague contributed to that upheaval (Lieberman 2011; Hymes 2014, in this issue).

In the field of climate and environmental history, a search for consilience among different kinds of historical evidence is openly embraced

31 Ansari (1994, also citing from Jahangir) says that the emperor first reported the disease not in 1619 but in 1615, noting that "the king wrote that it was the first time that the disease had occurred in India." Catanach (2001: 141) similarly identifies the seventeenth century as the time of the first outbreak of plague in India, when he notes an outbreak in 1631 among handloom weavers in Gujarat.

32 Granted, at this point we cannot rule out another possible narrative, unlikely though it may be given the distances involved and the fact that shipping of trade goods was not a factor: that plague reached East Africa via the Portuguese, who arrived in 1498. On the experience of plague in Portugal, see da Costa Roque 1979. The chronicles of Fernão Lopes, a fifteenth-century chronicler, are due to be published soon in English translation. My thanks to Iona McCleery for this information.

(McCormick 2011). A multidisciplinary approach to disease history, in contrast, might be more immediately served by focusing not just on points where the narratives of different disciplinary approaches converge (as, for example, in the case of the genetics, historical, and bioarcheological work on the London Black Death cemetery),[33] but also on areas where they seem to be in utter disagreement. As Altman and his colleagues have warned us, we should beware of "cherry picking those milestones in human history that are [already] best recorded." A study of *Y. pestis* strains in just three areas of India in 2009 showed three very different lineages (Kingston 2009), making it likely that plague has been imported there more than once. Much more research on the genetics of the modern African and Indian strains of plague, in addition to much more combing of historical archives and sampling of archeological evidence to look for extinct *Y. pestis* strains, will be necessary to confirm whether the suggestions I have made here about a late medieval impact of plague in India and sub-Saharan Africa are plausible. But we would have never seen this as a possible line of research had there not been a convergence of many different disciplines on questions of plague's histories in recent years.

Reclaiming Retrospective Diagnosis: Sources, Methods, and Goals for a Global History of Health

> If we want to understand what health and illness meant for past sufferers, we have to accept their labels, not impose ours. (McCleery 2013: 90)
>
> What was invisible to the [peoples of the past] need not remain invisible for us as well. (Stathakopoulos 2011: 95)

These two statements about what is called "retrospective diagnosis" capture the historian's dilemma: is our task to reconstruct the world as historical participants perceived it (what anthropologists would call an *emic* approach) and reject modern (biomedical) understandings of disease? Or, in a positivist mode, is our task to use the methods and categories of modern science to find out what "really" happened, as judged from an external frame of reference, that of modern science (an *etic* approach)? This question haunts the historian working with cultural remains in a way it would not haunt the microbiologist reconstructing aDNA fragments. For the historian, both of these perspectives are "real," since human experience and

33 See DeWitte (2014, in this issue) for a review of research on the London Black Death cemetery at East Smithfield.

the motives for human actions are major objects of our quest.[34] But among historians, too, there are different motives and different objectives.

"Plague," as Andrew Cunningham has most incisively pointed out, is a construct of modern biomedicine, built on a foundation of laboratory science, epidemiological studies, entomology, and zoology which together have contributed to our understanding that "plague" is a disease caused by an infectious microorganism (*Yersinia pestis*), transmitted by flea bites or other means, presenting certain characteristic clinical signs and affecting the human body through physiological processes known through countless clinical observations and laboratory studies of afflicted humans and animals both pre- and postmortem. Absent that laboratory, there is no "plague" in this sense (Cunningham 1992; cf. Arrizabalaga 2002 and Cunningham 2002). All we have are texts that describe various kinds of suffering, experiences that even those suffering might not have put into a single category of a namable disease. The "linguistic turn" that has affected most Anglophone historiographical traditions over the past thirty years has reinforced a sense that we can never fully break free of the conceptual categories of our historical texts and reconstruct a "real," unfiltered past.

I do not contest this interpretation; on the contrary, I accept it wholeheartedly in so far as it *applies to histories drawn from human cultural products* like written documents or works of art (cf. Green, Walker-Meikle, and Müller 2014, in this issue). But here is where the challenge, and the possibilities, of a multidisciplinary history face us. Microbiologists have broken through the nineteenth-century barrier of laboratory medicine. Nearly all modern laboratory samples of plague and other pathogens have been collected in just the past 150 years. But aDNA research reaches beyond that chronological limit, reconstructing and identifying old organisms in a way that microbiologists themselves now believe is possible (even if they still argue among themselves about best methods) and that connects plausibly with the narratives of pathogen evolutionary history created by genome-based phylogenetics. "Retrospective diagnosis," in other words, now has a completely new meaning, one based on assessment of a material substrate of the past rather than cultural products alone.[35]

---

34 The bioarcheologist, who draws on both cultural and material remains, stands somewhere in between these poles, a point I address below.

35 I have foregrounded here the diagnostic possibilities of molecular microbiology, but in diseases other than plague (most notably, leprosy as caused by *Mycobacterium leprae*, discovered by Armauer Hansen in 1873), the older field of paleopathology also has methods to draw plausible "retrospective diagnoses." See Green 2012 and forthcoming for an overview.

So, to return to the skeptic's "So what?" question about the significance of the new plague science posed at the beginning of this essay. My response is: "Because it gives us something to think with." The broadened narrative of plague I have sketched out in this essay suggests the possible significance of animal species and human populations and areas of the world that have never before been part of Black Death narratives. And the other essays in this special issue push those boundaries of new thinking on the histories of plague even further. In a typical anti-retrospective diagnostic stance, historian Iona McCleery says that "If we want to understand what health and illness meant for past sufferers, we have to accept their labels, not impose ours." But what if those sufferers are populations of the destroyed African civilizations of Zimbabwe or possibly Jenne-Jeno and Akrokrowa? What "labels" have we to interpret when these vanished societies left no written records? As Anna Colet and her colleagues make clear in their study of the communal graves of Tàrrega (2014, in this issue), it is sheer chance that we now have both documentary records and physical evidence for the slaughter of the Jewish community of that town in 1348. For so many victims of the Black Death—both those who died of plague and those who died at others' hands—we have no testimony of their suffering other than their physical remains or other traces. And even those are rare, especially in parts of the world where archaeological traditions are still nascent (Campana et al. 2013).

Reconstructing the history of the Black Death can proceed from many motives, and methodologies will be chosen according to the objectives that various researchers wish to achieve as well as their training and resources. Some possible methods for exploring plague's histories have not even been discussed here, such as the use of historical linguistics, which has already proven a powerful ally to both archaeological and genetics work (e.g., de Luna, Fleisher, and McIntosh 2012). Plague is an "elephant" that demands the efforts of many blind men and women to assess its full, huge, and awful expanse. *Yersinia pestis* has established itself as a worldwide pathogen not because (like, say, measles or tuberculosis) it is continually circulating in human bodies. Rather, it exists today in every continent save Australia and Antarctica because it was carried far from its apparent site of origin in the Tibet-Qinghai Plateau by combinations of human and animal carriers who recreated microenvironments in which *Y. pestis* could thrive.[36] It was then able to establish foci in new areas, moving from com-

36 Plague did reach Australia during the Third Pandemic (if not before), but it did not establish permanent foci thanks to aggressive public health measures. See Curson and McCracken 1989.

mensal rodent populations (transported by humans) into new, rural species where the organism could find permanent hosts.

This essay presents the new face of the Black Death, a medieval pandemic that may have spared Oceania and North and South America only because those areas had not yet been brought tightly into the networks of Afroeurasian trade.[37] A global approach to the disease's history—thinking across time and space and our own methodological perspectives, taking in the full evolutionary history of the pathogen and the full human impact of the disease—will give us a mechanism to explain how plague reached those last corners of the world, what it did when it got there, and how its many stories compare to those of other global diseases.[38] A "global" approach will also facilitate greater understanding of a disease that still affects several thousand people every year and could threaten many more (Ziegler 2014, in this issue). Much of the genetics work described above has been based on modern samples collected in China, and on the efforts of Chinese, Russian, and North American scientists, who for many decades have prioritized plague research because it exists as an enzootic (and even bioterrorist) threat in their own countries. But very little comparable genetics work has yet been done in other areas where plague is enzootic: in India, Southeast Asia, South America, and most parts of Africa. Johanna T. Crane (2011), among others, has noted the effects of such an imbalance in molecular research infrastructure on the study of another global disease, HIV/AIDS. This examination of the Black Death suggests that framing pandemics both widely (in geography) and deeply (in time) may not simply broaden our historical knowledge, but help us reconceive the world we live in today.

---

37 Though here, too, tracing commensal rodents shows medieval human movements. See Wilmshurst et al. 2008.

38 As this essay will have made plain, it will be necessary to gauge the hows and whys of plague's global history not in terms of human witnesses alone, but from other kinds of evidence. Moreover, all of the methods and perspectives surveyed here can be applied to other conundra in disease history, for example, the still mysterious case of the cocoliztli epidemic of 1544–50 in Central America (see Warinner et al. 2012). As outlined in Green 2012 and Green forthcoming, a global approach to the history of disease is not simply multidisciplinary but deliberately seeks out parallels and interactions between different diseases.

Bibliography

Achtman, M., K. Zurth, G. Morelli, G. Torrea, et al. 1999. "*Yersinia pestis*, the Cause of Plague, is a Recently Emerged Clone of *Yersinia pseudotuberculosis*," *Proceedings of the National Academy of Science* 96, no. 24: 14043–48

Achtman, M., G. Morelli, P. Zhu, T. Wirth, et al. 2004. "Microevolution and History of the Plague Bacillus, *Yersinia pestis*," *Proceedings of the National Academy of Sciences* 101, no. 51: 17837–42

Akasoy, A. and R. Yoeli-Tlalim. 2007. "Along the Musk Routes: Exchanges between Tibet and the Islamic World," *Asian Medicine: Tradition and Modernity* 3, no. 2: 217-40

Altmann, D. M., F. Balloux, R. J. Boyton. 2012. "Diverse Approaches to Analysing the History of Human and Pathogen Evolution: How to Tell the Story of the Past 70,000 years," *Philosophical Transactions of the Royal Society of London. B: Biological Sciences* 367, no. 1590: 765–69

Amann, Sabine. 2007. "Untersuchung zur Klassifizierung, Identifizierung und Differenzierung von *Yersinia* Arten" (master's thesis, Universität Wien)

Anandavalli, Lakshmikanthan. 2007. "The Black Death in Medieval India: A Historical Mystery," *Tangents: The Journal of the Master of Liberal Arts Program at Stanford University* 6: 20–25

Anisimov, A. P., L. E. Lindler, and G. B. Pier. 2004. "Intraspecific Diversity of *Yersinia pestis*," *Clinical Microbiology Reviews* 17, no. 2: 434–64

Ansari, B. M. 1994. "An Account of Bubonic Plague in Seventeenth Century India in an Autobiography of a Mughal Emperor," *Journal of Infection* 29: 351–52

Arrizabalaga, J. 2002. "Problematizing Retrospective Diagnosis in the History of Disease," *Asclepio* 54: 51–70

Ayyadurai, S., F. Sebbane, D. Raoult, and M. Drancourt. 2010. "Body Lice, *Yersinia pestis Orientalis*, and Black Death," *Emerging Infectious Diseases* 16, no. 5: 892–93

Beaujard, Philippe. 2005. "The Indian Ocean in Eurasian and African World-Systems before the Sixteenth Century," *Journal of World History* 16: 411–65

Beaujard, Philippe. 2012. *Les mondes de l'Ocean Indien*, 2 vols. (Paris: Colin)

Beckwith, Christopher. 2009. *Empires of the Silk Road: A History of Central Eurasia from the Bronze Age to the Present* (Princeton, NJ: Princeton University Press)

Biswas, S., S. Lal, V. Mittal, M. Malini, et al. 2011. "Detection of Enzootic Plague Foci in Peninsular India," *Journal of Communicable Diseases* 43, no. 3: 169–76

Bitam, I., S. Ayyadurai, T. Kernif, M. Chetta, et al. 2010. "New Rural Focus of Plague, Algeria," *Emerging Infectious Diseases* 16, no. 10: 1639–40

Boivin, N., A. Crowther, R. Helm, and D. Q. Fuller. 2013. "East Africa and Madagascar in the Indian Ocean World," *Journal of World Prehistory* 26: 213–81

Bos, K. I., V. J. Schuenemann, G. B. Golding, H. A. Burbano, et al. 2011. "A Draft Genome of *Yersinia pestis* from Victims of the Black Death," *Nature* 478, no.7370: 506–10

Buell, Paul D. 2012. "Qubilai and the Rats," *Sudhoffs Archiv* 96, no. 2: 127–44

Bulliet, Richard W. 1975. *The Camel and the Wheel* (Cambridge, MA: Harvard University Press)

Cabanel, N., A. Leclercq, V. Chenal-Francisque, B. Annajar, et al. 2013. "Plague Outbreak in Libya, 2009, Unrelated to Plague in Algeria," *Emerging Infectious Diseases* 19, no. 2: 230–36

Campana, M. G., M. A. Bower, P. J. Crabtree. 2013. "Ancient DNA for the Archaeologist: The Future of African Research," *African Archaeological Review* 30: 21–37

Carmichael, Ann G. 2014. "Plague Persistence in Western Europe: A Hypothesis," *The Medieval Globe* 1: 157–191

Cartwright, Frederick Fox, with Michael D. Biddiss. 1972. *Disease and History* (London: Hart-Davis)

Catanach, I. J. 2001. "The 'Globalization' of Disease? India and the Plague," *Journal of World History* 12: 131–53

Chouin, Gérard L., and Christopher R. DeCorse. 2010. "Prelude to the Atlantic Trade: New Perspectives on Southern Ghana's Pre-Atlantic History (800–1500)," *Journal of African History* 51: 123–45

Christie, A. B., T. H. Chen, and Sanford S. Elberg. 1980. "Plague in Camels and Goats: Their Role in Human Epidemics," *Journal of Infectious Diseases* 141, no. 6: 724–26

Colet, Anna, Josep Xavier Muntané i Santiveri, Jordi Ruíz Ventura, Oriol Saula, et al. 2014. "The Black Death and its Consequences for the Jewish Community in Tàrrega: Lessons from History and Archeology," *The Medieval Globe* 1: 63–96

Costa Roque, Mário da. 1979. *As Pestes Medievais Europeias e o Regimento Proveytoso contra a Pestenença, Valentim Fernandes (1495–1496): Tentativa de Interpretação à Luz dos Conhecimentos Pestológicos Actuais* (Lisbon: Fundação Calouste Gulbenkian)

Crane, J. T. 2011. "Viral Cartographies: Mapping the Molecular Politics of Global HIV," *BioSocieties* 6: 142–66

Cui, Y., C. Yu, Y. Yan, D. Li, et al. 2013. "Historical Variations in Mutation Rate in an Epidemic Pathogen, *Yersinia pestis*," *Proceedings of the National Academy of Science* 110, no. 2: 577–82

Cunningham, A. 1992. "Transforming Plague: The Laboratory and the Identification of Infectious Disease," in *The Laboratory Revolution in Medicine*, ed. Andrew Cunningham and Perry Williams, 209–44 (Cambridge: Cambridge University Press)

Cunningham, A. 2002. "Identifying Disease in the Past: Cutting the Gordian Knot," *Asclepio* 54: 13–34

Curson, P. H., and K. McCracken. 1989. *Plague in Sydney: The Anatomy of an Epidemic* (Kensington: New South Wales University Press)

Davis, D. H. S. 1953. "Plague in Africa from 1935 to 1949: A Survey of Wild Rodents in African Territories," *Bulletin of the World Health Organization* 9: 665–700

DeWitte, Sharon N. 2014. "The Anthropology of Plague: Insights from Bioarcheological Analyses of Epidemic Cemeteries," *The Medieval Globe* 1: 97–123

Dols, Michael W. 1977. *The Black Death in the Middle East* (Princeton: Princeton University Press)

dos Santos Grácio, A. J., and Maria Amélia A. Grácio. 2011. "Plague in Angola," *Acta Parasitológica Portuguesa* 18, no. 1/2: 1–10

Ducène, Jean-Charles. 2005. "Le commerce des fourrures entre l'Europe orientale et le Moyen-Orient à l'époque médiévale (IXe–XIIIe siècle): pour une perspective historique," *Acta Orientalia Academiae Scientiarum Hungaricae* 58: 215–28

Dutt, A. K., R. Akhtar, and M. McVeigh. 2006. "Surat Plague of 1994 Re-Examined," *Southeast Asian Journal of Tropical Medicine and Public Health* 37, no. 4: 755–60

Echenberg, Myron J. 2001. *Black Death, White Medicine: Bubonic Plague and the Politics of Public Health in Colonial Senegal, 1914–1945* (Portsmouth, NH: Heinemann)

Echenberg, Myron J. 2007. *Plague Ports: The Global Urban Impact of Bubonic Plague, 1894–1901* (New York: New York University Press)

Fedorov, V. N. 1960. "Plague in Camels and its Prevention in the USSR," *Bulletin of the World Health Organization* 23: 275–81

Franz, K., O. Riha, and C. Schubert, organizers. 2010. "Plagues in Nomadic Contexts: Historical Impact, Medical Responses and Cultural Adaptations in Ancient to Medieval Eurasia," conference held in Leipzig, 7–9 October <http://hsozkult.geschichte.hu-berlin.de/tagungsberichte/id=3431> [accessed February 15, 2014]

Goitein, S. D., and M. Friedman (eds. and trans.). 2008. *India Traders of the Middle Ages: Documents from the Cairo Geniza ('India Book')* (Leiden: Brill)

Green, Monica H. 2012. "The Value of Historical Perspective," in *The Ashgate Research Companion to the Globalization of Health*, ed. Ted Schrecker, 17–37 (Aldershot: Ashgate)

Green, Monica H. 2014. "Editor's Introduction to *Pandemic Disease in the Medieval World*: Rethinking the Black Death," *The Medieval Globe* 1: 9–26

Green, Monica H. Forthcoming. "The Globalisations of Disease," in *From Colonisation to Globalisation: Species Movements in Human History*, ed. Michael Petraglia and Nicole Boivin (Cambridge: Cambridge University Press)

Green, Monica H., Kathleen Walker-Meikle, and Wolfgang Müller. 2014. "Diagnosis of a 'Plague' Image: A Digital Cautionary Tale," *The Medieval Globe* 1: 309–326

Guérin, Sarah M. 2013. "Forgotten Routes? Italy, Ifrīqiya and the Trans-Saharan Ivory Trade," *Al-Masaq: Islam and the Medieval Mediterranean* 25: 70–91

Guiyoule, A., F. Grimont, I. Iteman, P. A. D. Grimont, et al. 1994. "Plague Pandemics Investigated by Ribotyping of *Yersinia pestis* Strains," *Journal of Clinical Microbiology* 32, no. 3: 634–41

Harbeck, M., L. Seifert, S. Hänsch, D. M. Wagner, et al. 2013. "*Yersinia pestis* DNA from Skeletal Remains from the 6th Century AD Reveals Insights into Justinianic Plague," *PLoS Pathogens* 9, no. 5: e1003349

Ho, S. Y. W., and G. Larson. 2006. "Molecular Clocks: When Times are A-Changin," *Trends in Genetics* 22, no. 2: 79–83

Horden, Peregrine. 2005. "Mediterranean Plague in the Age of Justinian," in *The Cambridge Companion to the Age of Justinian*, ed. Michael Maas, 134–60 (Cambridge: Cambridge University Press)

Horton, M. 1996/2012. "Coastal Towns of East Africa," in *The Oxford Companion to Archaeology*, ed. Brian M. Fagan and Charlotte Beck, 187–88; 2nd ed. Neil Asher Silberman (Oxford: Oxford University Press Online [accessed May 28, 2014])

Horton, M. 2004. "Artisans, Communities, and Commodities: Medieval Exchanges between Northwestern India and East Africa," in "Communities and Commodities: Western India and the Indian Ocean, Eleventh-Fifteenth Centuries," *Ars Orientalis* 34: 62–80

Horton, M., and J. Middleton. 2000. *The Swahili: The Social Landscape of a Mercantile Society* (Oxford: Blackwell)

Huffman, T. N., and J. C. Vogel. 1991. "The Chronology of Great Zimbabwe," *South African Archaeological Bulletin* 46: 61–70

Hymes, Robert. 2014. "A Hypothesis on the East Asian Beginnings of the *Yersinia pestis* Polytomy," *The Medieval Globe* 1: 285–308

Jones, E. P., H. M. Eager, S. I. Gabriel, F. Jóhannesdóttir, et al. 2013. "Genetic Tracking of Mice and Other Bioproxies to Infer Human History," *Trends in Genetics* 29, no. 5: 298–308

Kingston, J. J., U. Tuteja, M. Kapi, H. S. Murali, et al. 2009. "Genotyping of Indian *Yersinia pestis* Strains by MLVA and Repetitive DNA Sequence Based PCRs," *Antonie van Leeuwenhoek* 96: 303–12

Larson, G. 2013. "Testing the Chronology of Domestication Genes Using Ancient DNA," paper presented at the conference "Ancient DNA: The First Three Decades," held at the Royal Society, London, 18–19 November, podcast at <http://royalsociety.org/events/2013/ancient-dna/> [accessed January 17, 2014]

Le Roy Ladurie, Emmanuel. 1973. "Un concept: l'unification microbienne du monde (XVIe–XVIIe siècles)," *Schweizerische Zeitschrift für Geschichte*, 23, no. 4: 627–96 (An abbreviated English translation is also available: Emmanuel Le Roy Ladurie. 1981. "A Concept: The Unification of the Globe by Disease," trans. Sian Reynolds and Ben Reynolds, in *The Mind and Method of the Historian*, 28–83 [London: Harvester])

Li, Y., Y. Cui, Y. Hauck, M. E. Platonov, et al. 2009. "Genotyping and Phylogenetic Analysis of *Yersinia pestis* by MLVA: Insights into the Worldwide Expansion of Central Asia Plague Foci," *PLoS ONE* 4, no. 6: e6000

Lieberman, Victor. 2011. "Charter State Collapse in Southeast Asia, ca. 1250–1400, as a Problem in Regional and World History," *American Historical Review* 116: 937–63

Little, Lester K. ed. 2007. *Plague and the End of Antiquity: The Pandemic of 541–750* (Cambridge: Cambridge University Press)

Little, Lester K. 2011. "Plague Historians in Lab Coats," *Past and Present* 213: 267–90

Luna, K. M. de, J. B. Fleisher, J. B., and S. K. McIntosh. 2012. "Thinking across the African Past: Interdisciplinarity and Early History," *African Archaeological Review* 29, no. 2/3: 75–94

McCleery, Iona. 2013. "Medicine and Disease: The Female 'Patient' in Medieval Europe," in *A Cultural History of Women in the Middle Ages*, ed. Kim M. Phillips, 85–104 (London: Bloomsbury)

McCormick, Michael. 2007. "Toward a Molecular History of the Justinianic Pandemic," in *Plague and the End of Antiquity: The Pandemic of 541–750*, ed. Lester K. Little, 290–312 (Cambridge: Cambridge University Press)

McCormick, Michael. 2011. "History's Changing Climate: Climate Science, Genomics, and the Emerging Consilient Approach to Interdisciplinary History," *Journal of Interdisciplinary History* 42: 251–73

McDougall, E. Ann. 1990. "Salts of the Western Sahara: Myths, Mysteries and Historical Significance," *International Journal of African Historical Sources* 23, no. 2: 231–57

McIntosh, Roderick James. 1998. *The Peoples of the Middle Niger: The Island of Gold* (Oxford: Blackwell)

McNeill, William H. 1976. *Plagues and Peoples* (New York: Anchor)

Mengel, David. 2011. "A Plague on Bohemia? Mapping the Black Death," *Past and Present* 211: 3–34

Mitchell, P. 2012. "Linking Up East Africa: East Africa in the Indian Ocean World II, Oxford, 22–23 March 2012," *Azania: Archaeological Research in Africa* 47, no. 2: 226–30

Mitchell, Stephen. 2014. *A History of the Later Roman Empire, AD 284–641*, 2nd ed. (New York: Wiley-Blackwell)

Morelli, G., Y. Song, C. J. Mazzoni, M. Eppinger, et al. 2010. "*Yersinia pestis* Genome Sequencing Identifies Patterns of Global Phylogenetic Diversity," *Nature Genetics* 42, no. 12: 1140–45

Neerinckx, S. B., A. T. Peterson, H. Gulinck, J. Deckers, et al. 2008. "Geographic Distribution and Ecological Niche of Plague in Sub-Saharan Africa," *International Journal of Health Geographics* 7: art. no. 54

Neerinckx, S., E. Bertherat, and H. Leirs. 2010. "Human Plague Occurrences in Africa: An Overview from 1877 to 2008," *Transactions of the Royal Society of Tropical Medicine and Hygiene* 104, no. 2: 97–103

Pechous, R. D., V. Sivaraman, P. A. Price, N. M. Stasulli, et al. 2013. "Early Host Cell Targets of *Yersinia pestis* during Primary Pneumonic Plague," *PLoS Pathogens* 9, no. 10: e1003679

Pikirayi, Innocent. 2001. *The Zimbabwe Culture: Origins and Decline in Southern Zambezian States* (Walnut Creek, CA: Alta Mira Press)

Polo, Marco [and Rustichello of Pisa]. 1298–99/2003. *Le devisement du monde, édition critique, vol. II*, ed. Jeanne-Marie Boivin, Laurence Harf-Lancner, and Laurence Mathey-Maille (Geneva: Droz)

Prange, Sebastian. 2011. "'Measuring by the Bushel': Reweighing the Indian Ocean Pepper Trade," *Historical Research* 84, no. 224: 212–35

Riehm, J. M., G. Vergnaud, D. Kiefer, T. Damdindorj, et al. 2012. "*Yersinia pestis* Lineages in Mongolia," *PLoS ONE* 7, no. 2: e30624

Sallares, Robert. 2007. "Ecology, Evolution, and Epidemiology of Plague," in *Plague and the End of Antiquity: The Pandemic of 541–750*, ed. Lester K. Little, 231–89 (Cambridge: Cambridge University Press)

Sarris, Peter. 2007. "Bubonic Plague in Byzantium: The Evidence of the Non-Literary Sources," in *Plague and the End of Antiquity: The Pandemic of 541–750*, ed. Lester K. Little, 119–32 (Cambridge: Cambridge University Press)

Seifert, L., M. Harbeck, A. Thomas, N. Hoke, et al. 2013. "Strategy for Sensitive and Specific Detection of *Yersinia pestis* in Skeletons of the Black Death Pandemic," *PLoS ONE* 8, no. 9: e75742

Seland, Eivind Heldaas. 2008. "The Indian Ocean and the Globalisation of the Ancient World," *Ancient West and East* 7: 65–77

Seland, Eivind Heldaas. 2010. *Ports and Political Power in the Periplus: Complex Societies and Maritime Trade on the Indian Ocean in the First Century AD* (Oxford: Archaeopress)

Seland, Eivind Heldaas. 2014. "Archaeology of Trade in the Western Indian Ocean, 300 BC–AD 700," *Journal of Archaeological Research*, Published online: 2 April 2014, 10.1007/s10814-014-9075-7 <http://link.springer.com/article/10.1007/s10814-014-9075-7/fulltext.html> [accessed April 4, 2014]

Sibon, Juliette. 2012. "Travailler dans une autre communauté de la diaspora au XIVe siècle: corailleurs et médecins juifs entre Provence, Catalogne et Sardaigne," *Cahiers de la Méditerranée* 84: 19–37

Simpson, William John Ritchie. 1905. *A Treatise on Plague, Dealing with the Historical, Epidemiological, Clinical, Therapeutic and Preventive Aspects of the Disease* (Cambridge: Cambridge University Press)

Stathakopoulos, Dionysios. 2011. "Invisible Protagonists: The Justinianic Plague from a Zoocentric Point of View," in *Animals and Environment in Byzantium (7th–12th c.)*, ed. Ēlías Anagnōstákēs, Taxiarchēs G. Kollas, and Eutychia Papadopoulou, 87–95 (Athens: Centre for Byzantine Research, National Hellenic Research Foundation)

Stearns, Justin K. 2011. *Infectious Ideas: Contagion in Premodern Islamic and Christian Thought in the Western Mediterranean* (Baltimore: Johns Hopkins University Press)

Strauch, Ingo. 2012. *Foreign Sailors on Socotra: The Inscriptions and Drawings from the Cave Hoq* (Bremen: Hempen)

Sussman, G. D. 2011. "Was the Black Death in India and China?," *Bulletin of the History of Medicine* 85: 319–55

Talbi, Mohamed. 1981. "Laws and Economy in Ifrīqiya (Tunisia) in the Third Islamic Century: Agriculture and the Role of Slaves in the Country's Economy," in *The Islamic Middle East, 700–1900: Studies in Economic and Social History*, ed. Abraham Udovitch, 209–49 (Princeton: Darwin)

Tsiamis, C., E. Poulakou-Rebelakou, and E. Petridou. 2009. "The Red Sea and the Port of Clysma: A Possible Gate of Justinian's Plague," *Gesnerus* 66, no. 2: 209–17

Varlık, Nükhet. 2014. "New Science and Old Sources: Why the Ottoman Experience of Plague Matters," *The Medieval Globe* 1: 193–227

Veracx, A., R. Rivet, K. D. McCoy, P. Brouqui, et al. 2012. "Evidence That Head and Body Lice on Homeless Persons Have the Same Genotype," *PLoS ONE* 7, no. 9: e45903

Wagner, D. M., J. Klunk, M. Harbeck, A. Devault, et al. 2014. "*Yersinia pestis* and the Plague of Justinian, 541–543 AD: A Genomic Analysis," *Lancet Infectious Diseases* 14, no. 4: 319–26

Warinner, C., N. Robles García, R. Spores, and N. Tuross. 2012. "Disease, Demography, and Diet in Early Colonial New Spain: Investigation of a Sixteenth Century Mixtec Cemetery at Teposcolula Yucundaa," *Latin American Antiquity* 23: 467–89

Wilmshurst, J. M., A. J. Anderson, T. F. G. Higham, and T. H. Worthy. 2008. "Dating the Late Prehistoric Dispersal of Polynesians to New Zealand using the Commensal Pacific Rat," *Proceedings of the National Academy of Sciences* 105, no. 22: 7676–80

Wölfel, Hans. 1939. *Das Arzneidrogenbuch "Circa instans" in einer Fassung des XIII. Jahrhunderts aus der Universitätsbibliothek Erlangen. Text und Kom-*

mentar als Beitrag zur Pflanzen und Drogenkunde des Mittelalters (Berlin: Preilipper)

World Health Organization. 2008. *Interregional Meeting on Prevention and Control of Plague*. Geneva: World Health Organization.

Wray, Shona Kelly. 2009. *Communities and Crisis: Bologna during the Black Death* (Leiden: Brill)

Wu, L. 1924. "The Original Home of Plague," in *Far Eastern Association of Tropical Medicine, Transactions of the Fifth Biennial Congress Held at Singapore, 1923*, ed. A. L. Hoops and J. W. Scharff, 286–304 (London: Bale & Danielsson)

Wynne-Jones, S. 2013. "The Public Life of the Swahili Stonehouse, 14th–15th Centuries AD," *Journal of Anthropological Archaeology* 32: 759–73

Yan, Y., H. Wang, D. Li, X. Yang, et al. 2014. "Two-Step Source Tracing Strategy of *Yersinia pestis* and its Historical Epidemiology in a Specific Region," *PLoS ONE* 9, no. 1: e85374

Ziegler, Michelle. 2014. "The Black Death and the Future of the Plague," *The Medieval Globe* 1: 259–283

Monica H. Green (Monica.Green@asu.edu) is a historian of medieval European medicine and global health. In 2009 and 2012, she ran a National Endowment for the Humanities Summer Seminar in London on "Health and Disease in the Middle Ages," which had as its central goal the exploration of ways that the scientific and humanistic disciplines could engage in productive dialogue about the history of disease and health-seeking behaviors. During this same period, she has also argued for the development of a new field, "Global History of Health," which explores the evolution of the major pathogens that have afflicted the human species since its origin up to the present day, and the ways that human cultural changes have facilitated or hindered those pathogens' trajectories. In addition to many works on the cultural history of medieval medicine, she is the author of "The Value of Historical Perspective," in *The Ashgate Research Companion to the Globalization of Health*, ed. Ted Schrecker (Aldershot: Ashgate, 2012), pp. 17–37; and "The Globalisations of Disease," which will be published in 2015.

Abstract This essay introduces the inaugural issue of *The Medieval Globe*, "Pandemic Disease in the Medieval World: Rethinking the Black Death". It suggests that the history of the pathogen *Yersinia pestis*, as it has now been reconstructed by molecular biology, allows for an expanded definition of the Second Plague Pandemic. Historiography of the Black Death has hitherto focused on a limited number of vector and host species, and on Western Europe and those parts of the Islamicate world touching the Mediterranean littoral. Biological considerations suggest the value of a broadened framework, one that encompasses an enlarged range of host species and draws on new archeological, genetic, and historical researches to look for the presence of plague in the premodern Indian Ocean basin and East Africa, areas where it has previously not been suspected.

Keywords Afroeurasia, Indian Ocean, zoonotics, retrospective diagnosis, Black Death, Justinianic Plague, global history of health.

THE BLACK DEATH AND ITS CONSEQUENCES FOR THE JEWISH COMMUNITY IN TÀRREGA: LESSONS FROM HISTORY AND ARCHEOLOGY*

ANNA COLET, JOSEP XAVIER MUNTANÉ I SANTIVERI, JORDI RUÍZ VENTURA, ORIOL SAULA, M. EULÀLIA SUBIRÀ DE GALDÀCANO, and CLARA JÁUREGUI

In March 2014, an exhibit opened at the Museu Comarcal de l'Urgell in Tàrrega, commemorating a tragedy that had occurred in that Catalan town nearly seven hundred years earlier.[1] This tragedy—the murder of a large number of the town's Jewish inhabitants—has been acknowledged for centuries. Reports of the events that transpired in the summer of 1348 reached the ruler of the Crown of Aragon almost immediately. Legal proceedings continued for several years thereafter, not so much to identify and prosecute the murderers as to restore property and financial instruments that had been destroyed or stolen in the rioting.[2] Meanwhile, contemporary reports of the events in Tàrrega circulated among the Jewish communities of Catalonia. Stories of the event were also handed down among subsequent generations of Jews when they emigrated to Italy after their general expulsion from Spain in 1492. All of this, too, has been known for some time.

---

* This essay, originally drafted in Catalan, has been translated and revised for publication by Monica H. Green and Carol Symes.

1 Museu Comarcal de l'Urgell-Tàrrega, "Tragèdia al Call. Tàrrega 1348" <http://museutarrega.cat/exposicions-permanents/tragedia-al-call-tarrega-1348> [accessed April 23, 2014]. A catalogue of the exhibition is available at <http://museutarrega.cat/documents>. All skeletal samples referenced in this study derive from the medieval Jewish cemetery of Les Roquetes and are curated at the Museu Comarcal de l'Urgell-Tàrrega. There is no identifying information associated with any of these individuals (i.e., there are no burial records for this cemetery or coffin plates that identify interred individuals by name), and thus this research does not constitute any risk to living descendants. All the research at the site has been conducted in accordance with the *Llei 9/1993, de 30 de setembre, del Patrimoni Cultural Català* and the *Decret 78/2002, de 5 de març, del Reglament de protecció del patrimoni arqueològic i Paleontològic.*

2 Much of this local documentation, created by Christian authorities, was assembled and published by López (1956); see below.

But written accounts tend to take on a certain abstraction, which is why the discovery of the Jewish cemetery in Tàrrega in 2007 occasioned such interest. Within it were found six communal graves that seemed to hold the victims of the 1348 uprisings (Muntané 2007b, 2009, 2012a).[3] These graves are the only material evidence of the violent acts perpetrated against the town's Jewish minority. In the following essay, a team of archeologists, historians, and scientists lays out the evidence for the events of 1348 from a new perspective: first, we reassemble the historical documentation and examine it for evidence of the exact timing and circumstances of the events; then, we turn to the material evidence from the cemetery, examining it, too, to confirm the date of the events that produced these communal graves; and finally, in more detail, we look for evidence of the nature of the attack, the identities of the victims, and the circumstances in which they were laid to rest in this cemetery.

Part I: The Documentary Evidence

One of the acknowledged consequences of the plague epidemic of 1348–51 was an escalation in attacks on social minorities, including clerics, beggars, persons suffering from leprosy, and foreigners, who were blamed for the inexplicable mortality. In Catalonia, as in many other regions of Western Europe, Jews stood out as being the most powerful minority group and, as such, suffered disproportionally when the Black Death reached the area. What makes the Catalan case distinctive is that we now have an example of the documentary record being confirmed and extended by archeological data of an uprising against the Jewish community of Tàrrega in July 1348,[4] making it one of the first communities to suffer such an assault directly related to the Black Death.[5] The brutality of those uprisings is witnessed in various reports written by contemporary Jews.

3 Here and elsewhere, the Catalan term *fossa comuna* has usually been translated as "communal grave" rather than "mass grave." As the evidence summarized in this article indicates, aspects of the burials discovered at Les Roquetes were carefully planned, if hasty. This was not a haphazard disposal of bodies. That said, the editors' decision to render this ambiguous term as "communal grave" should not mask the fact that those buried in these graves were victims of a massacre.

4 In the original Catalan version of this essay, the authors used the term *avalot*, a "popular uprising" or "seditious tumult" (cf. *Diccionari de la llengua catalana de l'Institut d'Estudis Catalans*). The exact motivations behind these attacks may have been more complicated than the epithet "popular" can adequately capture, and yet the term *pogrom* seems too heavily freighted to be used unproblematically. Therefore, we have settled on the term "uprising."

5 Earlier attacks in April of 1348 occurred in Toulon, Hyères, and several other

With respect to the uprising in Tàrrega, we have the testimony of a contemporary rabbi, Hayyim Galipapa (b. Montsó, *c.* 1310–d. Pamplona, *c.* 1380), then living in the town of Huesca, in Aragón. His account has survived due to its incorporation into the historical narrative of an Italian Jew, Joseph ha-Kohen (1496–1578), who commemorated the sufferings of the Jewish people during the Black Death in his *Emeq ha-Bakha* (*Valley of Grief*, 1557–58) (ha-Kohen 1557–58/1981: 27).[6] Two points of information provided by Galipapa help to contextualize the attack on the Jews of Tàrrega and correlate it with the spread of the plague epidemic. The first has to do with the route connecting the three Catalan towns he mentions, in the following order: Barcelona, Cervera, Tàrrega. This same order is confirmed by several official documents from the royal chancery of Pere III (r. 1336–87) of Barcelona (Pere IV of Aragon), documents which also record attacks on Jews in each of these towns. Barcelona, Cervera, and Tàrrega were connected by the main east-west road, and the order thus reflects the direction that the plague took, moving westward from the coast toward the interior of the principality (López 1956, 1959a, 1959b). Galipapa's second informative contribution helps to establish the date of these three incidents. According to the rabbi, there was an uprising at Barcelona on a Saturday afternoon, followed by another at Cervera on an unspecified date, and by yet another at Tàrrega three days after the second. For this last, he assigns a specific date: the 10th of the month of Av.[7]

Establishing the link between the arrival of plague and the attacks on these three Jewish communities is not straightforward. First of all, we must accept that our sources will only record *human* cases of plague, and not the actual spread of the pathogen through rodent populations or contaminated foodstores. What we can see from the documented human cases is that plague seems to have arrived in Catalonia only recently, in the spring of 1348, having been reported first at Perpignan in April, and then by May at Girona, to the northeast of Barcelona. It also reached Tarragona and Valencia (other port cities to the southwest) as well as the

small towns in Provence. See Crémieux 1930–31; Shatzmiller 1974. The more widely known attacks in Savoy and the Rhineland did not start until later in the year 1348. On the latter, see most recently Cohn 2007.

6 Ha-Kohen also incorporated Galipapa's narrative into another work, *Dibre ha-Yamim le-Malke Zarfat we-'Otoman* (Chronicles of the Kings of France and Turkey), published in Venice in 1554: see Barzilay 2011. The authors thank Mr. Barzilay for sharing his work with them, and also Susan Einbinder for alerting them to this (and other) pertinent publications.

7 See ha-Kohen 1557–58/1981: p. מז line טו and p. מח line כה.

island of Mallorca in the month of May (López 1956: nos. 2 and 5; see also Guilleré 1984: 106).[8] By mid-May, at the latest, deaths are documented in Barcelona (Gyug 1983; Guilleré 1993–94, 1:171–72). The uprising against the Barcelonan Jewish quarter (*call*) therefore took place shortly after the arrival of the plague, since it seems that Jewish-Christian relations remained stable up through May 15 (Nirenberg 1996: 237–38).[9] According to the information we can extract from the royal chancery documents, the attack was vicious: "On Saturday last, some people incited by an evil temper, having set their fear of God and our dominion aside, gathered as a riotous mob and entered into the *call* of the Jews of Barcelona. And there they destroyed and despoiled many dwellings and they killed many Jews." That was on May 17, 1348. Just five days later, Pere III ordered the capture of the perpetrators of the uprising and the strengthening of security around the Jewish quarter in Barcelona.[10] A week later, on May 29—concerned lest there be further attacks – the king issued an order of protection to officers of the Jewish quarters in Montblanc, Tàrrega, Vilafranca del Penedès, and Cervera.[11] Almost two months after these precautions were taken, however, a document completed on 24 July shows their ineffectuality, as uprisings had already reached the towns of Cervera and Tàrrega.[12]

8 In Tarragona, the plague began the first of May: see Trenchs 1969.

9 The historian Esteve Gilabert Bruniquer (c. 1608/1915, 4: 319) claimed, confusingly, that there was "a great procession of many priests from the cathedral and parishes and monasteries and many other people" on May 2, but he then linked that ceremony to the great mortality in June.

10 "Die sabbati proxime preterita, nonnulli maligno spiritu concitati, Dei timore postposito at in nostre dominationis conceptum per modum aualoti intrarunt in Callem Judaycum Barchinone et inibi, plura hospitia fregerunt et disraubarunt ac multos judeos inibi occiderunt"; see López 1956: no. 8 (May 22, 1348).

11 "The king ordered his officials that 'you are to maintain and protect and defend each and every Jew of the Jewish quarter of the city and of his realm and their possessions and goods vigorously and earnestly from all disturbances, molestations, injuries, inconveniences and offenses'" ("El rei manava als seus oficials que 'omnes et singulos Judeos aljame Judeorum ville eiusdem et collectorie sue ac res et bona eorum quecumque, manuteneatis, protegatis et deffendatis viriliter et potenter, ab infestationibus, molestiis, injuriis, grauaminibus et offensis indebitis quorumcumque nec ipsos uel eorum aliquos in personis et bonis ipsorum, per modos supra specifficatos uel aliter, permittatis a quo quam contra jus et justitiam agrauari seu etiam molestari'"); see López 1956: no. 9 (May 29, 1348).

12 "Hiis diebus proxime lapsis, propter rumores nobis subito venientes, qualiter per nonnullos civitatis Barchinone et villarum Cervarie, Tarrage, contra aljamas et singulares dictarum civitatum et villarum, casu fortuito et inopinato, concitato populo, extitit suscitata occasione cuius strages seu neces, percussiones et vulnera

Like Galipapa's Hebrew account, these official documents offer no precise date for the attack on the Jewish quarter of Cervera. For Tàrrega, however, we have Galipapa's date: 10 Av of the year 5108, which would fall in the first half of July, probably around 6 July.[13] Since we have already seen that Pere III was reacting to the assaults on all three communities by 24 July, the date we can deduce from Galipapa's testimony seems credible.

This causal relationship between the occurrence of the epidemic and attacks on Jewish quarters is even clearer in a document of early 1362, during what is generally seen as the second wave of the plague in Western Europe (see Carmichael 2014, in this issue). Trying to pre-empt the alarm caused by the arrival of a new outbreak of the plague, the secretary of the Tàrrega Jewish community requested protection from the king. For "as in the time of deaths, by divine judgment, which took place long ago, the Jewish community and its members were despoiled and many of them put to a sword by some people of this town and others, so now [...] because of the deaths that have occurred and are still occurring in some parts of the kingdom, they fear that they will again be damned and plundered and killed as fiercely as before."[14]

Obviously, the same degree of alarm did not exist in the minds of Catalan Jews before 1348, so we find no documents (contemporaneous with the arrival of the plague) that indicate a fear of attack by Christians. However, understanding of this causal relationship was rapidly discerned by

varia et diversa rapinie ad destructiones domorum, adversas aliamas predictas et quampluribus singularibus ex ea fuerunt diversimode subsecuta"; see López 1959b: no. 5 (July 24, 1348). This document is addressed to the authorities of Lleida, who wanted to avoid an attack similar to the one in Cuirassa (one of the two Jewish neighborhoods of Lleida). It was of no use, as a document dated August 11, 1348 (included in one of July 18, 1349, no. 12) indicates that the wave of attacks spread elsewhere: "And especially recently, first in the city of Barcelona and now in the towns of Cervera, Tàrrega, and in the city of Lleida and other places" ("Et specialiter nuper primo in civitate Barchinone et nunc noviter in villis Cervarie et Tarrege et in civitate Ilerde et in aliis etiam locis").

13 See "Hebcal Jewish Calendar", online at <http://www.hebcal.com> [accessed March 1, 2014].

14 "Pro parte aljame Judeorum dicte uille, fuit nobis humiliter suplicatum ut cum tempore mortalitatum que, Dei juditio temporibus preteritis viguerunt, aljama ipsa et eius singulares, per aliquas personas uille eiusdem et aliunde, fuerint disraubati et plures ex ipsis gladio trucidati, timeantque nunc occasione mortalitatum que jam viguerunt vigentque nunc in aliquibus partibus regni nostri iterato dampnificari, depredari et interfici et immaniter prout prius dignaremur eisdem super hiis de nostri regia clementia subuenire"; see López 1956: no. 150 (January 12, 1362).

the survivors of that uprising. A few years later, the influential Tàrregan Jew Moixé Nathan wrote:

> On the day that any plague or famine occurs which threatens the earth, the people cry 'All this happens because of the sins of Jacob! Destroy this nation, kill them!' And during the disaster [...] they undertake in a violently thoughtless way to destroy the unfortunate Jews.[15]

Pope Clement VI (1342–52) and his successor expressed similar views.[16] So did Galipapa, who describes news of the plague spreading throughout Catalonia and Aragon, in conjunction with false accusations against Jews: "'For the sin of Jacob all this has passed, because they have taken a deadly poison into the world. From them is the fault and it is the cause of the great misfortune that afflicts us now!'" (ha-Kohen 1557–58/1981: מח). Whether Galipapa was accurately voicing contemporaneous concerns about well-poisoning or projecting later concerns back onto the past, he captures a sense of radical changes occurring in Catalonia and Aragon.[17]

One final point of information gleaned from Galipapa's account (as reported by ha-Kohen) needs to be assessed here: his claim that the number of Jews killed in Tàrrega exceeded three hundred.[18] The royal chancery's references to the death toll are often vague.[19] At one point, it is stated that almost all of Tàrrega's Jewish citizens were exterminated:

---

15 Nathan, *Accords* § 1b, signed in the month of Tevet of the year 5115 (between December 16, 1354 and January 13, 1355). For an edition of the original Hebrew text, see Baer (1929: no. 253). For a Catalan translation and introduction, see Feliu and Riera i Sans (1987). See also Pieters (2006), which includes a photographic reproduction of the manuscript Oxford, Bodleian Library, MS Bodley 2237, fols. 270v–272v.

16 See Clement's letter to prelates of the Church in Simonsohn 1998: no. 373 (November 26, 1348). See also a surviving Spanish translation of the papal bull issued by Innocent VI at Avignon on January 21, 1356 (Simonsohn 1998: no. 378).

17 Ha-Kohen 1557–58/1981: מז. Nirenberg (1996: 236–37) argues that there were no *contemporaneous* accusations of poisoning in Catalonia in 1348. In other words, Galipapa's temporal distance from the events of 1348 may be significant.

18 See the excerpt from Galipapa's testimony provided in the documentary appendix below.

19 E.g. (emphasis added) "ratione seu occasione necium in personis *plurium* judeorum ipsius ville nequiter perpetratarum et aliorum criminum et excessum": López 1959b: no. 11 (June 26, 1249); "et *plures* ex ipsis glaudio trucidati": López 1956: no. 150 (January 12, 1362). Compare (emphasis added) "*non pauci* Judei [de Tàrrega] crudeliter interfecti et disraubati fuerunt" with "*aliqui* Judei ville Cervarie interfecti et disrobati fuerunt": López 1959b: no. 29 (May 31, 1352).

"the greater part of the Jews, men and women both, of the said town were ferociously slaughtered in the invasion of the Jewish quarter."[20] Another report mentions "uprisings, murders, and despoiling done and perpetrated against the Jews of Barcelona and Cervera and especially those in the town of Tàrrega, of whom more than three hundred were viciously murdered."[21] The stress placed on Tàrrega (*specialiter ville Tarrage*) suggests that most of the deaths occurred there. This accords closely with Galipapa's account, which gives specific mortality figures for each of the uprisings: twenty dead in Barcelona, eighteen in Cervera, and three hundred in Tàrrega. Although, as we will see, the archeological evidence cannot fully support this large number, we must remember that the cemetery in Tàrrega has not been fully excavated.

Archival research is also allowing us to refine and understand another side effect of the plague that is often forgotten, because it almost exclusively affected the economic status of a social minority. In Catalonia, an ongoing crisis was already being felt some decades before the arrival of the plague. By the time the Black Death struck, the region had suffered a long period of famine and economic instability starting in 1333 ("the first bad year"). This crisis, in turn, led to a substantial growth in loans made by Jews, with borrowers increasingly drowning in debt while trying to overcome their continued losses (Abad 1999). In other words, the disease struck at a time when the population was already weakened, both physically and financially. It is therefore significant that Jewish sources, as well as the official records of the chancery, corroborate the fact that assaults on local Jewish communities were accompanied by the looting of their homes and property and the extensive destruction of documentation relating to these debts. In all three of the cases noted above, the violence was not only focused to greater or lesser degree on the Jewish population, but also on the financial instruments in Jewish archives.

For the summer of 1349, furthermore, there is extensive notarial evidence of Jewish citizens filing claims to recover debts that remained

---

20 López 1959: no. 18 (15 April 1350): "judeos et iudeas aljame ville pretacte in *maxima ipsorum parte* atrociter trucidarunt in quorum Judeorum invasione" (emphasis added). The magnitude of this number depends on the number of people living in Tàrrega at the time, which we cannot know with any certainty according to Riera i Sans (1987).

21 López 1959b: no. 10 (document of March 23, 1349 found in one of June 13, 1349): "in facto concitationum, necium et raubariarum factarum et perpetratarum contra judeos Barchinone et Cervarie et specialiter ville Tarrage, ex quibus ultra trecentos fuerint nequiter interempti."

unpaid after the plague and the attack on the Jewish quarter of Barcelona.[22] The fact that most of these claims specify the amount to be repaid without factoring in accrued interest suggests that these are references to debt instruments that were destroyed or lost, the intention being to recover at least the capital that had been initially invested. Among these we can also find instruments held by Jews from Cervera and Tàrrega, who were trying to recover investments they had made while living in these towns, but who were registering their claims in Barcelona—probably because they did not yet dare to do so at home.[23] (Among them was Moixé Nathan, who moved to Barcelona after the attacks.) Indeed, the claims that begin to appear in mid-1349 are supported by a royal mandate (dated September of the same year) that absolves Jews from fines or possible errors incurred in collecting debts for which they do not possess the original instruments (López 1959a: 335). By contrast, references to debt instruments do not appear in the documentation for Tàrrega until the years 1352–54 (López 1959a: 354). The atmosphere in Barcelona and Tàrrega could not have been more different: while the attack on the Jewish community in Barcelona was not as brutal, and there was clear legal recourse for the recovery of Jewish property, the magnitude and memory of the Tàrrega massacre may have continued to frighten survivors for many years, delaying any such claims to what was their own.

---

22 Arxiu Capitular de Barcelona (hereinafter ACB), Notaris de la ciutat, Jordi de Vilarrubia, vol. 221 (1347–51). In this volume, between pages 97 and 128, there are over sixty debt instruments which allow us to glimpse legal actions undertaken by survivors of the attacks on the *call* of Barcelona. Other similar documents (although not so many) can be found at ACB, Notaris de la ciutat, Francesc de Puig, vol. 233 (1348–49).

23 ACB, Notaris de la ciutat, Jordi de Vilarrubia, vol. 221 (1347–51), fols. 99r, fol. 128v, and fol. 166v.

DOCUMENTARY APPENDIX

Description of the Uprising according to the Secretaries of the Tàrrega Jewish Community, as Documented by the Crown of Aragon

The following is an excerpt from a longer document created in the chancery of Pere III which lays out the formal complaints of the Jewish community of Tàrrega, whose survivors were seeking restoration of property seized or destroyed in the attack of 1348. This passage summarizes the events as reported to royal officials. Arxiu Reial de Barcelona (ARB), reg. 658, fol. 52r–v (December 2, 1349); excerpted from López 1959b: no. 14.[24]

> *Anno proxime lapso, nonnulli ipsius ville, populum eiusdem fortiter concitando, Dei timore et nostre correctionis postposito, nostram magestatem offendere non verentes, diabolico spiritu incitati, manu armata et mente deliberata ad callum ipsius aljame hostiliter accesserunt et ausibus indebitis violenter ostias ipsius callis tamen securibus et allis* [sic] *armorum generibus fregerunt et etiam destruxerunt ipsumque callum intrarunt unanimiter et potenter clamosis vocibus emittentes "Muyren los traydors" et, hiis non contenti, sed mala peyoribus comulantes, hospitia ipsorum judeorum nequiter dimitarunt lanceis, lapidibus et sagitis et demum in eis intrantes, res et bona omnia eorumdem tamquam raptores secum perperam asportarunt et plura instrumenta ac scripturas ipsorum judeorum diversorum contractuum laniarunt et etiam conburserunt et plures judeos ipsius aljame inaniter occiderunt et quosdam alios atrociter percusserunt et etiam vulnerarunt et plura alia dampna gravia et inmensa, injurias, ofensas, raubarias molestias et violentias ipsis judeis fecerunt.*

> (In the year just passed [i.e. 1348], some individuals of this town strongly aroused its people to put aside the fear of God and our authority, not hesitating to offend our majesty. Incited by a diabolical spirit, with armed hand and deliberate intent, they came maliciously to the *call* of the Jewish community [*aljama*] and with unwarranted recklessness they violently broke down and destroyed the gates of this *call* with axes and other types of weapons, and they even destroyed the *call* itself, entering into it all together and shouting loudly with raised voices, "Kill the traitors" [*Muyren los traydors*]. And not satisfied with that, but rivaling terrible acts with even worse things, they ruthlessly raided Jewish homes with spears, stones, and arrows. And, finally entering the said houses, they took away all the goods and property of the Jews, just as if they were

24 The quoted passage is couched as a reported speech clause (introduced with *quod*), which explains the verb forms used here. Note that the incendiary cry "Kill the traitors" is quoted in Catalan, not in Latin. A different English translation of a longer selection from this document can be found in Aberth (2005: 142-43).

thieves, and lawlessly they tore and burned many legal instruments and various written contracts of the Jews and they senselessly murdered many Jews in this community, and others were beaten mercilessly and were wounded, and they inflicted many terrible evils, grave injuries, offenses, robberies, harms, and atrocities and on these Jews.)

Description of the Uprisings of Barcelona, Cervera, and Tàrrega by Hayyim Galipapa, as Preserved in the Chronicle of Joseph ha-Cohen

Excerpted from ha-Kohen 1557–58/1981: מח–מז.

ויהי ביום השבת לעת ערב ויקומו על עם ה' אשר בבארצילונה ויהרגו מהם כעשרים נפש ובביזה שלחו את ידם ואין אומר השב עודם נלחמים וה' נתן קולות ומטר וגשם שוטף ואש מתלקחת ויתבהלו הקמים עליהם בלל ה' שפתם וילכו גם שרי העיר וגדוליה ויצלו הנשארים מידם ולא עצרו כח להצילם בטרם היות הקולות והמטר כי רבו הקמים עליהם האומרים נכחידם מגוי ולא יזכר שם ישראל עוד ייטיב ה' לטובים והמטים עקלקלותם יוליכם את פועלי האון אמן ואמן. ויהי לימים עוד ויקומו על היהודים אשר בעיר צירבירה וירגו כשמנה עשרה נפש ובביזה שלחו את ידם והנשארים ברחו לנפשם ויענו בצום חייתם ושק ואפר הציקו לרבים ויהי לימים עוד שלשה ביום העשירי לחדש אב ביום ענות נפשם ויקומו גם יושבי טאריגה ויכו ביהודים ואבד יותר משלש מאות נפש ויסחבום אל בור רק ובביזה שלחו את ידם ודנשארים ברחו לנפשם אל בית מכריהם במתן בסתר עד עבור הזעם וישארו ערומים מכל קנינם ולא יתבוששו ביום הנמהר ההוא.

(He arrived Saturday evening, which was when the Lord rose against the people who were in Barcelona. About twenty people were killed and despoiled[a] and nobody said "Hold back!"[b] The uprising was continuing when a storm broke out[c] and then, before the rain fell and lightning struck, those who had risen up against the Jews took fright. The Lord confused their speech.[d] Then came the elders of the city and the leading men and they rescued the survivors. Before the thunder and the rain had scared them, there were many who were rioting against the Jews and saying "Exterminate them from among the nations! Let the name of Israel be remembered no more."[e] May the Lord reward the good and may he torment those who turned themselves into malefactors.[f] Amen, Amen.

After some days, people in the town of Cervera rose up against the Jews, killing about eighteen of them and despoiling them.[g] The survivors fled, mortifying their souls with fasting and sack cloth and ashes and suffering greatly.[h]

And after three more days, in the tenth day of the month of Av, which is a day of mortification, the inhabitants of Tàrrega also rose up against the Jews. They killed more than three hundred people and dragged them to an empty cistern, and despoiled them.[i] The survivors fled to the homes of acquaintances and remained hidden until the fury subsided.[j] On that rash day, they remained naked of all their possessions but without shame.[k])

[a] Esther 9. 10, 15, 16 [b] Isaiah 42. 22 [c] 1 Samuel 12. 11 [d] Genesis 11. 7
[e] Psalms 83. 4 [f] Psalms 125. 4 [g] Esther 9. 10, 15, 16 [h] Esther 4. 1, 2
[i] Esther 9. 10, 15, 16 [j] Isaiah 26. 20 [k] Genesis 2. 25

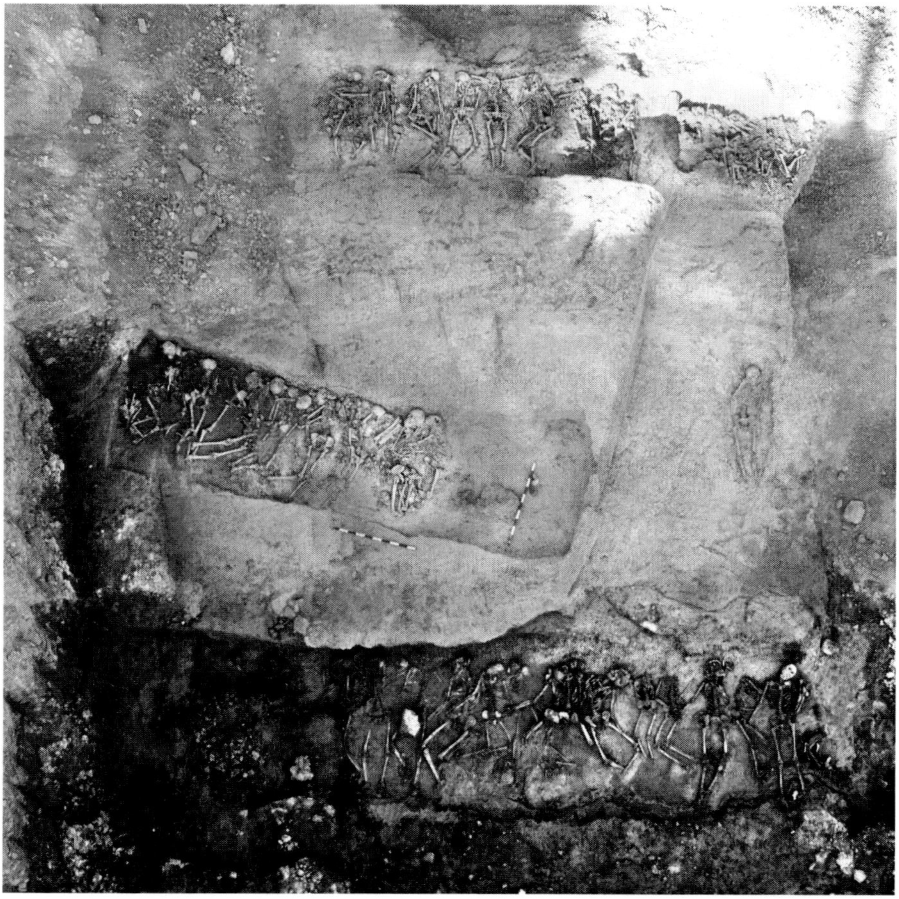

Figure 1. Overview of the Communal Graves

Part II: The Material Evidence

The Site

In 2007, in preparation for the construction of a housing development in an area classified as an historic site, excavations began at the Maset hill in the town of Tàrrega. It had already been reported that skeletons had been found in the area, during prior work on the street leading to the development, so an anthropologist was present when the archeological dig began. In conjunction with this investigation, historian J. X. Muntané (2007b) conducted an assessment of the *Llibres d'estimes* for the year 1501,[25] from

25 In medieval Catalan municipalities, the property registers called *llibres d'estimes* (books also known as *del manifest* or *de valies*) were used to assess taxes on their

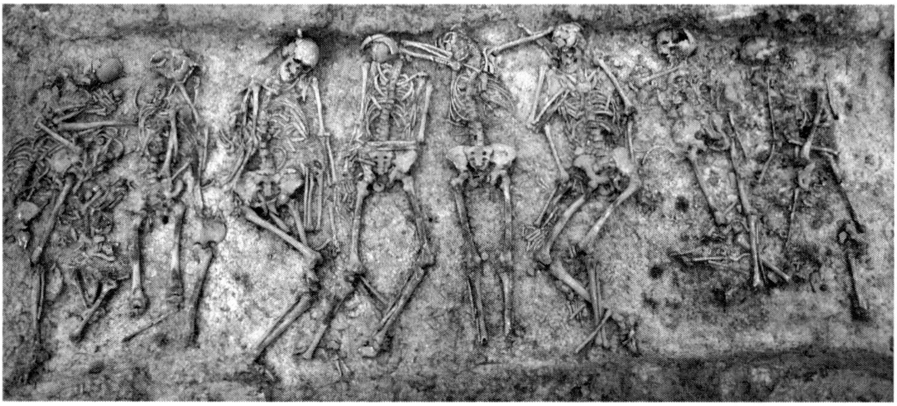

Figure 2. Communal Grave (FS) 161

which he deduced the possible location of a medieval Jewish cemetery on that same site, which is known as "Les Roquetes." This hypothesis was confirmed by the discovery of two rings bearing Hebrew inscriptions and other remains indicative of Jewish burial customs (Colet at al. 2009; Colet and Ruíz 2014), as evinced by similar findings in the Jewish cemeteries of Valladolid (Moreda and Serrano 2009), Barcelona (Duran and Millas 1947), and the street of Nové Město in Prague (Wallisová 2011).

The archeological excavations in the western sector of the cemetery revealed a concentration of anthropomorphic tombs, of a kind resembling sunken baths, covered with slabs of rock. This may be considered the oldest part of the cemetery, based on the typology of similar tombs found on Montjuic in Barcelona and in Girona (Casanovas Miró 2003). Also uncovered were six communal graves containing the remains of at least sixty-nine individuals (**Figure 1**). The total number of individuals interred in all of these graves cannot be determined at the present time, because the graves clearly extend to the south, beyond the excavated area.

The Graves

The communal grave shown in **Figure 2** (designated FS [fossa comuna] 161) is located furthest to the west of the excavated area. Its shape, like that of the other graves, is roughly rectangular. The north and south walls of this particular pit have been lost, perhaps due to erosion of the hillside's steep northern slope; erosion could also account for the destruction of the

inhabitants' property (houses, gardens, mills, fields, vineyards, etc.). Each owner made a detailed declaration, under oath, of real estate held in the municipality, and a value was then established as the basis for calculating the tax owed.

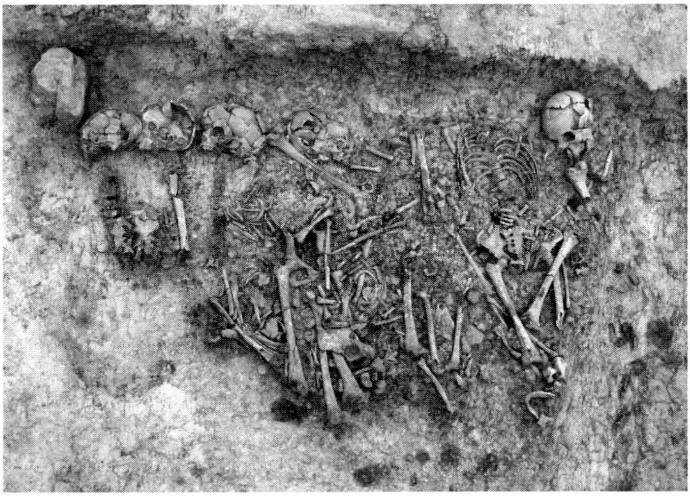

Figure 3. Communal Grave (FS) 163

south wall. However, there is another possible explanation for the absence of the grave's north wall: it could be that this grave and FS 163 (situated immediately to north: see below) formed a single pit, and that there was originally an empty space between the groups of bodies interred here.

One feature evident in this comunal grave is the limited breadth of the east-west axis. (This is the case in all of the graves except for FS 54: see below.) In this grave, the shaft is only about 1.5 meters wide, constraining the bodies contained within it. Placement of the bodies in the pits therefore involved either bending the legs or forcing the heads downward, to adapt them to this narrow space. The position of these bodies is suggestive of the speed with which they were buried.

In this particular grave, at least ten individuals were interred, among them a child aged between seven and twelve, an individual of indeterminate sex between seventeen and twenty-five years old, three men and a woman all aged between twenty-five and thirty-five years, two men aged forty and fifty, and one adult individual of indeterminate sex. One of the bodies (EU[26] 1173) was found with a set of five buttons located under the right collarbone. (See the further discussion of this evidence below.)

The grave shown in **Figure 3** (FS 163) is unusual when compared to the others. In the first place, a wooden cover was found beneath the landfill. This cover was made of pine,[27] in accordance with Jewish burial prac-

26 In Catalan, EU is the acronym for the stratigraphic unit associated with every individual in a communal grave (FS).

27 Dr. Raquel Piqué, of the Universitat Autònoma de Barcelona, has made a study of these remains.

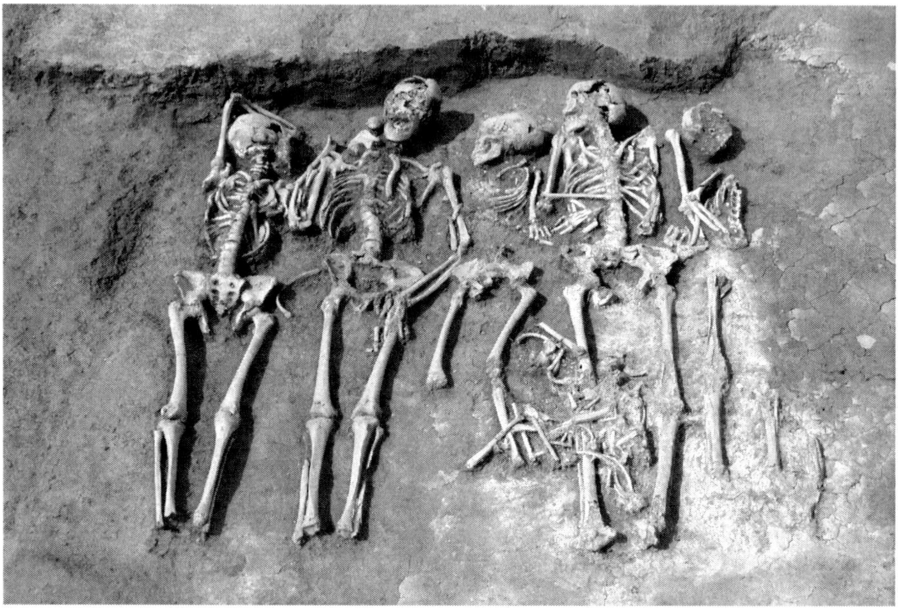

Figure 4. Communal Grave (FS) 54

tices (de Vries 1929/2001: 253). Another special feature of this grave is the degree of anatomical disarticulation exhibited by the human remains within it. Of the (at least eight) distinct individuals whose remains have been found in this grave,[28] only one has remained partially articulated. Analysis of the skulls yields the following information about the victims: one child aged three or four, two young women between twenty and thirty years of age, a man and a woman between the ages of thirty and forty, a woman aged between forty and forty-four years, a woman aged between fifty and sixty years, and an adult woman of undetermined age.

Also found in this grave were artifacts that might constitute the pieces of a necklace associated with the child buried here (EU 1185). Such artifacts might be considered amulets, either on the basis of the material from which they are made or the manner of their production (Colet et al. 2010). The child in question appears to have suffered from a slight malformation of the lower limbs, which may account for the necklace of protective charms, meant to safeguard or heal the child.

The communal grave shown in **Figure 4** (FS 54) has retained only its west wall. Unlike the rest of the graves, the breadth of its east-west axis suited the heights of the individuals buried there, since their legs

28 In Catalan, the NMI or minimum number of individuals.

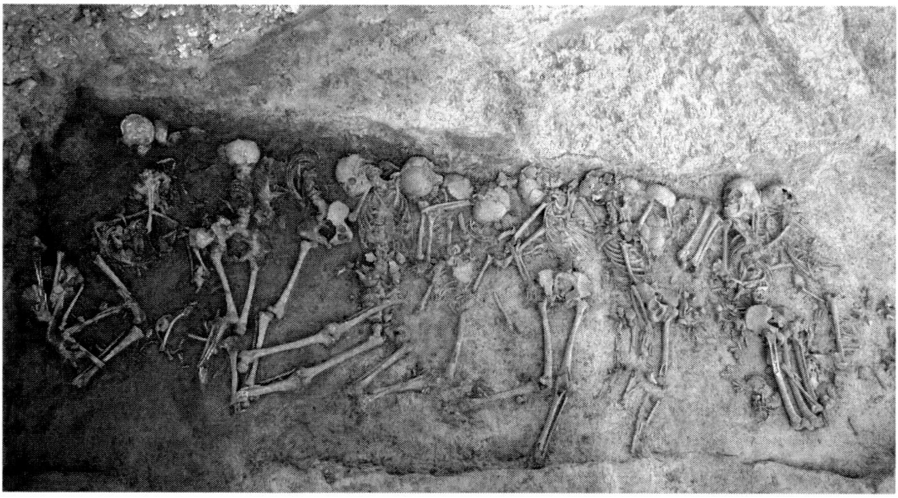

Figure 5. Communal Grave (FS) 162

are unbent and their skulls intact. It contains the remains of at least five individuals whose body were carefully prepared for burial. However, the bodies of individuals EU 1051 and 1053 appear to have been moved, causing disarticulation of the skeletons and depositing some remains atop the right leg of the individual EU 1052. Individual EU 1055 also appears to have been moved slightly. All of these movements could be interpreted as the result of successive burials or the later reopening of the graves, actions which (voluntarily or involuntarily) displaced the remains.

This grave contains two individuals of indeterminate sex, one between ten and twelve years old and the other around seventeen, a young woman aged between seventeen and twenty-five, a man aged between twenty-five and thirty-five years, and a woman aged between thirty-three and forty-five years.

The grave shown in **Figure 5** (FS 162) has a north-south axis measuring 5.4 meters, while the east-west axis ranges between 1.3 and 1.51 meters. Due to the limited breadth of the latter axis, those burying the individuals contained in it had to force their bodies into the grave. Yet these burials do not fill the entire grave, which extends about a meter and a half further to the north. Noteworthy features of this grave are the discoveries of a white glazed ceramic jar, buried near the bottom and almost intact, and also part of a white glazed ceramic lid, found on the north side. Interestingly, a fragment of the same lid was discovered in the landfill of another grave (FS 166: see below). This proves that both graves were covered over at the same time, but the unusual presence of these ceramic materials in the graves has not yet been explained.

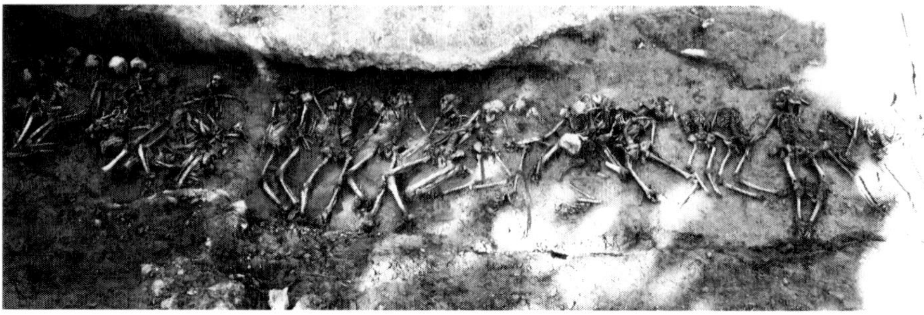

Figure 6. Communal Grave (FS) 164

This grave, FS 162, contains the remains of at least twenty individuals. As in the case of FS 161 (see Figure 2 above), the mangled positions of the bodies indicate the speed with which burial was performed. Identifiable remains include those of a perinatal or newborn child of indeterminate sex, a child who was about six months old, two children aged between two and three years, a child of five to six years, two children of indeterminate sex between the ages of six and seven, a boy and a girl between thirteen and fifteen years of age, two young men and two young women between eighteen and twenty-five years old, two men and a woman between twenty-five and thirty years of age, and four adult individuals of indeterminate sex.

The communal grave shown in **Figure 6** (FS 164) has yielded, so far, the largest number of remains. However, it has not been excavated in its entirety, because it extends to the south of the area that could be accessed in 2007. Moreover, the north side has been destroyed, possibly by erosion. The excavated length of the north-south axis measures 7.74 meters in length. The east-west axis measures approximately 1.56 meters. The most obvious of this grave's noteworthy features is the fact that the bodies placed further to the south display a lower degree of anatomical articulation than those to the north. While the latter are clearly individualized, those in the sourthern edge of the grave have been jumbled together, although they maintain a certain uniform orientation, with the heads placed toward the west.

In this grave, buttons have been recovered among the remains of two individuals: a female of undetermined age (EU 1201) and an adult male (EU 1211). A number of coins and the key to a chest have also been found (designated MCUT[29] 4653). A minimum of twenty-five individuals can be

29 The acronym denoting the artifact's number in the inventory of the Museu Comarcal de l'Urgell-Tàrrega.

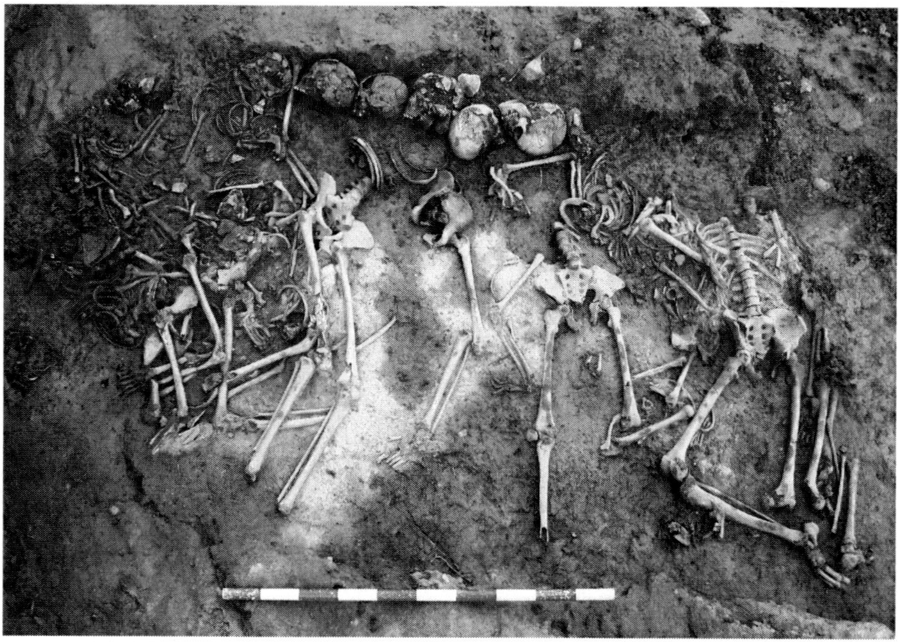

Figure 7. Communal Grave (FS) 166

identified. Among them are a child aged approximately six years, six children aged between seven and twelve, a girl between thirteen and fifteen years of age, three young women and two young men between twenty and thirty years of age, a woman and two men aged between thirty and forty years, two women and three men aged between forty and sixty years, a man in his sixties, and three individuals of indeterminate age (two men and an individual of indeterminate sex).

The grave shown in **Figure 7** (FS 166) is located farthest to the east of the area excavated at Les Roquetes. As with FS 164, the southern arm of the grave extends beyond the range of the archaeological dig and was not fully excavated. The north wall has been destroyed, either due to erosion or previous human efforts to prevent water from leaking into the area (a problem that persists today). The breadth of the grave's east-west axis varies between 1.42 and 1.57 meters. In addition to the fragment of pottery noted above, identifed as part of the lid to the ceramic jar found in FS 162, another set of coins was also found.

FS 166 contains the remains of at least twelve individuals of both sexes, as in FS 161 and 162. Among them are a child aged five to six years, two children between the ages of seven and twelve, two adolescents between twelve and twenty years of age, three individuals aged between twenty and thirty, and four aged between thirty to forty.

Summary Analysis of the Archeological Evidence

The excavation of these communal graves and the findings described above have allowed us to draw up the following hypotheses.

The fact that one of the skeletons in FS 161 (Figure 2) has retained a set of five buttons (located under the right collarbone), and the discovery of additional buttons in FS 164 (Figure 6), indicates that these bodies may have been clothed at the time burial. This possibility is reinforced by the discovery of sets of coins in two graves (FS 164 and FS 166: Figures 6 and 7). The way these coins were found, clustered together, indicates that they were contained in receptacles of perishable material, such as purses, that could have been hidden within outer garments.

All of the burials in these communal graves conform to the orientation characteristic of Jewish ritual, with the heads to the west and the feet to the east. We wish to highlight that this was so in all cases, even in those graves where decomposition has caused the skeletons to fall apart. Certain care can also be discerned in the placing of individuals' remains: efforts were taken to avoid piling them up. We believe that the careful orientation and disposition of the bodies indicates that they were buried by the surviving members of the Jewish community.

In one of the graves (FS 164: Figure 6), the bones show evidence of violent trauma visible to the naked eye. The later anthropological study of the remains (summarized below) showed that over half the bodies in the six communal graves show signs of violent trauma as the cause of death, which occurred either immediately or in the hours following the attack.

The demographic distribution of the people buried in these communal graves reveals that they include all age groups—from a newborn to adults over the age of sixty—and that both sexes are equally represented: evidence that suggests an indiscriminate attack on those interred in this section of Les Roquetes.

A numismatic study of the two sets of coins found in graves FS 166 and FS 164 proposes a date no later than the mid-fourteenth century (Clua 2009). This chronology is backed by the Carbon-14 dating of one of the skeletons (EU 1220) found in grave FS 164, which is datable to the years 1280–1391 CE (CNA1644 cal 2σ[30]). The dating obtained from these assessments accords with what is known about the uprising in Tàrrega.

---

30 This has been established by the Centro Nacional de Aceleradores attached to the Universidad de Sevilla–Junta de Andalucía and the Spanish *Consejo Superior de Investigaciones Científicas (CSIC).*

All of these indications lead us to propose that the 1348 uprising against the Jewish community of Tàrrega, which is well documented in written sources, is now documented, too, in the communal graves found in Tàrrega's Jewish cemetery. The survivors of the uprising—who, as the historical documentation implies, were almost all from the Jewish community—had to bury their dead. But the magnitude of the violence must have generated considerable fear among the survivors, making it difficult to lay the slain members of their community to rest immediately. At the same time, the massacre had occurred at high summer and in the context of the plague epidemic, which means that the survivors would have worked quickly once it seemed safe to do so. All of this explains the decision to bury a large number of bodies in communal graves that were not always of a suitable size.

Communal burial is not common in Jewish burial rites, under most documented conditions. There are, however, notable exceptions.[31] In the medieval Christian territories of the Iberian Peninsula, a contemporary example can be found in Valencia, where the Jewish community was also the target of violence (Calvo Gálvez 2003). But in this case, the shape of the mass grave was roughly polygonal and it contained forty bodies, heaped up and mixed together. As can be inferred from the disposition of those bodies that have retained anatomical articulation, the dead were gathered and buried within a brief period of time, since rigor mortis had not yet set in, in the majority of cases. A significant percentage of the individuals buried in the Valencia gravesite (30%) also display traumatic lesions. These lesions are especially discernible in skeletons of ten male adults, and were caused by fatal and intentional wounds. The other individuals in this grave may have died of plague, as their bodies show no signs of violence. The majority were adult males, and only one child and one adolescent have been identified.

Unlike the uprising in Tàrrega, the attack on the Jews in Valencia is not documented in either Christian or Jewish sources. However, the discovery of two coins among a pile of materials dumped into the upper part of the grave suggests that the most feasible date for this mass burial is 1348 (Calvo Gálvez and Lerma 1998). Comparing the Valencian grave with those at Les Roquetes highlights several important differences between them. In Tàrrega, the attack on the Jewish community was indiscrimate, since representatives of the entire Jewish population (men and women of all ages) are found in the communal graves. In Valencia, the attack was

31 Multiple burials have been found at Córdoba: see Larrea and Hiedra 2010. See also the study of the medieval Jewish cemetery in Prague by Wallisová (2011).

selective and most of the individuals in the grave were adult men, some of whom may have been victims of the plague and not of violence. The differences between the distribution of the bodies in the two sites also shows that the Jewish burial customs were observed (to at least a certain extent) at the Tàrrega site, where it is highly likely that survivors of the attack there buried their own dead.

Elsewhere in Europe, evidence for the mass or communal burial of Jews also tends to confirm that such burials result from violence. In 2004, a well containing seventeen skeletons was dicovered in Norwich, England: the remains of eleven children (between the ages of two and fifteen) and six adults, all dated between the twelfth and thirteenth centuries. Although the initial identification of these individuals as Jews was controversial, and the results of ancient DNA testing generated much debate, subsequent analyses suggest that they were indeed the victims of violence, and they have since been given a Jewish burial.[32] Excavations at the Jewish cemetery of Jewbury (York, England) have revealed contemporaneous evidence of communal burials: in this case, a series of tombs hold more than one body, and this may be interpreted as a solution to the burial of family members who died at the same time, or of people who died on the same day. Although it is unclear whether such unusual measures were taken as a result of an attack on the Jews of York, it is undeniable that there was a marked increase in violence there during the late twelfth and thirteenth centuries (Lilley et al. 1994: 338–39 and 380–81).[33]

Other communal and mass burials dating from the fourteenth century have been found in the lands of Christian Europe, mostly connected (as shown by aDNA analysis) with the arrival of plague. The fact that no signs of violence are discernible on the remains of those buried in these graves makes it plausible (in cases where DNA studies have not been carried out) that they died from infectious disease (Ollich 2012; Kacki and Castex 2012). Yet attacks on Jewish communities occurred in places other than Tàrrega and Valencia during 1348. The first documented assaults

32 See the summary "Bodies in Norwich Well Buried in Jewish Cemetary, published online at *The History Blog* <http://www.thehistoryblog.com/archives/24175> [accessed May 13, 2014].

33 Violence against the Jewish communities of both Norwich and York (in particular) has been very well documented, and this violence escalated toward the end of the twelfth century. On the slaughter of the Jewish communty at York in the pogrom of 1190, see Jones and Watson (2013). It should be noted that violent attacks on the Jews of England did not occur during the Black Death; Jews had already been expelled from the realm in 1290.

occurred in Toulon, in April, and then in other places in Provence.[34] The wave of attacks later spread to Swiss and German cities (Cohn 2007). The archeological evidence from Tàrrega thus helps to substantiate the documentary records of all these events.

Anthropological Field Analysis

This section will focus on the particular features of the bodies buried in the six communal graves at Les Roquetes. As noted above, the archeological excavation uncovered the remains of at least sixty-nine individuals interred in this section of the Jewish cemetery and revealed the careful arrangement of the bodies in these graves. The bodies were oriented with the heads to the west and the feet to the east, in accordance wth Jewish burial practices. The individuality of the bodies was maintained insofar as was possible, by avoiding the piling of corpses. These facts, again, make it likely that the surviving members of the Jewish community took charge of the burial, despite the tense atmosphere that no doubt prevailed in Tàrrega after the uprising. However, the condition of those human remains which do not maintain anatomical articulation suggests that the period between the time of death and final burial must have been long. This evidence allows for differentiation among the graves, depending on the degree of articulation displayed by certain bodies. This field study accordingly offers some hypotheses about events that occurred at the time of death and burial, based on this data.

Graves containing primary deposits—that is, bodies that have remained intact up to the time of excavation (e.g., FS 54: Figure 4)—indicate that the decomposition process took place entirely on site, after burial. Once deposited, these bodies would not have been shifted, aside from the normal movement caused by natural taphonomic processes. If there had been any outside intervention, these displacements would be reflected in the excavated skeletal material, which would then be considered secondary deposits.

Graves that contain bodies displaying significant joint disarticulation suggest that these bodies had started to decompose prior to burial, probably in a different place, before they were brought to the site. The graves FS 163 and FS 166 (Figures 3 and 7) contain remains with little or no discernible anatomical articulations. The burial of these remains would therefore have taken place some time after the death of the victims. This period would have been long enough to allow the process of decompo-

34 See note 5.

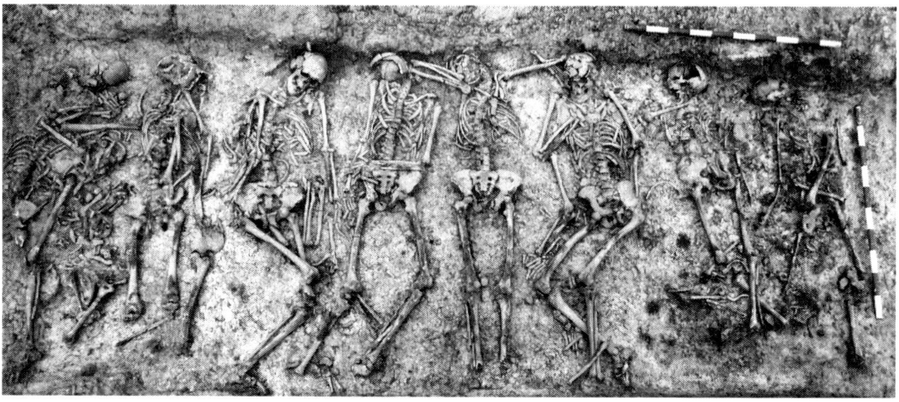

Figure 8. Detail of a Communal Grave Containing Primary and Secondary Deposits

sition to begin, thus explaining the loosened joints leading to disarticulation. Despite the difficulty of establishing the amount of time that had elapsed before burial, it is important to note that the remains found in this secondary state were still carefully disposed. Special care was taken to arrange the skulls of the victims, and to align all heads and feet on the west-east axis. This further demonstrates the intention to follow the precepts of Jewish burial in laying out these remains, as well as the intention to avoid overcrowding.

Graves of a mixed type, containing the remains of both primary and secondary deposits, are represented by FS 161, FS 162, and FS 164 (**Figure 8**). These graves are characterized by the burial of a core group of individuals whose remains display relatively good anatomical articulation (primary deposits), accompanied on one side or both ends of the grave by secondary deposits of bones. Although skulls and limbs have often become disconnected, the disposition of these remains still adheres to Jewish burial customs. As already noted, the differing degrees of joint articulation exhibited in all cases is remarkable and provides information that allows for study of the time elapsed between the death of an individual and his or her final burial.

Although the reasons for this variety in the burial pattern are still unknown, the two decisive variables are the location of an individual corpse during the interval between death and burial as well as the amount of time elapsed during that interval. During the time of chaos and insecurity immediately following the uprising and the assault on the Jews of Tàrrega, it is difficult to imagine that survivors would have dared to bury the victims. They would have had to wait for a certain degree of security to be re-established by royal authorities before preparations for ritual

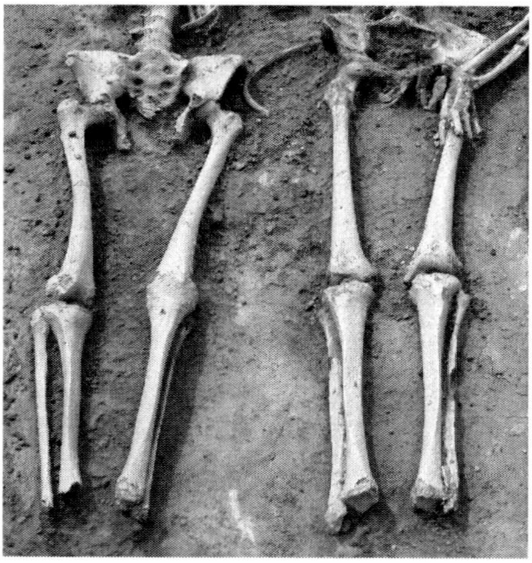

Figure 9. Bodies Lacking Feet (Detail of Figure 4)

burial could begin. During this period, the bodies of victims could have been kept in a secluded place away from the town, so as to prevent the spread of disease and also to protect the bodies. In fact, Galipapa's testimony refers to a cistern where bodies might possibly have been stored until the moment of the burial (Muntané 2009: 175). Thus, both the time between death and final burial, and the conditions in which bodies were preserved during this period, are likely to explain the different degrees of anatomical articulation found in the bodies of several graves.

Before we move to assess evidence for the circumstances of the victims' deaths, it is important to emphasize that the feet of many individual bodies were missing at the time of their interment (see **Figure 9**). Of the seventy-one recovered legs displaying good overall anatomical preservation and articulation, only thirty-six retain the foot connected with the rest of the limb. The explanation for this phenomenon is not related to the attack itself, since the affected limbs do not show any evidence of violence: that is, the missing feet were not amputated during the assault on the *call*. On the contrary, the disappearance of the feet occurred after death and probably before the corpses' final disposal in the graves. The distal regions of the legs in question do not show signs that would lead us to infer that the feet were removed by a cutting tool. Rather, the perfectly preserved state of anatomical articulation could suggest that the feet were accidentally pulled off when those preparing the corpses for burial attempted to remove shoes by tugging at them: an action that would not have severed the connective tissues, were they still intact. Moreover, the fact that no isolated foot bones were recovered during the excavation indicates that feet were removed when the bodies were already skeletonized, and that this occurred before the time of burial.

We can offer possible hypotheses that relate this phenomenon to the time elapsed between death and burial. As previously mentioned, this period must have been relatively long, and some of the bodies were clearly affected by advanced decomposition. It may well be, then, that some of these individual bodies lost their feet in the course of their transfer to the grave. We might also consider the possibility that it was necessary to reuse footwear in a time of crisis, such as that which prevailed after the uprising, provided that the removal of shoes from severely decomposed bodies did not affect the rest of the skeleton. Alternatively, the removal of shoes (and feet) could be interpreted as a posthumous act of revenge by Christians of the town,[35] but performed so skillfully so as to leave no anatomical evidence of damage to the distal part of the legs. In any case, no separate foot skeletons were retrieved, and we await further evidence that might lead to the resolution of this mystery.

Anthropological Laboratory Analysis

This section summarizes the results of the laboratory analysis of human remains recovered from the Tàrrega cemetery at Les Roquetes, data that helps to reconstruct the events that occurred during the assault on the Jewish *call* in July of 1348. This study accounts for all of the individuals—at leasy sixty-nine in number—whose remains have been recovered so far and from which a demographic reconstruction could be made (with the proviso that the cemetery has still not yet been completely excavated). Those individuals represent all age groups and both sexes, and present a demographic profile very similar to that of the people buried in other parts of the cemetery. Therefore, it seems clear that the attack was perpetrated against the Jewish population as a whole, without any apparent intentional selection of victims.

Focusing on the age of the victims, we find that 32% are subadult individuals (i.e., individuals below the age of approximately twenty years) and 67% are individuals of adult age, leaving a remainder of 1% whose age has not yet been determined due to the poor preservation of those remains. The pattern of mortality shows that young adults (aged twenty to thirty) are in the majority, making up 30% of the people buried in the communal graves.

---

35 For example, the narrative account of the pogrom against the Jews in the Provençal town of Toulon, an event which occurred during April 1348, notes that the massacred Jews, who had been left dead in the streets, were stripped of their clothes ("et suis vestibus spoliatos projessiaverunt"). See Cremieux 1931: 59.

Figure 11. Example of Skeletal Injury

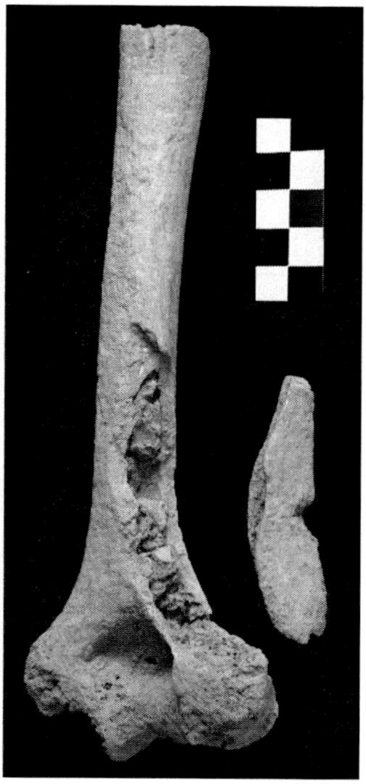

Figure 10. Example of Cranial Injury

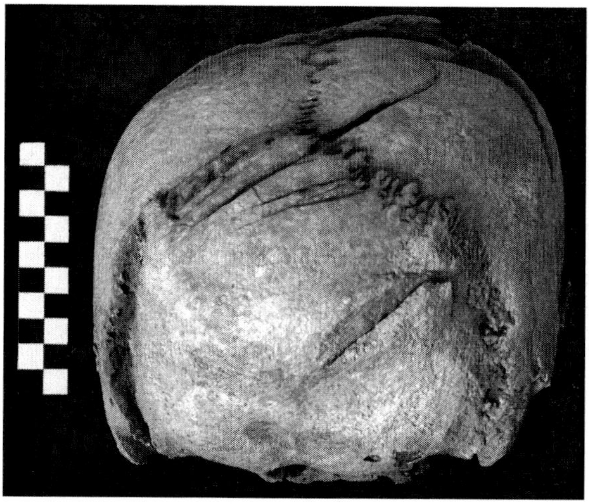

Regarding the distribution of sexes, we should highlight the imbalance found between the proportion of males (31%) and females (50%). Perhaps the 19% of individuals whose sex could not be determined figures in this disparity, but poor preservation of some remains and the difficulty of diagnosing the sex of subadult individuals prevent further identifications at this time. Indeed, individuals for whom it was not possible to determine either age or sex constitute 32% of the total number of buried in the communal graves. This means that we cannot establish whether individuals of a particular sex or age group were targeted during the uprising. However, the evidence overall suggests that the attack was perpetrated against the community at large, with no discrimination as to age or sex.

Laboratory analysis strengthens this hypothesis because it shows that the majority of individuals buried in the graves (at least thirty-seven out of sixty-nine) suffered injuries traumatic enough to mark the bone. We counted 155 injuries in total, both cranial (105 cases: see **Figure 10**) and skeletal (fifty cases: see **Figure 11**). The characteristics of these lesions and the number of injuries identified in each case (up to twenty-two injuries were afflicted on a single individual) further establishes the brutality of the attack, which seems to have been intended to eradicate the Jewish community of Tàrrega. As for the thirty-two individuals for whom no injury of this type can be discerned, this lack of evidence may be due (on the one hand) to the poor state of preservation of some remains or (on the other) to cases where the fatal injury occurred in soft tissue without penetrating to the bone, thus leaving no visible traces on the skeleton. Moreover, this hypothesis is supported by the fact that individuals who exhibit no such markings were buried simultaneously and alongside those whose wounds are evident, thus indicating that all those buried in the communal graves died within the same period of time. In addition, some of those without evident wounds could have died of plague or other infectious diseases during that time, and would then have been buried with the rest of the victims. Unfortunately, no aDNA tests have been performed, but comparison of the paleodemography of Les Roquetes with other cemeteries bearing witness to catastrophic episodes may hint at the effects of plague on the pattern of mortality here (Margerison and Knüsel 2002; Gowland and Chamberlain 2005). The demographic profile of a community's plague victims is often closely aligned with that of the population at large, because all the individuals have an approximately equal probability of dying, irrespective of age or sex (Keckler 1997). However, the simultaneity of the uprising in Tàrrega and the plague epidemic masks the effects of each.

Of the thirty-seven individuals who were detected to have injuries caused by violence, ten are children and the remaining twenty-seven are adults. As for the distribution by gender, twelve female and fifteen male individuals could be identified with this type of injury, maintaining the same equity mentioned in the demographics of those buried in the mass graves. Thus, there is no discernible difference between the injuries inflicted on any age group or sex, demonstrating once again the indiscriminate attack that the Jewish inhabitants of Tàrrega suffered. It is important also to acknowledge the evidence of cruelty towards the defenseless, such as the male individual EU 1215, found in grave FS 164. This man sustained at least twenty-two injuries, twelve inflicted on the skull and ten on the rest of the body (**Figure 12**). A careful study of the remains revealed that this individual had an old fracture in his right leg that had healed poorly, with osteomyelitis in the right tibia and fibula. This old injury would have made escape difficult, since the victim would not have been able to run and thus would have been an easy target. This is further evidenced by the extensive leg injuries that he apparently suffered during the attack.

The detailed study of such trauma and speculation about the weapons and tools used during the attack enable us to fill an important gap in the exisiting scholarship and to begin reconstructing the events that occurred. Examining the types of imprints left on the bones—cuts, fractures, fissures, and so forth—allows us to extrapolate information about the types of weapon that were used during the assaults on each individual, pro-

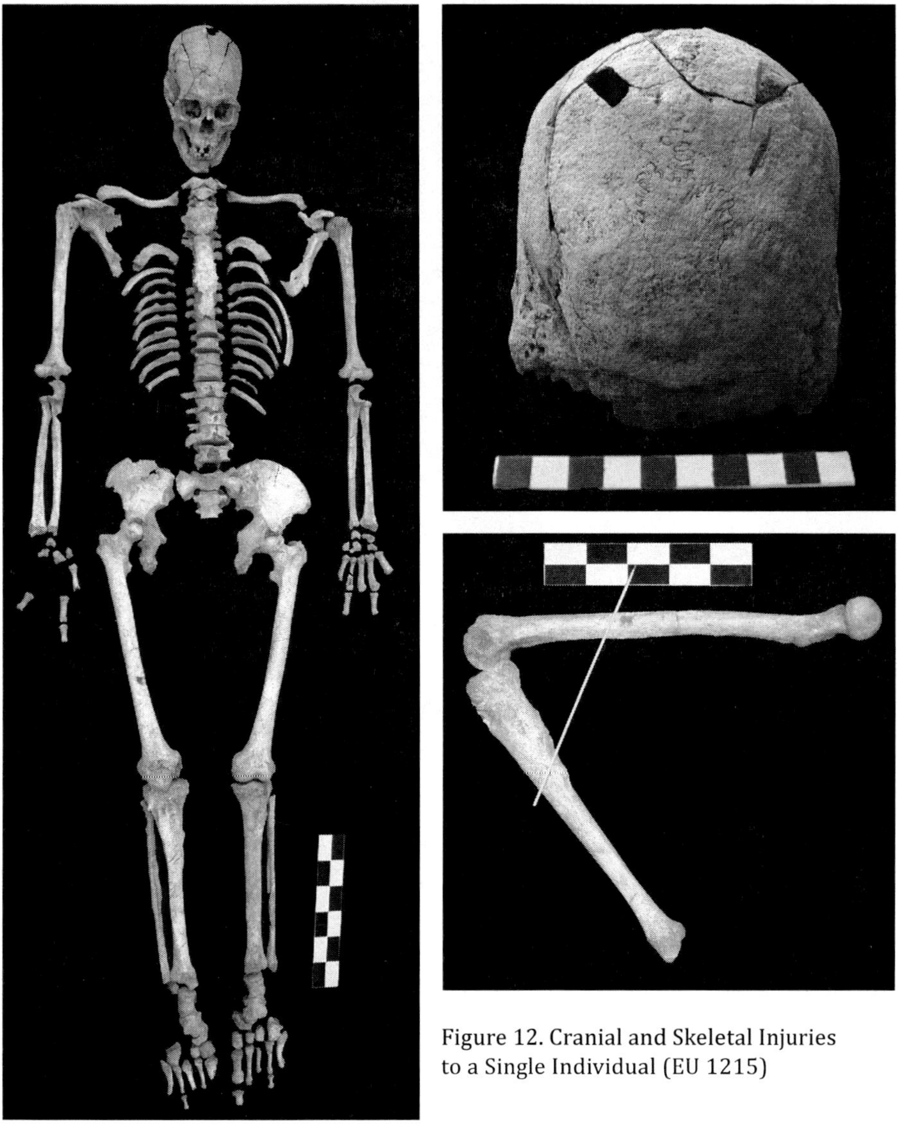

Figure 12. Cranial and Skeletal Injuries to a Single Individual (EU 1215)

vided that the mark has not been degraded by the passage of time and the conditions of burial. Thus, in the case of perimortem trauma (i.e., injuries sustained around the time of death that could be the cause of death), the most common injuries are those made by sharp objects such as swords, axes, and sickles, all of which produced a clean cut to the bone. These appear in 153 cases (out of 155 visible injuries), representing 98.7% of all the injuries documented. In these cases, the cut is seen to follow a more or less straight line, indicating the energy and skill behind the blow. Based on the cuts observed both on the skull and the rest of the skeleton, it can be determined that such injuries were incurred by sharp blows inflicted with a lot of energy, using tools that were quite sharp. In some cases, the force of the blows was so great that all the bone was sectioned, amputating a limb. We also find crush injuries or fractures. These are caused by the impact of a blunt instrument, again with considerable weight behind the blow, but made at a slower speed that fails to penetrate the bone. These objects could be stones or heavy objects that were thrown, causing injury that radiated widely and resulted in contusions. In the graves of Les Roquetes, there is only one such case: an injury to the skull. There was also a unique case of a skull injury caused by the impact of a rectangular object wielded with so much strength and energy that it penetrated the bone, leaving a characteristic mark. This injury can be seen in the skull of the individual EU 1215 (Figure 12) and was dealt with a force sufficient to shatter the skull. The shape and position of the lesion (just on the cranial vault) allows us to surmise that the weapon could have been an ax handle or the handle of a sword. In this case, the bone fragment resulting from the impact was recovered inside the skull.

In conclusion, therefore, we can say that laboratory analysis has allowed us to clarify and confirm the archeological evidence and the results of the anthropological analysis undertaken on site. It also corroborates the existing documentary narratives of the events that occurred during the uprising and proves that many of those buried at Les Roquetes lost their lives during that bloody attack.

Part III: Conclusions

The significance of the Tàrrega site is clear. It is an exceptional archeological record of events previously documented only by written accounts. To date, the attack against the Jewish citizens of Tàrrega is the first for which both documentary and archeological evidence have been found, helping to substantiate reports that many Jewish communities suffered atrocities between 1348 and 1349.

The excavation of the communal graves has enabled us to reconstruct, in part, the events that occurred during the attack on the Jewish quarter and to compare archeological evidence with that of the documentary sources. As the remains show and the sources explain, not all of the victims were buried immediately after the uprising. The sources mention that some of the dead were tossed into a cistern—a fact that the archeology and anthropology cannot substantiate, but that is consistent with the varying degrees of anatomical articulation exhibited by the bodies recovered so far. We think that all of the individuals found in the communal graves were victims of the attack on the Jewish quarter in 1348, but those whose remains exhibit a higher degree articulation were buried first, while those whose remains are disarticulated remained unburied for a period of time, long enough for the process of decomposition to advance.

During the archeological excavation, it was not possible to document the different phases of the burial process. However, the evidence of graves FS 161 and 163 (Figures 2 and 3) is suggestive in this regard. During the initial excavations, these were interpreted as two different structures; but given the fact that they are adjacent—and the fact that field work did not uncover the north wall of FS 161 or the south wall of FS 163—they could correspond to two different initiatives. The first of these would have been the burial of the bodies in FS 161. Having been partially filled with earth, this grave was then used to bury the bodies we initially assigned to FS 163. This suggests that a prudent gap was left between the first set of burials and the second set. (The space between the individuals in FS 161 and FS 163 is 1.5 meters.)

The same hypothesis is plausible for the grave FS 164 (Figure 6): here, the remains displaying a high degree of anatomical articulation are separated by 50 cm from those that had begun to decompose. The former group of bodies could have been placed in the grave and covered with earth. The rest of the bodies were then added, towards the southern end of the structure, when they had already begun to decompose.

In general, the care with which all of these individuals were originally interred leads us to surmise that they were buried by the surviving members of the Jewish community in Tàrrega. Although full observance of all funeral rites was impossible, bodies were arranged with the heads to the west and care was taken not to heap the bodies on top of one another.

Study of the written sources referring to the medieval Jewish community of Tàrrega reveals evidence that could not be gleaned from archaeology or anthropology (Muntané 2007a and 2012b; Ruíz and Subirà 2009). The study of the documentation also enabled the location of the Jewish quarter and its cemetery to be determined (Muntané 2014a). The latter has now been confirmed by the excavation in Les Roquetes, and archeological evidence and anthropological analysis have supplied further information about aspects of Jewish funeral rites and beliefs (Colet 2014; Colet and Ruíz 2014). Perhaps most importantly, our combined efforts have made it possible to confirm both the occurrence of the uprising, its connection with the Black Death and the ongoing economic crisis within the Crown of Aragon (Garcia Biosca 2014), and the resulting severity of the attack on Tàrrega's Jews in 1348.

Bibliography

Abad, Anna Rich. 1999. "La comunitat jueva de Barcelona (segle XIV)," *Butlletí de la Societat Catalana d'Estudis Històrics* 10: 53–56

Aberth, John. 2005. *The Black Death: The Great Mortality of 1348–1350. A Brief History with Documents* (New York: Palgrave MacMillan)

Baer, Fritz. 1929. *Die Juden im Christlichen Spanien, Erster Teil: Urkunden und Regesten I. Aragonien und Navarra* (Berlin: Akademie)

Barcelona, Arxiu Capitular de Barcelona (ACB), Notaris de la ciutat, vol. 221 (Jordi de Vilarrubia, 1347–51) and vol. 233 (Francesc de Puig, 1348–49)

Barcelona, Arxiu Reial de Barcelona (ARB), reg. 658

Barzilay, Tzafrir. 2011. "The Black Death in Aragon: A Look at a Jewish Chronicle," *Hayo Haya: A Young Forum for History* 8, no. 1: 53–71

Bruniquer, Esteve Gilabert. [*c.* 1608]/1912–16. *Rúbriques de Bruniquer: Ceremonial dels Magnífichs Consellers y Regiment de la Ciutat de Barcelona*, 5 vols (Barcelona: Impr. d'Henrich)

Calvo Gálvez, Matías. 2003. "Necrópolis judía de Valencia, nuevos datos," in *Juderías y sinagogas de la Sefarad medieval*, ed. Eloy Benito Ruano et al., 583–612 (Cuenca: Ediciones de la Universidad de Castilla-La Mancha)

Calvo Gálvez, Matías, and Josep Vincente Lerma. 1998. "Peste negra y pogrom en la ciudad de Valencia: La evidencia arqueológica," *Revista de Arqueología* 19, no. 206: 50–59

Carmichael, Ann G. 2014. "Plague Persistence in Western Europe: A Hypothesis," *The Medieval Globe* 1: 157–191

Casanovas Miró, Jordi. 2003. "Las necrópolis judías hispanas: Las fuentes y la documentación frente a la realidad arqueológica," in *Juderías y sinagogas de la Sefarad medieval*, ed. Eloy Benito Ruano et al., 493–532 (Cuenca: Ediciones de la Universidad de Castilla-La Mancha)

Clua, Maria. 2009. "Les fosses comunes del fossar dels jueus de Tàrrega, testimoni de la realitat monetària de mitjan segle xiv," *Urtx* 23: 140–55

Cohn, Samuel K., Jr. 2007. "The Black Death and the Burning of Jews," *Past and Present* 196: 3–36

Colet, Anna. 2014. "Creences i supersticions de la comunitat jueva a través dels seus objectes," in *Tragèdia al call*, 181–88 (Tarrega: Museu Comarcal de l'Urgell, Exhibit Pamphlet)

Colet, Anna, and Jordi Ruíz. 2014. "El fossar dels jueus de Tàrrega i el ritual funerari jueu," in *Tragèdia al call*, 135–42 (Tarrega: Museu Comarcal de l'Urgell, Exhibit Pamphlet)

Colet, Anna, Jordi Ruíz, Oriol Saula, M. Eulàlia Subirà, et al. 2009. "Les fosses comunes de la necròpolis medieval jueva de les Roquetes, Tàrrega," *Urtx* 23: 103–23

Colet, Anna, Jordi Ruíz, Oriol Saula, M. Eulàlia Subirà, et al. 2010. "Els amulets de la necrópolis medieval hebrea de les Roquetes, Tàrrega (L'Urgell)," in *Actes del IV Congrés d'Arqueologia Medieval i Moderna a Catalunya* 2: 1021–24 <http://museutarrega.cat/download/pdf/Amulets.pdf> [accessed August 30, 2014]

Crémieux, Adolph. 1930–31. "Les juifs de Toulon au moyen âge et le massacre du 13 avril 1348," *Revue des études juives* 79, no. 1–2: 33–72; 80, nos. 1–2: 43–64

Duran, Agustí, and Josep Maria Millas. 1947. "Una necrópolis judaica en el Montjuich de Barcelona," *Sefarad* 7: 231–59

Feliu, Eduard, and Jaume Riera i Sans. 1987. "Els acords de Barcelona de 1354," *Calls* 2: 145–79

Garcia Biosca, Joan. 2014. "Condicionants polítics i econòmics del pogrom del 1348 a Tàrrega," in *Tragèdia al call*, 117–21 (Tarrega: Museu Comarcal de l'Urgell, Exhibit Pamphlet)

Gowland, R. L., and A. T. Chamberlain. 2005. "Detecting Plague: Palaeodemographic Characterisation of a Catastrophic Death Assemblage," *Antiquity* 79, no. 303: 146–57

Guilleré, Christian. 1984. "La peste noire à Gerone (1348)," *Annals de l'Institut d'estudis Gironins* 27, no. 1: 87–161

Guilleré, Christian. 1993–94. *Girona al segle XIV*, trans. Núria Mañé, 2 vols (Girona: Ajuntament de Girona; Barcelona: Publicacions de l'Abadia de Montserrat)

Gyug, Richard Francis. 1983. "The Effects and Extent of the Black Death of 1348: New Evidence for Clerical Mortality in Barcelona," *Mediaeval Studies* 45: 385–98

ha-Kohen, Joseph. 1557–58/1981. *Sefer 'Emeq ha-Bakha (The Vale of Tears), with the Chronicle of the Anonymous Corrector*, ed. Karin Ambladh (Uppsala: Almqvist & Wiskell)

Jones, Sarah Rees, and Sethina Watson (eds.). 2013. *Christians and Jews in Angevin England: The York Massacre of 1190. Narratives and Contexts* (Woodbridge: Boydell)

Kacki, Sacha, and Dominique Castex. 2012. "Réflexions sur la variété des modalités funéraires en temps d'épidémie. L'exemple de la Peste noire en contextes urbain et rural," *Archéologie médiévale* 42, no. 1: 1–22

Keckler, C. N. W. 1997. "Catastrophic Mortality in Simulations of Forager Age-at-Death: Where Did All the Humans Go?," in *Integrating Archaeological Demography: Multidisciplinary Approaches to Prehistoric Population*, ed. Richard R. Paine, 205–28 (Carbondale, IL: Center for Archaeological Investigation)

Larrea Castillo, Isabel, and Enrique Hiedra Rodríguez. 2010. "La lápida hebrea de época emiral del Zumbacón: Apuntes sobre arqueología funeraria judía en Córdoba," *Anejos de Anales de Arqueología Cordobesa* 2: 327–42

Lilley, J. M., G. Stroud, D. R. Brothwell, and M. H. Williamson. 1994. *The Jewish Burial Ground at Jewbury* (York: York Archeological Trust)

López de Meneses, Amada. 1956. "Documentos acerca de la peste negra en los dominios de la Corona de Aragón," *Estudios de Edad Media de la Corona de Aragón* 6: 291–447 (repr. as *Documentos acerca de la peste negra en los dominios de la corona de Aragón* [Saragossa: Heraldo de Aragón])

López de Meneses, Amada. 1959a. "Una consecuencia de la peste negra en Cataluña: el Pogrom de 1348," *Sefarad* 19: 92–131

López de Meneses, Amada. 1959b. "Una consecuencia de la peste negra en Cataluña: el Pogrom de 1348: Apéndices (Documentos inéditos)," *Sefarad* 19: 321–64

Margerison, Beverly J., and Christpher J. Knüsel. 2002. "Paleodemographic Comparison of a Catastrophic and an Attritional Death Assemblage," *American Journal of Physical Anthropology* 119, no. 2: 134–43

Moreda Blanco, Javier, and Rosalía Serrano Noriega. 2009. *La necrópolis judía del Paseo de la Acera de Recoletos (Valladolid)* (Valladolid: Junta de Castilla y León)

Muntané i Santiveri, Josep Xavier. 2007a. "La Pràctica del lloguer de bèsties entre els jueus targarins a la fi del segle XV," *Tamid* 11: 65–85

Muntané i Santiveri, Josep Xavier. 2007b. "Proposta d'ubicació del fossar dels jueus de la vila de Tàrrega a partir dels testimonis documentals continguts en els llibres d'estimes (1501-1510)," *Urtx* 20: 104–18

Muntané i Santiveri, Josep Xavier. 2008. "L'alimentació a l'Aljama medieval de Tàrrega," *Urtx* 22: 105–28

Muntané i Santiveri, Josep Xavier. 2009. "Itinerari pels documents relatius a l'assalt al call de Tàrrega de l'any 1348," *Urtx* 23: 158–79

Muntané i Santiveri, Josep Xavier. 2012a. "Aproximació a les causes de l'avalot de Tàrrega de 1348," *Tamid* 8: 103–29

Muntané i Santiveri, Josep Xavier. 2012b. "Metges jueus contractats pel govern municipal de Tàrrega durant els segles XIV i XV," *Urtx* 26: 135–47

Muntané i Santiveri, Josep Xavier. 2014a. "Identificació del fossar dels jueus a través de la documentació," in *Tragèdia al call,* 131–34 (Tarrega: Museu Comarcal de l'Urgell, Exhibit Pamphlet)

Muntané i Santiveri, Josep Xavier. 2014b. "Localització i estructura del call jueu de Tàrrega," in *Tragèdia al call*, 87–96 (Tarrega: Museu Comarcal de l'Urgell, Exhibit Pamphlet)

Nirenberg, David. 1996. *Communities of Violence: Persecution of Minorities in the Middle Ages* (Princeton, NJ: Princeton University Press)

Ollich i Castanyer, Imma. 2012. "La necròplis medieval de l'Esquerda (segles VII–XIV DC): Cronologia i noves perspectives de recerca," in *Arqueologia funerària al nord-est peninsular (segles VI–XII)*, ed. Núria Molist and Gisela Ripoll, 275–86 (Olèrdola-Barcelona: Museu d'Arqueologia de Catalunya-MAC)

Pieters, Bert. 2006. *De Akkorden van Barcelona (1354): historische en kritishe analyse*: (Barcelona: PPU)

Riera i Sans, Jaume. 1987. *Catalunya i els jueus* (Barcelona: Departament de Comerç, Consum I Yurism de la Generalitat de Catalunya)

Ruíz Ventura, Jordi, and Eulàlia Subirà de Galdàcano. 2009. "Reconstrucció antropològica del pogrom de 1348 a Tàrrega," *Urtx* 23: 126–37

Simonsohn, Shlomo. 1998. *The Apostolic See and the Jews: Documents, 492–1404* (Toronto: Pontifical Institute of Mediæval Studies)

Shatzmiller, Joseph. 1974. "Les juifs de Provence pendant la Peste Noire," *Revue des etudes juives* 133, nos. 3–4: 457–80

Trenchs, J. 1969. "La archidiócesis de Tarragona y la Peste Negra: los cargos de la catedral," in *La Corona de Aragón en el siglo XIV*, VIII Congreso de Historia de la Corona de Aragón, 2:59–60 (València: Caja de Ahorros y Monte de Piedad de Valencia)

Vries, Simon Philip de. 1929/2001. *Ritos y símbolos judíos*, trans. Jamie Mestre (Madrid: Caparrós)

Wallisová, Michaela Selmi. 2011. "Le cimetière juif médiéval du quartier de Nové Město a Prague," in *L'archéologie du judaïsme en France et Europe*, ed. Paul Salmona and Laurence Sigal, 273–84 (Paris: La Découverte)

Anna Colet (acoletm@gmail.com) graduated from the Universitat de Lleida in 2000, with a degree in History. She has led many archaeological digs in the province of Lleida, and in 2007 she directed the excavation of Les Roquetes. She is currently a member of the research team created around this site and a technician at the Museu Comarcal de l'Urgell-Tàrrega

Josep Xavier Muntané i Santiveri holds a BA from the Pontificio Istituto Biblico (Roma) and a PhD in Hebrew Philology from the Universitat de Barcelona (2010). He has published two books related to the Jews of Tàrrega and forms part of the research team created by the Museu Comarcal de l'Urgell-Tàrrega on the occasion of the discovery of the Jewish cemetery. He has held a postdoctoral research fellowship at the Maison des Sciences de l'Homme Ange Guépin in Nantes (France), for a project entitled "The Legal Status of Religious Minorities in the Euro-Mediterranean World (5th–15th centuries)," funded by the "Ideas" program of the European Research Council's Seventh Framework (FP7/2007-2013/ERC). He currently works as a researcher at the Institut d'Estudis Món Juïc, on a project devoted to the transcription, edition, and study of documents related to the Catalan Jewish communities of Tàrrega and Verdú (1295–1492).

Jordi Ruíz Ventura earned an MSc in Physical Anthropology from the Universitat Autònoma de Barcelona. He directed the fieldwork and laboratory analyses of anthropological evidence during the excavation at Les Roquetes.

Oriol Saula graduated with degrees in Geography and History (specializing in prehistory and ancient history) from the Universitat de Barcelona in 1989. He is currently the technical director of the Museu Comarcal de l'Urgell-Tàrrega. Since 1990, he has led different archeological digs in the province of Lleida, and his research focuses on medieval Jewish society in Iberia. In 2007, he coordinated the excavation of the Jewish cemetery in Tàrrega and is a member of the research team that has formed around this site. He has participated in various congresses and scientific meetings related to this project, and he has also worked on several publications. He is the co-director of the journal *Urtx: revista d'humanitats de l'Urgell.*

M. Eulàlia Subirà de Galdàcano holds a PhD in Biological Science and an MS in Human Biology, and is Professor of Human Biology in the Unitat d'Antropologia Biològica at the Universitat Autònoma de Barcelona. Her areas of specialization include field and laboratory anthropology (the morphological and chemical analysis of human remains). From 2001 to 2005, she was First Vice-President and then President of the Associació Catalano-Balear de Paleopatologia de l'Acadèmia de Ciències Mèdiques de Catalunya i Balears. She is the author of many books and articles.

Clara Jáuregui holds a BA in History from the Universitat Autònoma de Barcelona and an MA in Medieval Cultures from the Universitat de Barcelona. She is currently writing a doctoral dissertation on Jewish medical practice in Barcelona during the fourteenth century at the Universitat de Barcelona, where she is affiliated with the Institute for Medieval Cultures. She has also researched and curated an exhibition for the Museu d'Història de L'Hospitalet de Llobregat.

Abstract In 2007, excavations in a suburb of the Catalan town of Tàrrega identified the possible location of the medieval Jewish cemetery. Subsequent excavations confirmed that multiple individuals buried in six communal graves had suffered violent deaths. The present study argues that these communal graves can be connected to a well-documented assault on the Jews of Tàrrega that occurred in 1348: long known as one of the earliest episodes of anti-Jewish violence related to the Black Death, but never before corroborated by physical remains. This study places textual sources, both Christian and Jewish, alongside the recently discovered archeological evidence of the violence.

Keywords Pogrom, anti-Jewish violence, Catalonia, Jewish cemeteries, communal graves, bioarcheology, Black Death.

THE ANTHROPOLOGY OF PLAGUE: INSIGHTS FROM BIOARCHEOLOGICAL ANALYSES OF EPIDEMIC CEMETERIES

SHARON N. DEWITTE

THE BLACK DEATH, the first outbreak of medieval plague that swept through Eurasia and Northern Africa in the mid-fourteenth century, was one of the most devastating epidemics in human history.[1] The epidemic killed tens of millions of people in Europe alone within a very short period of time (Benedictow 2004; Cohn 2002; Dols 1977; Wood, Ferrell, and DeWitte-Avina 2003). This disease initiated or enhanced social, demographic, and economic changes throughout Western Eurasia and Northern Africa (see, for example, essays by Borsch 2014, Carmichael 2014, Colet et al. 2014, and Green 2014—all in this issue), and thus has attracted the interest of a variety of researchers for decades. In addition to its importance in shaping events hundreds of years ago, the Black Death continues to be of interest today, in part because the epidemic was caused by the same pathogen that causes modern plague, the bacterium *Yersinia pestis*. Given molecular evidence that the Plague of Justinian (*c.* sixth to eighth centuries CE) was also caused by *Y. pestis* (Harbeck et al. 2013; Wagner et al. 2014; Wiechmann and Grupe 2005), the Black Death was a terrible manifestation of a disease that has affected humans for nearly fifteen hundred years. The continued existence and threat of plague means that it is crucial to understand the extent of the geographic and temporal variation of the disease so that we might best be prepared for its effects on our species in the future.

This paper focuses on the reconstruction of medieval Black Death mortality patterns, particularly those patterns that have been estimated using

I am grateful to Jelena Bekvalac and Rebecca Redfern at the Museum of London's Centre for Human Bioarchaeology for providing access to the East Smithfield skeletons; and to Jesper Boldsen, Syddansk Universitet Odense, for providing access to the Danish cemetery samples. I am also grateful to Monica Green and the two anonymous reviewers for reading and providing comments on an earlier version of this manuscript. Funding for my research, which is summarized in this paper, was provided by the National Science Foundation (grant number BCS-0406252) and the Wenner-Gren Foundation for Anthropological Research (grant number 7142).

1 Here, and throughout this paper, the "Black Death" refers only to the first outbreak of the Second Pandemic of plague during the mid-fourteenth century.

the skeletal remains of victims of the epidemic in the mid-fourteenth century. Such research is essential for several reasons. Though it is now clear from molecular evidence, particularly the results of recent whole genome sequencing studies, that the Black Death was caused by *Y. pestis* (Bos et al. 2011; Drancourt and Raoult 2002; Haensch et al. 2010; Raoult et al. 2000; Schuenemann et al. 2011), this is a relatively recent discovery. The most convincing and least controversial molecular studies, which have yielded sequences specific to *Y. pestis* and used samples clearly dated to the fourteenth-century epidemic (rather than merely suspected victims or victims of more recent historic epidemics), have all been published since 2009 (Bos et al. 2011; Haensch et al. 2010; Schuenemann et al. 2011). Prior to these new molecular insights, the cause of the Black Death was much more hotly debated, and researchers were motivated to clarify in exacting detail how the historic and modern diseases differed epidemiologically. The ultimate goal was determining whether Black Death was, in fact, plague (and if so, whether the strain of *Y. pestis* that caused it was of exceptionally heightened virulence), or whether it was caused by some other disease, such as anthrax or viral hemorrhagic fever (Scott and Duncan 2001; Twigg 1984).

The exciting nature of the molecular findings has made many people forget why the identification of the specific causative agent of medieval plague matters at all. Now that we know (insofar as anything is truly known in scientific research) that it was caused by *Y. pestis*, research can clarify the temporal and geographic variation associated with the disease, to further broaden and improve our understanding of: first, plague virulence (e.g., why was mortality during the Black Death so high?); second, host-pathogen interactions (e.g., how did host population dynamics affect the disease dynamics during medieval plague epidemics?); and third, how this particular disease might manifest in the future (e.g., is it possible that future outbreaks of *Y. pestis* will ever approximate medieval patterns of mortality and transmission?).

Clarifying the human context of the Black Death via bioarcheological research is essential to these goals. Bioarcheology is the study of human skeletal remains excavated from archeological sites with the aim of furthering our understanding of the demography, health, and ways of life of people in past populations. Bioarcheologists examine these remains to determine the ages at which people died, whether they were male or female, what foods they regularly consumed, how healthy or unhealthy they were prior to their deaths (based on the presence or absence of certain markers of physiological stress on the skeleton), whether they experienced interpersonal violence, and other phenomena that leave evidence on or in the skeleton. Through the direct observation and analysis of human skeletal remains, bioarcheological research can provide demographic data that are crucially important for contextualizing the results of the ongoing molecular analyses (e.g., DNA and immunological studies) of both *Y. pestis* and the humans affected by historic plague epidemics. Such context is particularly important given recent evidence that the medieval and modern strains lack significant functional differences in regions of the genome associated with virulence. This suggests that factors other than genetic changes in the causative pathogen are responsible, at least in part, for changes in plague epidemiology (see also Ziegler 2014, in this issue), who argues that research should focus on factors other than a genetic "smoking gun" to further our understanding of plague virulence).

The combination of demographic and molecular data will allow for a disentanglement of the factors that affected medieval health and demography—that is, a determination of whether it was the biological effects of plague or the social and economic consequences of the epidemic that primarily shaped demographic and health patterns in the surviving population. Such interdisciplinary research on the Black Death also has the potential to clarify population dynamics and human biological responses to disease episodes in general, and thus can contribute to our understanding of precisely how and why diseases shape human demography (including age and sex structures, and population density and growth) and human evolution (e.g., acting as forces of natural selection resulting in relatively robust immune responses or genetic resistance to disease). Regarding the latter phenomenon, Crespo and Lawrenz (2014, in this issue) detail how heterogeneity in immune competence during the Black Death might have affected risks and levels of mortality during the epidemic, and how Black Death mortality might have shaped variation in immune function in the surviving population.

In addition to improving our understanding of the dynamics of the Black Death in particular, bioarcheological studies of the epidemic are relevant to current concerns about emerging diseases. Emerging diseases are those that increase in frequency after being introduced into a new, immunologically naïve host population. More than fifty diseases have emerged in the past thirty years, including HIV/AIDS, West Nile Virus, and SARS, and new diseases will emerge in the future (Cleaveland, Haydon, and Taylor 2007; Morens, Folkers, and Fauci 2004; Morse 1995). The Black Death was an emerging disease in the fourteenth century, and the persistence of this ancient emerging disease to the present day provides an ideal opportunity to examine, from an anthropological perspective, long-term trends in emerging disease dynamics, and thereby understand the effects such diseases have had on human populations and predict how they can affect us in the future. In addition to improving our understanding of plague, bioarcheological research on the Black Death can provide much needed data to evaluate models of the evolution of virulence in emerging pathogens (Ebert and Bull 1999; Frank 1996) and help to resolve questions about whether changes in emerging disease epidemiology are the result of human adaptation, changes in human or non-human host demography or behavior, or evolution of the causative pathogens (Alizon et al. 2009; André and Hochberg 2005; Grenfell et al. 2004).

Furthermore, Black Death bioarcheological research contributes to efforts to understand the phenomena of heterogeneous frailty (an individual's risk of death, relative to other members of the population: Vaupel, Manton, and Stallard 1979) and selective mortality (disproportionate deaths of those with highest frailty), and how they shape population dynamics in living and past populations. Because individuals differ in their susceptibility to disease and death as a result of genetic, biological, environmental, socioeconomic, or other causes, differences in frailty exist among individuals within a population (Aalen 1994; Wood et al. 1992). Mortality is expected to be selective, at least under normal, non-catastrophic conditions; that is, because of differences in frailty, the individuals who die at each age will not be a random sample of all the individuals living at that age, but rather will be disproportionately selected from among those with the highest risk of dying (the highest frailty).

Many researchers are interested in revealing the sources and consequences of heterogeneous frailty in living populations so that health and mortality disparities can potentially be ameliorated or eliminated (Olden and White 2005). It is just as important to understand these processes in the past, particularly in the context of parasitic and infectious disease (which were the most common causes of death for most of human history and continue be the most significant causes of death for many living populations), in order to understand modern human biology. By revealing how biological factors such as age, sex, and history of physiological stress (such as malnutrition or infectious disease) affected risks of mortality during one of the most dramatic disease epidemics in human history, Black Death research has the potential to clarify why and how affected populations have changed in the intervening centuries. The Black Death also offers a case study of how heterogeneous frailty and selective mortality operate during times of crisis mortality, which characterized much of the mortality experience of pre-industrial populations throughout the world (Gage 2005).

Documentary Evidence of Black Death Mortality Patterns

Studies using data from historical documents have confirmed the devastating nature of the Black Death and have shown that mortality during the epidemic was perhaps even higher than previously thought (Benedictow 2004; Cohn 2002; Dols 1977; Scott and Duncan 2001; Wood, Ferrell, and DeWitte-Avina 2003). Using data from court records of payments made by residents, Poos (1991) estimated the annual totals of males ages twelve years and older living on manors in Essex. He found that several manors lost as much as 54% of their male residents during the Black Death. Wood, Ferrell, and DeWitte-Avina (2003) analyzed data on deaths of beneficed priests in the Lincoln diocese in England. In the eighteen months before the Black Death, the mean mortality rate for priests was 38.9 per 1000, but during the twelve-month period beginning with the outbreak of the Black Death in Lincoln, the mean mortality rate increased to 463.6 per 1000. During the Black Death, annual mortality rates for priests were eleven times higher and, more dramatically, *monthly* mortality rates were about thirty-five to forty-five times higher than in the pre-epidemic period. Total mortality from the Black Death was typically 30% to 50% of the total population in affected regions of Europe. Following the Black Death, plague mortality decreased steeply and steadily with subsequent outbreaks (Carpentier 1971; Cohn 2002; Hatcher 1977), which might indicate that the population was generally less frail, that there were changes in susceptibility to plague following the epidemic, or that there were factors involving nonhuman animal hosts that affected plague epidemiological patterns in humans.

It is clear that the mortality caused by the Black Death was extraordinarily high. What has not been as clear is how this excess mortality was distributed by age, sex, socioeconomic status, and other biological and social factors. Several medieval European chroniclers suggest that the Black Death killed people indiscriminately, irrespective of age or sex. For example, Matteo Villani (Florence, d. 1363) described the Black Death as "a pestilence among men of every condition, age and sex" (cited and translated in Cohn 2002: 126). According to the chronicler Michele da Piazza (Sicily, fourteenth century), the mortality from the Black Death was "so heavy that sex and age made no difference, but everyone died alike" (cited and translated in Horrox 1994: 41). Both of these statements suggest indiscriminate mortality, at least with respect to age and sex. Some contemporaries, however, believed that the epidemic was selective, and, for example, killed more women than men, and that in subsequent outbreaks of plague (which are believed to be the same disease) men were killed in greater numbers than were women (Cohn 2002: 210–12; Horrox 1994: 85). According to Jean de Venette (1307–70), a French Carmelite friar and chronicler, "the young were more likely to die than the elderly" (cited and translated in Horrox 1994: 54). Many chroniclers noted that the age pattern of subsequent outbreaks was quite different from that of the Black Death. For example, the 1361 outbreak was called the "Pestilence of Children," as young people were more severely affected than were adults (Cohn 2002: 212–15; Cohn 2008: 86–87; Holmes 1971: 92).

Reconstruction of age-specific mortality patterns during the Black Death has been attempted using historical data. Based on information from inquisitions post mortem, Russell (1948) produced life-table estimates of age-specific mortality among high-status individuals during the Black Death in England.[2] These were royal inquisitions into the cause of death of tenants-in-chief, people who held land directly from the king. The inquisitions provide a wide sample of the highest rank of landholders. When a tenant died, if the heir was underage, the king assumed guardianship of the property until the heir came of age. Such guardianships were quite lucrative, and it was in the interest of all parties to establish accurately the age of the heir; thus, the age estimates provided by the inquisitions are supported by multiple documents (Russell 1948). Unfortunately, the samples are too small to provide useful life-table estimates, particularly for intervals below the age of twenty; indeed, for some age intervals, the 95% confidence intervals for probability of death include negative values (Wood et al. 2002a). Despite the limitations of the available data, Russell concluded from the life-table estimates that age did have an effect on Black Death mortality. He argued that older men were particularly susceptible (although individuals over the age of sixty apparently fared better than those in their late fifties), and children between the ages of ten and fifteen were at a reduced risk of dying from the disease compared to other age groups. Ohlin (1966), however, has criticized Russell's approach and argued that the data do not support the conclusion that mortality varied by age during the Black Death.

Using manorial court records from the English village of Halesowen (West Midlands), Razi (1980) estimated ages at death among the peas-

---

2 Life tables are frequently used in demography to display the numbers of deaths at each age or age interval, age-specific mortality rates, survival rates at various ages, and other related demographic measures for a particular population. Model life tables are constructed using data from living populations and can be applied to small samples obtained from living or past populations to compensate for missing data.

antry during the epidemic. Individuals appear in the manorial court rolls multiple times, and the last appearance of each individual is the death duty (*heriot*) payment made by heirs to the lord of the manor before taking possession of the deceased's property. Razi assumes that each individual appeared for the first time in the court rolls at the age of twenty years and counted forward from this first appearance to the death-duty payment in order to estimate ages at death. His age estimates are therefore imprecise, and by definition no information is available for individuals younger than twenty. Estimating age-specific mortality rates for males during the Black Death, he finds, similar to Russell (1948), that for males between twenty and fifty-nine years of age, mortality rates increased with age, but that age-specific mortality rates for those over sixty years were lower than those of younger men. Such a pattern of mortality is typical under conditions of normal mortality, though a plateau in mortality is usually observed at later adult ages in living populations (Gage 1988). Given the small samples available for Razi's study, the results might not be generalizable to the entire English population.

As limited as the reconstructions of Black Death age-patterns have been using historic documents, such sources are even less forthcoming with respect to the effects of other biological or social factors. For example, the determination of whether one sex was disproportionately affected or both sexes faced equal risks of death during the epidemic is even more problematic than that of age patterns given that there is very little documentary data on age-at-death for women and children at the time of the Black Death (Razi 1980; Russell1948). Though there are data on sex ratios during the medieval period (see, e.g., Kowaleski 2013), these data do not allow reconstruction of sex differences in mortality across the lifespan. There is also no information, as far as I am aware, from any documentary sources about whether pre-existing health conditions had any effect on an individual's risk of death during the epidemic. Historical records, therefore, do not provide a clear and complete picture of Black Death mortality patterns. Without such data, our ability to learn more about the ways in which the Black Death, and other diseases, have the power to shape human demography, biology, and evolution is severely hindered.

Fortunately, skeletal material exists that provides empirical evidence about mortality patterns that is not available in written records. Though human skeletal samples are not without their own limitations, they can, when analyzed properly, reveal much more (and more direct) information about the individuals who died during the Black Death.

Black Death Cemeteries

During the Black Death, existing cemeteries proved inadequate to accommodate the overwhelming numbers of people killed by the epidemic, and providing normal burials for all the victims of the epidemic became difficult (Horrox 1994: 21, 64, 268–71). Though many victims of the disease were buried in existing cemeteries, mass burial grounds were established across Europe during the Black Death to accommodate the excess mortality. One such mass burial ground was the East Smithfield cemetery in London.

The Black Death was apparently introduced to England during the summer of 1348 via the Dorsetshire port of Melcombe Regis, and it reached the suburbs of London as early as September 1348 (the disease was recorded in the suburb of Stepney, two miles east of the city walls, in December 1348). The epidemic ravaged the city throughout 1349 and ended by the spring of 1350 (Gasquet 1977; Hawkins 1990). Aware that the Black Death was spreading towards London, "substantial men of the city" ordered that emergency burial grounds be established prior to its arrival (Grainger et al. 2008; Hawkins 1990). The East Smithfield cemetery was established in late 1348 or early 1349 just outside the city walls in East London, northeast of the Tower of London, on land that had previously been used as a vineyard. The exact dimensions and location of the cemetery are provided by the cartulary of the priory of Holy-Trinity-without-Aldgate, and it was originally called the Churchyard of the Holy Trinity, as the land was acquired from the priory (Grainger et al. 2008; Hawkins 1990).

East Smithfield was partially excavated in the 1980s, as part of the larger Royal Mint Site, by the Museum of London's Department of Greater London Archaeology (now Museum of London Archaeology [MOLA]). The burials in East Smithfield were concentrated in two areas: first, a western area with two mass burial trenches, a mass burial pit, and individual graves arranged in several parallel north-south rows; and second, an eastern area with one mass burial trench and individual graves arranged in several parallel rows (Hawkins 1990). Over six hundred skeletons were excavated from the cemetery, a fraction of the estimated twenty-four hundred individuals originally buried in East Smithfield, and they are now curated by the Museum of London Centre for Human Bioarchaeology. The cemetery could have accommodated many more burials, but the epidemic waned before it was necessary to use all the available space. Excavation of the cemetery revealed that the individuals interred in East Smithfield were buried carefully. Almost without exception, the bodies were buried in standard medieval Christian fashion: extended on their backs with their heads oriented west and feet oriented east. Some of the skeletons were missing limbs at the time of excavation, indicating that these individuals had been partly disarticulated as a result of putrefaction before burial (Grainger et al. 2008; Hawkins 1990). However, even these bodies were buried in the standard Christian fashion and were treated with apparent care, rather than tossed hastily into a burial trench.

East Smithfield was one of two known emergency burial grounds established in London (Grainger et al. 2008; Hawkins 1990). The other burial ground was at West Smithfield, which later became the site of the London Charterhouse. The West Smithfield site is now beneath Charterhouse Square and thus will not be excavated in its entirety (or even in large part) in the foreseeable future, though a few individuals from the cemetery were recently uncovered during construction of a new London Underground line (Palmer 2013). The East Smithfield site, which yielded several hundred individuals, is thus one of a very few large *excavated* cemeteries in all of Europe with unambiguous documentary and archeological evidence linking it to this outbreak of the medieval disease. At the time of writing, to my knowledge, the only other large, excavated burial grounds that are clearly associated with the Black Death are the Hereford Cathedral cemetery in England (Gowland and Chamberlain 2005) and the Heiligen-Geist Hospital mass burial in Lübeck, Germany (Lütgert 2000). Of these, East Smithfield has been investigated most extensively by various researchers, according to the number of publications recorded in the Wellcome Osteological Database.[3]

The ability to study the skeletal remains of victims of the Black Death and subsequent plagues that have been recovered from East Smithfield and other medieval plague burial grounds yields insights that are simply not supported by existing historical documents. The advantage of bioarcheological research is that the information derived from skeletal remains of victims is not subject to the same biases that are inherent in historical documents, thereby allowing bioarcheologists not only to reveal what is missing from historical data, but also to challenge narratives based on those conventional sources (Perry 2007).

3 WORD Database (Wellcome Osteological Research Database) 2013: <www.museumoflondon.org.uk/Collections-Research/LAARC/Centre-for-Human-Bioarchaeology/Resources/Medievaldatadownloads.htm> [accessed August 31, 2014].

Previous Bioarcheological Studies of the Black Death

Several researchers have analyzed the East Smithfield Black Death cemetery to discern the mortality patterns of the Black Death (Gowland and Chamberlain 2005; Margerison and Knüsel 2002; Waldron 2001). The aim of some of these inquiries was to determine whether Black Death cemeteries are more representative of the demographics of a living population than is generally true of mortality samples derived from other cemeteries. As discussed above, normal causes of mortality are expected to be selective, targeting the weakest individuals in a population, such as infants, the elderly, and those with immune systems compromised by disease or malnutrition (Milner, Wood, and Boldsen 2008). Because of this selective mortality, skeletal assemblages are inherently biased samples of the once living populations from which they derived. For each age group, the individuals within a cemetery are not a representative sample of all the individuals who were once alive at that age, but rather those individuals who were at the highest risk of dying at that age. This makes it difficult to infer the characteristics of the once-living population in a straightforward manner based on observations of the cemetery assemblage. However, some researchers have suggested that the Black Death might have been so virulent that it killed indiscriminately, rather than selectively, such that mortality samples resulting from the epidemic would contain relatively healthy, robust individuals not usually found in normal cemeteries. If this were the case, Black Death cemeteries might provide a true cross-section of the once-living population not typically available in normal mortality cemeteries (Chamberlain 2006; Margerison and Knüsel 2002).

Waldron (2001) compares the mortality profile from East Smithfield to that of the St. Mary Graces cemetery (*c.* 1350–1538), which was established in the same location as East Smithfield after the Black Death ended, and to the age distribution of the living population of medieval London as predicted from a model life table.[4] He finds no systematic differences between the mortality profiles of the two cemeteries. Furthermore, the profiles of both cemeteries differed from the expected living age structure. Waldron argues that the skeletal evidence does not support the idea that any particular age or sex was at an elevated risk of dying during the Black Death. Waldron also finds that the two cemeteries had generally similar frequencies of skeletal pathologies. He concludes that the East Smithfield

---

4 Model life tables are constructed using data from living populations and can be applied to small samples obtained from living or past populations to compensate for missing data.

cemetery is not representative of the once-living population, as one might expect if the Black Death killed people indiscriminately.

However, several researchers have found that the East Smithfield age-at-death distribution more closely resembles a model living population age distribution than the age-at-death distribution of a normal mortality sample. Margerison and Knüsel (2002) compare East Smithfield to the St.-Helen-on-the-Walls cemetery in York, northern England, a normal non-epidemic cemetery in use from the late twelfth century to 1550. The East Smithfield mortality profile differs significantly from that of the St.-Helen-on-the-Walls cemetery, but generally resembles the living age distribution from a model life table assumed to be representative of the age distribution of a living (poor) medieval urban population; in particular, that is, East Smithfield, like a living medieval population, contained many young people and few older individuals. Gowland and Chamberlain (2005) compare East Smithfield to a pre-Black Death sample from Blackgate cemetery in Newcastle, northeastern England. They also find that the East Smithfield distribution differs from the normal mortality sample and more closely resembles a model life table living age distribution, suggesting that all age groups were equally affected by the Black Death.

More recently, I have examined the age and sex patterns associated with the epidemic and the health of the victims, as evidenced by skeletal pathologies (or, more generally, skeletal stress markers, which are visible anomalies of the skeleton that indicate exposure to physiological stress, such as infection or malnutrition at some point in life) (DeWitte 2009; DeWitte and Hughes-Morey 2012; DeWitte and Wood 2008). My research, however, differs in several key ways from the studies described above. With the exception of Gowland and Chamberlain (2005), other studies of East Smithfield use comparison samples that partly or completely post-date the Black Death. This is potentially problematic because the Black Death itself initiated profound demographic changes throughout Europe. Paine (2000) finds, using population modeling, that episodes of catastrophic mortality may have effects on age-at-death distributions that last for several generations. Further, as my work has indicated, if the mortality during the Black Death was selective with respect to preexisting health conditions, it is possible that the epidemic altered patterns of health, as indicated by skeletal stress markers, in the surviving population. It is thus possible that post-Black Death samples, at least those dating to just after the epidemic, more strongly reflect the effects of the Black Death than they do typical medieval mortality patterns. Therefore, in order to determine whether the Black Death killed selectively and how its mortality patterns differ from normal medieval mortality, I have used an exclusively pre-Black Death comparison sample composed of people who died in the two centuries just before the Black Death arrived.

Another way in which my research has differed from most other investigations of East Smithfield (except for that of Gowland and Chamberlain) is my use of a relatively unbiased method of adult age estimation. Paleodemographic age estimation in adults is based on observations of the morphology of certain parts of the skeleton that change in fairly predictable ways with age (though the timing of such changes can be highly variable). These include changes to parts of the pelvis and to the skull. Studies of known-age-at-death reference samples have yielded various age-estimation methods (which I hereafter refer to as "traditional" methods) which involve assigning a skeleton to one of several stages based on the morphology of a particular skeletal feature. Each stage has a corresponding mean age at death and an age interval, both of which are estimated from known-age individuals in the reference sample who display the morphological features distinctive of each stage. Unfortunately, traditional paleodemographic age-estimation methods have a built-in bias. They tend to lead to underestimations of older adult ages because the age estimates are biased toward known-age reference samples, which are often composed predominantly of young individuals (Bocquet-Appel and Masset 1982; Buikstra and Konigsberg 1985; Milner and Boldsen 2012; Müller, Love, and Hoppa 2002; Van Gerven and Armelagos 1983). For example, the McKern-Stewart Korean War reference sample is made up primarily of young men (Milner, Wood, and Boldsen 2008). This "age mimicry" means that the numerous paleodemographic adult age-at-death distributions that have been estimated for cemetery samples are nearly identical regardless of their temporal or geographic context. Such biased distributions hinder informative comparisons of paleodemographic mortality profiles. Another potential limitation of traditional age-estimation methods is the use of broad terminal age intervals, for example, those fifty years or older, because of the difficulty of estimating age in older adults (Boldsen et al. 2002; Buikstra and Konigsberg 1985). These methods, therefore, are not capable of making distinctions between, for example, a fifty-year-old and a ninety-year-old, two ages for which one would expect very different morbidity and mortality regimes, at least in living populations.

Because of these limitations of traditional age-estimation approaches, I have estimated ages using the method of transition analysis described by Boldsen et al. (2002). Transition analysis resolves the problem of age estimates that are biased toward the known-age reference sample. It also yields point estimates of age and their corresponding 95% confidence intervals (rather than broad and fixed interval estimates), even for older adults. In transition analysis, data from a known-age reference collection are used to obtain the conditional probability that a skeleton will exhibit a particular age indicator stage, or suite of age indicator stages, given the individual's known age. Using Bayes's theorem and maximum likelihood estimation,[5] this conditional probability is combined with a prior distribution of ages at death to determine the posterior probability that an individual in the cemetery sample died at a particular age given that the skeleton displays particular age indicator stages. In transition analysis, the prior distribution of ages at death can either be an *informative prior* based on documentary data or a *uniform prior*, and I have used an informative prior based on data from seventeenth-century Danish rural parish records. By combining the conditional probability from a known-age reference sample with a prior distribution of ages at death, transition analysis avoids imposing the age distribution of the reference sample on the unknown-age cemetery sample (Boldsen et al. 2002). I have applied transition analysis to East Smithfield data using the Anthropological Database, Odense University (ADBOU) Age Estimation software (Boldsen et al. 2002).

Lastly, my research differs from that of others by incorporating hazard analyses (statistical assessment of risks of death) to examine mortality patterns, rather than using life tables as a standard of comparison. Life tables are typically constructed for living populations using huge datasets that include, among other things, the number of individuals alive at each age and the number who die within a particular interval. They have been used for several decades in paleodemography to examine intra- and inter-population demographic variation (Acsádi and Nemeskéri 1970; Wood et al. 2002b).[6] The construction of paleodemographic life tables is based on the assumption that the age-at-death distribution in a cemetery is equiva-

5 Bayes's theorem allows for the estimation of the probability of a trait (such as the unknown age of an individual in a cemetery) that cannot be directly observed, but which is associated with another trait that can be observed (such as a skeletal age indicator). In the case of age-estimation, this requires information about the association between age and skeletal indicators of age, which is derived from known-age reference samples in which both the ages of individuals and their skeletal age indicators are observable. The joint distribution of ages at death and the skeletal age indicators for all individuals in a reference sample is used to determine the probability that an individual in a cemetery sample (for whom only the skeletal age indicator can be observed) is a particular age given the skeletal age indicators observed for that individual (Milner, Wood, and Boldsen 2008).

6 Paleodemography is a subfield of bioarcheology that examines demographic patterns, such as mortality and fertility, in past populations using skeletal samples.

lent to the cohort age-at-death column in a life table;[7] however, this is true only under a set of stringent criteria that many past populations do not fulfill (e.g., no migration and no changes in age-specific fertility or mortality rates) (Milner, Wood, and Boldsen 2008). Further, the use of life tables in paleodemography is complicated by small sample sizes and a lack of quantitative information about the original population at risk of death. Life tables are considered by many researchers to be an inefficient way to make use of the data that are available from cemetery samples, as these samples are almost always too small to allow for unbiased estimates of the numerous parameters necessary to construct a life table (Buikstra 1997; Hoppa and Vaupel 2002; Konigsberg and Frankenberg 2002; Milner, Wood, and Boldsen 2008; Wood et al. 2002b). Some paleodemographers, including previous researchers of East Smithfield, have adopted a model life-table approach by applying a theoretical life table that matches or provides a baseline comparison for the age-at-death distribution observed in a cemetery (Weiss 1973; Wood et al. 2002b). Unfortunately, a single paleodemographic age-at-death distribution will often match more than one model life table, and uncertainty exists about which model life tables are most appropriate to use (Gage 1988; Milner, Wood, and Boldsen 2008; Wood et al. 2002b).

In light of these problems, many researchers argue that rather than using life tables, some form of hazard analysis is the most reliable way to derive information from the small samples typical of paleodemography (Buikstra 1997; Gage 1988; Hoppa and Vaupel 2002; Konigsberg and Frankenberg 1992; Konigsberg and Frankenberg 2002; Wood et al. 2002b). Most human age-at-death distributions can be described using five or fewer parameters, and parsimonious parametric models provide a useful alternative to life tables in paleodemographic studies (Holman, Wood, and O'Connor 2002). This is the approach I took in my research and examples of such models are described below.

Hazard Analysis of Black Death Mortality

Hazard analysis of Black Death mortality patterns has, for the most part, involved comparison of the East Smithfield cemetery to a normal (i.e., non-epidemic) mortality sample from the medieval Danish urban parish cemeteries of St. Albani Church, Odense, and St. Mikkel Church, Viborg (*c.* 1100s to mid-1500s), both of which form part of the current ADBOU collection (DeWitte and Hughes-Morey 2012; DeWitte 2010; DeWitte and

7 A cohort in this context refers to individuals who were all born at the same time.

Wood 2008). The advantages of using the Danish sample as a comparison for East Smithfield include its large size, which allows for estimation of the hazard model parameters; the generally good preservation of the Danish skeletons (which facilitates estimation of age and sex); and the ability to accurately date skeletons and, thus, to select a predominantly (if not exclusively) pre-Black Death sample. The Danish sample contains only individuals who died before the Black Death arrived in Denmark in 1350, and thus provides a baseline of normal, non-epidemic mortality patterns for comparison with East Smithfield. The populations of Denmark and Southern England at this time were similar economically, socially, and demographically (Benedictow 1996; Poulsen 1997; Roesdahl 1999; Sawyer and Sawyer 1993; Widgren 1997). However, the fact that the Black Death and Danish normal mortality samples were drawn from two different geographic regions means that possible population differences have to be considered when interpreting the results of these studies. An ideal comparison sample for East Smithfield should be drawn from England, and therefore, in future research I will use exclusively London samples, some of which have been made available to researchers only recently.[8]

I have previously examined the age patterns of Black Death mortality, and how they compared to those produced by normal mortality conditions, by using age-at-death data from each sample to estimate the parameters of a parsimonious model of human mortality: the Siler model. The Siler model of mortality describes the typical pattern of population-level risk of mortality across the lifespan, which begins relatively high at birth, drops rapidly during childhood before leveling off between late childhood and young adult ages, and then increasing again during later adult ages (Siler 1979). Though the absolute levels of mortality and timing of declines and increases in mortality can vary tremendously across populations, this same general pattern (the so-called "bathtub curve") has been observed in nearly all human populations (and even nonhuman animal populations) for which data are available (Gage 1989).[9]

The results of this research indicate that the Black Death did not kill indiscriminately with respect to age. The results of estimation of the Siler model in the East Smithfield and normal mortality samples indicates that

8 The Museum of London Centre for Human Bioarchaeology, which provides access to these samples, was established in 2003, and some of the samples that will be used in future research were made available for general research following the publication of the corresponding site report in 2012.

9 Further details about the Siler model can be found in Gage (1988 and 1989) and Wood et al. (2002b).

for both, the risk of death increased with advancing adult age. This means that elderly adults faced higher risks of death compared to their younger peers during times of both catastrophic Black Death mortality and under normal medieval mortality conditions (DeWitte 2010). However, use of the Siler model did not yield convincing estimates of the parameters of the juvenile component for the East Smithfield sample. Typically, in human populations, the juvenile risk of mortality is initially relatively high at birth, but it declines very rapidly with small changes in age for the first few years of life; this change might reflect increases in immune competence with age and thus consequent decreases in risks of infection (Gage 1989). The estimated juvenile risk for the normal mortality sample conforms to such expectations; however, for the East Smithfield sample, the juvenile risk was initially low at birth and increased slowly with age, with no drop in risk during early childhood. At face value, this might suggest that infants faced relatively low risks of mortality during the Black Death; however, the estimated juvenile pattern in East Smithfield might have been the result of the small sample of infants and children available, as they only made up 8% of the East Smithfield sample (which might reflect poor preservation of these bodies or different burial practices for children). Estimation of the juvenile component of mortality is based primarily on individuals in the sample who are between the ages of zero and five years, and it is difficult to estimate accurately the juvenile risk with small sample sizes (Wood et al. 2002b). Such small sample sizes in East Smithfield means that clarification of mortality for the youngest individuals in the population during the Black Death awaits further work with larger samples.

Assessment of whether the Black Death differentially affected one sex has been limited to adults, given the lack of current methods to accurately assess sex in immature individuals. Thus in my previous work, I modeled sex as a covariate affecting the parameters of the Gompertz-Makeham model, which fits the general human pattern of relatively low mortality during the young adult ages and an increasing risk of death with increasing adult age (Wood et al. 2002). The effect of the sex covariate was modeled in such a way that it was free to take on values indicating either an elevated or decreased risk of mortality for females compared to males, or a complete lack of differences in risk between males and females. The results indicate that, under both conditions of the Black Death and normal medieval mortality, males and females did not differ significantly in their risks of death (DeWitte 2009). It should be noted, however, that the way I modeled the covariate effect (i.e., the proportional hazard specification) does not allow for variation in differences in risk between the sexes across adult ages, and thus this approach cannot detect potential crossovers in mortality. It is possible that female mortality was higher than that of males during reproductive ages, as some diseases, such as malaria, disproportionately affect pregnant women. However, examination of such variation in sex differentials across adult ages requires further analysis using larger sample sizes.

To determine whether the Black Death disproportionately affected people already in poor health, I used the Usher model, which allows for variation in the risk of death between individuals with and without skeletal stress markers (see DeWitte and Wood 2008 for a description of these markers) (Usher 2000). The Usher model allows researchers to avoid making the conventional assumption that the presence of stress markers always indicates poor health and similar or identical levels of frailty for all individuals in a particular population, an assumption that might not be justified (Milner, Wood, and Boldsen 2008; Ortner 1991; Wood et al. 1992). Most detectable skeletal stress markers take a minimum of weeks to form. Thus, an individual must be minimally healthy to survive a physiological stressor long enough for an associated stress marker to develop. Some individuals in a skeletal sample might lack stress markers despite exposure to physiological stress because they were very frail and died before skeletal stress markers formed. Alternatively, individuals in the sample might lack stress markers because they were fortunate enough to avoid exposure to a particular stressor or had immune systems robust enough to fight off disease before stress markers formed, both of which reflect relatively low frailty. Under these circumstances, individuals who lack a particular stress marker might have had higher or lower levels of frailty compared to individuals who have them. Thus, the presence of skeletal stress markers might actually indicate relatively good health in some cases, but this will not be apparent in a simple dichotomous comparison of stress marker frequencies.

The Usher model allows for an explicit examination of the relationship between skeletal stress markers and risks of mortality, and thus the determination of whether, in a particular context, stress marker presence is indicative of good or poor health. The model has three non-overlapping states: State 1 includes people with no stress markers; State 2 includes people with stress markers; and State 3 is death. Individuals in a cemetery are observed after they have made the transition to State 3, and the presence or absence of visible stress markers indicates which of the two living states they were in just before they died. Transitions between the states are governed by age-specific hazard rates, and data on age and the presence of stress markers allow for the estimation of the model parameters. The model allows for differences in the risks of death associated with State 1 and State 2. The model thus enables one to estimate whether individuals with stress markers are at an elevated or decreased risk of dying compared to those without them.

I have applied the Usher model to data on a variety of nonspecific skeletal markers of physiological stress within the Black Death cemetery. Some of these stress markers reflect exposure to physiological stressors (such as malnutrition or infectious disease) strictly during childhood, and others can manifest in response to stressors at any point during the lifespan. (See DeWitte and Wood 2008 and DeWitte and Hughes-Morey 2012 for details about these stress markers.) Fitting the Usher model to data on age and the presence of these stress markers in the normal mortality sample reveals that these stress markers are, at least under normal medieval mortality conditions, indicative of frailty or poor health, and that the risk of mortality was higher for people with the markers compared to those without them. The results from East Smithfield indicate that the Black Death disproportionally killed people who had them. That is, people who experienced physiological stressors, and who developed stress markers in response to those stressors, at some point (perhaps even long) before the arrival of the epidemic were subsequently more likely to die during the Black Death compared to their peers who lacked the stress markers (DeWitte and Hughes-Morey 2012; DeWitte and Wood 2008).[10]

Together, the results of analysis of age and frailty reveal that contrary to the common assumption that the Black Death killed indiscriminately, there was variation in risks of dying during the epidemic. This means we should question any historical, molecular, or bioarcheological study that implicitly or explicitly assumes that the Black Death was not a selective killer. Further, the similarities between the East Smithfield and normal mortality cemeteries indicate that we should expect mortality to be selective and for people to differ in their risks of death under all mortality conditions, even in the event of catastrophic mortality. This has implications, not just for our understanding of the effects of disease in the past but also for our expectations of and preparedness for disease outbreaks in living populations.

---

10 Initial analysis, using the Usher model, of the effect of physical stature on risk of death found no effect in either the Black Death or the normal mortality sample (DeWitte and Wood 2008). However, the Usher model is an unnecessarily complicated approach to assess stature. Reanalysis using a more appropriate and simpler analytical approach did find an effect of short adult stature on risk of death (DeWitte and Hughes-Morey 2012).

Bioarcheological research on the Black Death has revealed not only the mortality patterns of this particular historical epidemic, but also more generally it demonstrates that bioarcheological research has important contributions to make to lines of inquiry that have traditionally been the purview of historians. The unique contribution of anthropology to medieval plague studies is that it allows the victims themselves (or, more precisely, their skeletal remains) to bear witness to their experiences while they were alive and to the context of their deaths—in this case, how an individual's age and health status elevated or reduced his or her risk of mortality during the Black Death. This is particularly important for our understanding of the experiences of those who are not typically included in the historical record: that is, the vast majority of people who lived in the past.

Future Directions in Black Death Bioarcheology

The results of bioarcheological research on the Black Death raise questions about the demographic and health consequences of the epidemic. The very high levels of Black Death mortality, and the results from hazard analysis which indicate that this mortality was selective and targeted frail people of all ages, means that the epidemic might have exerted a strong selective force on the European population, removing the frailest, unhealthiest individuals on a very large scale. If the post-Black Death population included individuals who were exposed to and survived the Black Death, this episode of selection might, at least in part, explain the very rapid apparent changes in medieval plague epidemiology. These changes include the apparent decline in plague mortality as described in contemporaneous historical documents. As explained by Carmichael (2014, this issue), patterns of human plague deaths might reflect the disease dynamics of nearby animal host populations, which can influence exposure of humans to plague. However, in the case of medieval plague, the lower estimated mortality rates in later outbreaks of plague (Carmichael 1986; Cohn 2008; Russell 1966) might reflect lower average frailty among people who survived the first outbreak, as well as among their descendants. Furthermore, health might have been strongly shaped by the apparent improvements in standards of living that occurred after the Black Death and that resulted primarily from the massive depopulation caused by the epidemic. Such changes in standards of living included improvements in diet for people of all social classes (Dyer 2002; Hatcher 1977; Poos 1991; Rappaport 1989; Stone 2006). Given the effects of nutrition on immune competence, dietary improvements and decreases in social inequities in access to food (which might have strongly benefitted the lower social echelons who made up the bulk of the English populace) might have acted to reduce average levels of frailty within affected populations.

There is some evidence to suggest improvements in survival and thus health following the Black Death. Russell (1966) found—based on comparisons of British and Spanish documentary data (tax records and inquisitions post mortem) to skeletal data from seventy-seven burial grounds primarily from Central Eastern Europe—that the ratio of individuals above the age of sixty relative to those between ages twenty to sixty increased after the Black Death in some areas. However, a comparison of pooled skeletal data from a wide geographic region (mostly Eastern Europe) to documentary data from Western Europe is not ideal. Among other potential problems, each source is subject to different sources of bias (e.g., poor skeletal preservation of children in some cemeteries, biased skeletal age estimates, or underrepresentation of the poorest individuals in some tax records) which complicates comparison. Thus, this line of inquiry needs to be further pursued using large skeletal samples from cemeteries that pre- and postdate the Black Death, preferably from one relatively circumscribed area, and the application of newer, unbiased age-estimation methods and rigorous quantitative approaches such as hazard analysis. Ongoing bioarcheological research is examining temporal trends in survival, risks of mortality, and patterns of skeletal stress markers using samples from London cemeteries that date to the pre-Black Death (1000–1300) and post-Black Death (1350–1540) periods. Thus far, initial results using these samples indicate improvements in survival and health in general following the Black Death (DeWitte 2014).

Not only is there much to learn about the ways in which the Black Death shaped the demographic and health characteristics within surviving populations, there are also questions about the epidemic itself that remain unresolved, and which could benefit from study of other Black Death burial grounds that have been excavated or that will potentially be excavated in the future. As mentioned above, the relatively small proportion of children in the East Smithfield cemetery has prohibited accurate reconstruction of the risk of death for infants and young children during the Black Death. Larger sample sizes of children would allow for the clarification of patterns of mortality for children during the Black Death. This is particularly important given evidence from historical sources that the second outbreak of plague in 1361 disproportionately targeted children. In order to understand precisely how and why mortality patterns might have changed between the first and second outbreak, it is essential to clarify what the risks for children were during the former.

As noted by Varlık (2014, in this issue), there is variation in the manifestation of plague based on local conditions. Thus, it is crucial to repeat and expand the bioarcheological work that has been done with the East Smithfield sample using samples from other areas to reveal how such variation might have produced geographic or temporal differences in the mortality patterns by age, sex, frailty, and other factors during medieval plague epidemics. Given the Eurocentric perspective common to Black Death scholarship highlighted by contributions to this issue of *The Medieval Globe*, it is particularly important to examine plague mortality using cemetery samples from regions outside of Europe if they become available.

Bioarcheological analysis also allows us to better understand the social responses to the Black Death. For example, Colet et al. (2014, in this issue) describe a cemetery containing the victims of violence perpetrated against the Jewish community of the Catalan town of Tàrrega following the epidemic's arrival in the region. This cemetery provides rare insights regarding the specific victims of the violence perpetrated against the Jewish minority (which was blamed for the disease) and how survivors dealt with the victims' burial. In the case of Black Death cemeteries, such as that of East Smithfield, the organization of the burial ground and the positions of the individuals interred therein are informative about how the living treated the victims of the epidemic and how this treatment might have differed from practices discernible during conditions of normal mortality (Grainger et al. 2008; Hawkins 1990; Kacki et al. 2011). In East Smithfield, for example, we have evidence that individuals were afforded a level of care similar to what they would have received during times of normal mortality (Grainger et al. 2008).

Black Death cemeteries, including and in addition to East Smithfield, also provide opportunities for expanding molecular analyses of the medieval plague pathogen. As mentioned above, the integration of bioarcheological research with paleomicrobiological approaches (e.g., ancient DNA analyses) will provide a powerful tool for understanding changes in plague epidemiology, the effects of other circulating diseases on the emergence and epidemiology of plague, and human-pathogen coevolution, thereby addressing questions of great interest to a variety of researchers, including historians, anthropologists, and evolutionary geneticists. Bioarcheology is ideally suited to bridge historical and molecular research on plague (or, indeed, on any important disease in human history). More than any other field, bioarcheology provides the human context that might be missing from other approaches, but which ultimately makes plague research relevant both to the study of human history as well as to the study of biological variation and responses to infectious disease among living people.

Bibliography

Aalen, O. O. 1994. "Effects of Frailty in Survival Analysis," *Statistical Methods in Medical Research* 3, no. 3: 227–43

Acsádi, G., and J. Nemeskéri. 1970. *History of Human Life Span and Mortality* (Budapest: Akadémiai Kiadó)

Alizon, S., A. Hurford, N. Mideo, and M. Van Baalen. 2009. "Virulence Evolution and the Trade-Off Hypothesis: History, Current State of Affairs and the Future," *Journal of Evolutionary Biology* 22, no. 2: 245–59

André J.-B., and M. E. Hochberg. 2005. "Virulence Evolution in Emerging Infectious Diseases," *Evolution* 59, no. 7: 1406–12

Benedictow, Ole J. 1996. *The Medieval Demographic System of the Nordic Countries* (Oslo: Middelalderforlaget)

Benedictow, Ole J. 2004. *The Black Death, 1346–1353: The Complete History* (Woodbridge: Boydell)

Bocquet-Appel, Jean-Pierre, and Claude Masset. 1982. "Farewell to Paleodemography," *Journal of Human Evolution* 11, no. 4: 321–33

Boldsen, J. L., G. R. Milner, L. W. Konigsberg, and J. W. Wood. 2002. "Transition Analysis: A New Method for Estimating Age from Skeletons," in *Paleodemography: Age Distributions from Skeletal Samples*, ed. R. D. Hoppa and J. W. Vaupel, 73–106 (Cambridge: Cambridge University Press)

Borsch, Stuart. 2014. "Plague Depopulation and Irrigation Decay in Medieval Egypt," *The Medieval Globe* 1: 125–156

Bos, K. I., V. J. Schuenemann, G. B. Golding, H. A. Burbano, et al. 2011. "A Draft Genome of *Yersinia pestis* from Victims of the Black Death," *Nature* 478, no. 7370: 506–10

Buikstra, J. E. 1997. "Paleodemography: Context and Promise," in *Integrating Archaeological Demography: Multidisciplinary Approaches to Prehistoric Population*, ed. R. R. Payne, 367–80 (Carbondale, IL: Center for Archaeological Investigations, Southern Illinois University)

Buikstra, J. E., and L. W. Konigsberg. 1985. "Paleodemography: Critiques and Controversies," *American Anthropologist* 87: 316–33

Carmichael, Ann G. 1986. *Plague and the Poor in Renaissance Florence* (Cambridge: Cambridge University Press)

Carmichael, Ann G. 2014. "Plague Persistence in Western Europe: A Hypothesis," *The Medieval Globe* 1: 157–191

Carpentier, E. 1971. "The Plague as a Recurrent Phenomenon," in *The Black Death: A Turning Point in History?*, ed. William M. Bowsky, 35–57 (New York: Holt, Rinehart and Winston)

Chamberlain, A. T. 2006. *Demography in Archaeology* (Cambridge: Cambridge University Press)

Cleaveland, S., D. T. Haydon, and L. Taylor. 2007. "Overviews of Pathogen Emergence: Which Pathogens Emerge, When and Why?," *Current Topics in Microbiology and Immunology* 315, no. 1: 85–111

Cohn, Samuel K. 2002. *The Black Death Transformed: Disease and Culture in Early Renaissance Europe* (London: Arnold)

Cohn, Samuel K. 2008. "Epidemiology of the Black Death and Successive Waves of Plague," *Medical History Supplement* 27, no. 1: 74–100

Colet, Anna, Josep Xavier Muntané i Santiveri, Jordi Ruíz Ventura, Oriol Saula, et al. 2014. "The Black Death and its Consequences for the Jewish Community in Tàrrega: Lessons from History and Archeology," *The Medieval Globe* 1: 63–96

Crespo, Fabian, and Matthew B. Lawrenz. 2014. "Heterogeneous Immunological Landscape and Medieval Plague: An Invitation to a New Dialogue between Historians and Immunologists," *The Medieval Globe* 1: 229–257

DeWitte, Sharon N. 2009. "The Effect of Sex on Risk of Mortality during the Black Death in London, A.D. 1349-1350," *American Journal of Physical Anthropology* 139, no. 2: 222–34

DeWitte, Sharon N. 2010. "Age Patterns of Mortality during the Black Death in London, A.D. 1349–1350," *Journal of Archaeological Science* 37, no. 12: 3394–400

DeWitte, Sharon N. 2014. "Health in Post-Black Death London (1350–1538): Age Patterns of Periosteal New Bone Formation in a Post-Epidemic Population," *American Journal of Physical Anthropology* 155, no. 2: 260–67

DeWitte, Sharon N., and James W. Wood. 2008. "Selectivity of the Black Death with Respect to Preexisting Health," *Proceedings of the National Academy of Sciences* 105, no. 5: 1436–41

DeWitte Sharon N., and Gail Hughes-Morey. 2012. "Stature and Frailty during the Black Death: The Effect of Stature on Risks of Epidemic Mortality in London, A.D. 1348–1350," *Journal of Archaeological Science* 39, no. 5: 1412–19

Dols, Michael W. 1977. *The Black Death in the Middle East* (Princeton: Princeton University Press)

Drancourt, M., and D, Raoult. 2002. "Molecular Insight into the History of Plague," *Microbes and Infection* 4, no. 1: 105–09

Dyer, Christopher. 2002. *Making a Living in the Middle Ages: The People of Britain 850–1520* (New Haven, CT: Yale University Press)

Ebert, D., and J. J. Bull. 1999. "The Evolution and Expression of Parasite Virulence," in *Evolution in Health and Disease*, ed. S. C. Stearns and J. C. Koella, 161–72 (Oxford: Oxford University Press)

Frank, S. A. 1996. "Models of Parasite Virulence," *Quarterly Review of Biology* 71, no. 1: 37–78

Gage, T. B. 1988. "Mathematical Hazard Models of Mortality: An Alternative to Model Life Tables," *American Journalof Physical Anthopology* 76, no. 4: 429–41

Gage, T. B. 1989. "Bio-Mathematical Approaches to the Study of Human Variation in Mortality," *Yearbook of Physical Anthropology* 32, no. 1: 185–214

Gage, T. B. 2005. "Are Modern Environments Really Bad for Us? Revisiting the Demographic and Epidemiologic Transitions," *American Journal of Physical Anthropology* 128, supp. 41: 96–117

Gasquet, Francis Aidan. 1977. *The Black Death of 1348 and 1349* (New York: AMS Press)

Gowland, R. L., and A. T. Chamberlain. 2005. "Detecting Plague: Palaeodemographic Characterisation of a Catastrophic Death Assemblage," *Antiquity* 79: 146–57

Grainger, Ian, Duncan Hawkins, Cowal Lynne, and Richard Mikulski. 2008. *The Black Death Cemetery, East Smithfield, London* (London: Museum of London Archaeology Service)

Green, Monica H. 2014. "Taking 'Pandemic' Seriously: Making the Black Death Global," *The Medieval Globe* 1: 27–61

Grenfell, B. T., O. G. Pybus , J. R. Gog, J. L. N. Wood, et al. 2004. "Unifying the Epidemiological and Evolutionary Dynamics of Pathogens," *Science* 303, no. 5656: 327–32

Haensch, S., R. Bianucci, M. Signoli, M. Rajerison, et al. 2010. "Distinct Clones of *Yersinia pestis* Caused the Black Death," *PLoS Pathogens* 6, no. 10: e1001134

Harbeck, M., L. Seifert, S. Hänsch, D. M. Wagner, et al. 2013. "*Yersinia pestis* DNA from Skeletal Remains from the 6th Century AD Reveals Insights into Justinianic Plague," *PLoS Pathogens* 9, no. 5: e1003349

Hatcher, John. 1977. *Plague, Population, and the English Economy, 1348–1530* (London: Macmillan)

Hawkins, D. 1990. "Black Death and the New London Cemeteries of 1348," *Antiquity* 64: 637–42

Holman, Daryl L., J. W. Wood, and K. A. O'Connor. 2002. "Estimating Age-at-Death Distributions from Skeletal Samples," in *Paleodemography: Age Distributions from Skeletal Samples*, ed. R. D. Hoppa and J. W. Vaupel, 193–201 (Cambridge: Cambridge University Press)

Holmes, G. A. 1971. "England: A Decisive Turning Point," in *The Black Death: A Turning Point in History?*, ed. William M. Bowsky, 91–99 (New York: Holt, Rinehart and Winston)

Horrox, Rosemary (ed. and trans.). 1994. *The Black Death* (Manchester: Manchester University Press)

Kacki, S., L. Rahalison, M. Rajerison, E. Ferroglio, et al. 2011. "Black Death in the Rural Cemetery of Saint-Laurent-de-la-Cabrerisse Aude-Languedoc, Southern France, 14th Century: Immunological Evidence," *Journal of Archaeological Science* 38, no. 3: 581–87

Konigsberg, L. W., and S. R. Frankenberg. 1992. "Estimation of Age Structure in Anthropological Demography," *American Jounral of Physical Anthropology* 89, no. 2: 235–56

Konigsberg, L. W., and S. R. Frankenberg. 2002. "Deconstructing Death in Paleodemography," *American Jounral of Physical Anthropology* 117 no. 4: 297–309

Kowaleski, Maryanne. 2013. "Gendering Demographic Change in the Middle Ages," in *The Oxford Handbook of Women and Gender in Medieval Europe*, ed. Judith M. Bennett and Ruth Mazo Karras, 181–96 (Oxford: Oxford University Press)

Lütgert, S. A. 2000. "Victims of the Great Famine or the Black Death? The Archaeology of the Mass Graves Found in the Former Graveyard of Holy Ghost Hospital, Lübeck (N. Germany), in the European Context," *Hikuin* 27, no. 1: 255–65

Margerison, B. J., and C. J. Knüsel. 2002. "Paleodemographic Comparison of a Catastrophic and an Attritional Death Assemblage," *American Journal of Physical Anthropology* 119, no. 2: 134–43

Milner, G. R., and J. L. Boldsen. 2012. "Transition Analysis: A Validation Study with Known-Age Modern American Skeletons," *American Journal of Physical Anthropology* 148, no. 1: 98–110

Milner, G. R., J. W. Wood, and J. L. Boldsen. 2008. "Paleodemography," in *Biological Anthropology of the Human Skeleton*, ed. M. A. Katzenberg and S. R. Sanders, 561–600 (New York: Wiley-Liss)

Morens, D. M., G. K. Folkers, and A. S. Fauci. 2004. "The Challenge of Emerging and Re-Emerging Infectious Diseases," *Nature* 430, no. 6996: 242–49

Morse, S. S. 1995. "Factors in the Emergence of Infectious Diseases," *Emerging Infectious Diseases* 1, no. 1: 7–15

Müller, H. G., B. Love, and R. D. Hoppa. 2002. "Semiparametric Method for Estimating Paleodemographic Profiles from Age Indicator Data," *American Journal of Physical Anthropology* 117, no. 1: 1–14

Ohlin, G. 1966. "No Safety in Numbers: Some Pitfalls of Historical Statistics," in *Industrialization in Two Systems*, ed. Henry Rosovsky, 68–90 (New York: Wiley)

Olden, K., and S. L. White. 2005. "Health-Related Disparities: Influence of Environmental Factors," *Medical Clinics of North America* 89, no. 4: 721-38

Ortner, D. J. 1991. "Theoretical and Methodological Issues in Paleopathology," in *Human Paleopathology: Current Syntheses and Future Options*, ed. D. J. Ortner and A. C. Aufderheide, 5–11 (Washington, D.C.: Smithsonian Institution Press)

Paine, R. R. 2000. "If a Population Crashes in Prehistory, and There Is No Paleodemographer There to Hear It, Does It Make a Sound?," *American Journal of Physical Anthropology* 112, no. 2: 181–90

Palmer, J. 2013. "'Black Death Pit' Unearthed by Crossrail Project," BBC News, March 14, 2013

Perry, M. A. 2007. "Is Bioarchaeology a Handmaiden to History? Developing a Historical Bioarchaeology," *Journal of Anthropological Archaeology* 26, no. 3: 486–515

Poos, L. R. 1991. *A Rural Society after the Black Death: Essex, 1350–1525* (Cambridge: Cambridge University Press)

Poulsen, B. 1997. "Agricultural Technology in Medieval Denmark," in *Medieval Farming and Technology: The Impact of Agricultural Change in Northwest Europe*, ed. Grenville Astill and John Langdon, 115–46 (Leiden: Brill)

Raoult, D., G. Aboudharam, E. Crubezy, G. Larrouy, et al. 2000. "Molecular Identification by 'Suicide PCR' of *Yersinia pestis* as the Agent of Medieval Black Death," *Proceedings of the National Academy of Sciences* 97, no. 23: 12800–03

Rappaport, Steve L. 1989. *Worlds within Worlds: Structures of Life in Sixteenth-Century London* (Cambridge: Cambridge University Press)

Razi, Zvi. 1980. *Life, Marriage, and Death in a Medieval Parish: Economy, Society, and Demography in Halesowen, 1270–1400* (Cambridge: Cambridge University Press)

Roesdahl, E. (ed.). 1999. *Dagligliv i Danmarks middelalder: En arkæologisk kulturhistorie* (Copenhagen: Nordisk Forlag)

Russell, Josiah Cox. 1948. *British Medieval Population* (Albuquerque: University of New Mexico)

Russell, Josiah Cox. 1966. "Effects of Pestilence and Plague, 1315–1385," *Comparative Studies in Society and History* 8, no. 4: 464–73

Sawyer, Birgit, and Sawyer, Peter. 1993. *Medieval Scandinavia: From Conversion to Reformation, circa 800–1500* (Minneapolis: University of Minnesota Press)

Schuenemann, V. J., K. I. Bos, S. N. DeWitte, S. Schmedes, et al. 2011. "Targeted Enrichment of Ancient Pathogens Yielding the pPCP1 Plasmid of *Yersinia pestis* from Victims of the Black Death," *Proceedings of the National Academy of Sciences* 108, no. 38: E746–52

Scott, S., and C. J. Duncan. 2001. *Biology of Plagues: Evidence from Historical Populations* (Cambridge: Cambridge University Press)

Siler, W. 1979. "A Competing-Risk Model for Animal Mortality," *Ecology* 60, no. 4: 750–57

Stone, D. J. 2006. "The Consumption of Field Crops in Late Medieval England," in *Food in Medieval England: Diet and Nutrition*, ed. C. M. Woolgar, D. Serjeantson, and T. Waldron, 11–26 (Oxford Oxford University Press)

Twigg, G.. 1984. *The Black Death: A Biological Reappraisal* (London: Schocken)

Usher, B. M. 2000. "A Multistate Model of Health and Mortality for Paleodemography: Tirup Cemetery" (PhD Dissertation, Pennsylvania State University)

Van Gerven, D. P., and G. J. Armelagos. 1983. "'Farewell to Paleodemography?' Rumors of its Death Have Been Greatly Exaggerated," *Journal of Human Evolution* 12, no. 4: 353–60

Varlık, Nükhet. 2014. "New Science and Old Sources: Why the Ottoman Experience of Plague Matters," *The Medieval Globe* 1: 193–227

Vaupel, J. W., K. G. Manton, and E. Stallard. 1979. "The Impact of Heterogeneity in Individual Frailty on the Dynamics of Mortality," *Demography* 16, no. 3: 439–54

Wagner, D. M., J. Klunk, M. Harbeck, A. Devault, et al. 2014. "*Yersinia pestis* and the Plague of Justinian, 541–543 AD: A Genomic Analysis," *Lancet Infectious Diseases* 14, no. 4: 319–26

Waldron, H. A. 2001. "Are Plague Pits of Particular Use to Palaeoepidemiologists?," *International Journal of Epidemiology* 30, no. 1: 104–08

Weiss, Kenneth M. 1973. *Demographic Models for Anthropology* (Washington, DC: Society for American Archaeology)

Widgren M. 1997. "Fields and Field Systems in Scandinavia during the Middle Ages," in *Medieval Farming and Technology: The Impact of Agricultural Change in Northwest Europe*, ed. Grenville Astill and John Langdon, 173–92 (Leiden: Brill)

Wiechmann, I., and G. Grupe. 2005. "Detection of *Yersinia pestis* DNA in Two Early Medieval Skeletal Finds from Aschheim (Upper Bavaria, 6th century A.D.)," *American Journal of Physical Anthropology* 126, no. 1: 48–55

Wood, J. W., R. J. Ferrell, and S. N. DeWitte-Avina. 2003. "The Temporal Dynamics of the Fourteenth-Century Black Death: New Evidence from English Ecclesiastical Records," *Human Biology* 75, no. 4: 427–48

Wood, J. W., R. J. Ferrell, S. N. DeWitte-Avina, and D. J. Holman. 2002a. "Mortality Differentials during the Black Death in England, 1349" (paper presented at the 27th Annual Meeting of the Human Biology Council, Buffalo, NY (11–14 April))

Wood, J. W., D. J. Holman, K. A. O'Connor, and R. J. Ferrell. 2002b. "Mortality Models for Paleodemography," in *Paleodemography: Age Distributions from Skeletal Samples*, ed. Robert D. Hoppa and James W. Vaupel, 129–68 (Cambridge: Cambridge University Press)

Wood, J. W., G. R. Milner, H. C. Harpending, and K. M. Weiss. 1992. "The Osteological Paradox: Problems of Inferring Prehistoric Health from Skeletal Samples," *Current Anthropology* 33, no. 4: 343–70

Ziegler, Michelle. 2014. "The Black Death and the Future of the Plague," *The Medieval Globe* 1: 259–283

Sharon N. DeWitte (dewittes@mailbox.sc.edu) is a biological anthropologist with interests in bioarcheology, paleodemography, paleoepidemiology, and infectious and epidemic diseases. For over a decade she has been investigating the mortality patterns, demographic context, and consequences of medieval plague epidemics, including the Black Death of 1347–51. By applying hazard analysis to large skeletal samples from Europe, Dr. DeWitte is able to examine population-level phenomena associated with past crisis mortality events, including the effects of biological factors like age and sex on risks of death during epidemics as devastating as the Black Death, how and why those risks change over time, and how epidemics shape demography and health. Her Black Death research is summarized in publications such as "Selectivity of Black Death Mortality with Respect to Pre-Existing Health," co-authored with James Wood in *Proceedings of the National Academy of Sciences USA* 105 (2008): 1436–41; and "Age Patterns of Mortality during the Black Death in London, A.D. 1349–1350," in *Journal of Archaeological Science* 37 (2010): 3394–3400. She is also interested in the molecular biology and evolution of the pathogen that caused the Black Death, *Yersinia pestis*, and is part of a collaborative project that has produced the first complete genome of the fourteenth-century bacterium (Bos et al. 2011). She is currently an associate professor in the Department of Anthropology at the University of South Carolina.

Abstract Most research on historic plague has relied on documentary evidence, but recently researchers have examined the remains of plague victims to produce a deeper understanding of the disease. Bioarcheological analysis allows the skeletal remains of epidemic victims to bear witness to the contexts of their deaths. This is important for our understanding of the experiences of the vast majority of people who lived in the past, who are not typically included in the historical record. This paper summarizes bioarcheological research on plague, primarily investigations of the Black Death in London (1349–50), emphasizing what anthropology uniquely contributes to plague studies.

Keywords Black Death, medieval London, paleodemography, osteology, hazard models, plague cemeteries, East Smithfield.

PLAGUE DEPOPULATION AND IRRIGATION DECAY IN MEDIEVAL EGYPT

STUART BORSCH

THE FIFTEENTH-CENTURY EGYPTIAN chronicler al-Maqrīzī provides us with a substantial account of the Black Death in his historical narrative of several thousand pages: the *Kitāb al-sulūk lī-ma 'rifa duwal al-mulūk* (*The Book of Methods for Understanding the Kingdoms [of the World]*). Al-Maqrīzī was a market inspector (*muhtasib*) as well as a prominent historian. His extensive works have therefore provided modern scholars with a great deal of information about Egypt's economic history. Concerning the plague's arrival in Egypt, al-Maqrīzī's narrative describes a sequence familiar to historians of the Black Death: how, in 1347 CE, a pestilence "worse than any seen before in the Islamic world" began with a ship full of corpses drifting into Alexandria. There were a few sailors still alive; they died soon after—and Egypt's experience with the Black Death began (al-Maqrīzī, *al-Sulūk*, 2: 772–73).

Al-Maqrīzī reports that in Alexandria the plague began killing a hundred people a day, and that the death toll subsequently doubled to two hundred a day. As the plague outbreak reached its peak, there were mass funerals for as many as seven hundred people. The plague then spread throughout the Nile Delta, where "no one was left to gather the crops." In the city of Bilbays at the eastern edge of the Delta, al-Maqrīzī reports that "mosques, shops and lodges were left empty" (al-Maqrīzī, *al-Sulūk*, 2: 777–79). When the plague struck Cairo, the sultan and leading members of the ruling regime fled the city, as mass prayers were held in the mosques and the cemeteries. When the plague reached its peak around December of 1348, it was reported that something like 7,000 people died per day. The plague finally abated the following February; in the quiet that followed, Cairo was like a graveyard, still and empty (al-Maqrīzī, *al-Sulūk*, 2: 780–84).

Scenes of devastation like that of Cairo in February 1349 were to become all too common in Egypt. Plague depopulation in the instance of the Black Death had a deep and long-term impact on Egypt's economy. This article examines the manner in which plague shaped the economic history of Egypt. It assesses the relative scale and scope of rural mortality and argues that plague depopulation led to the collapse of Egypt's economic infrastructure; the analysis that follows is intended to show exactly how and why this happened. In so doing, this essay illustrates an important lesson to be learned from the historical study of plague: the economic impact of massive depopulation could vary greatly from region to region throughout the affected areas of the medieval globe. These economic responses to exogenous demographic shocks were, moreover, shaped by and dependent upon diverse social, institutional, and environmental variables. In this case, emphasis falls on the dependent variable of geography; but other variables, such as political institutions rooted in social structures, also demand attention. While it might sound obvious that we should keep our theoretical expectations flexible, it is all too easy to fall into the comforting conceptual trap of familiar and well-established trajectories: that is, the well-known European pattern of falling prices, rising wages, social mobility, and improved nutrition discernible in the aftermath of the Black Death. Egypt offers a very different picture of the outcomes stemming from rapid, plague-induced demographic changes.

Studying the Economic Impact of the Black Death in Egypt

The Black Death of 1347–50—and the cycles of plague that followed it—brought depopulation and change not only to Egypt but also to the Middle East in general. While it is accurate to say that this process of transformation and evolution is only partially understood, it is worth examining what progress has been made; the following is a review of the scholarship (largely focused on Egypt) that pertains to economic developments influenced by plague depopulation. The work of Eliyahu Ashtor (1949, 1969, 1976, 1977) is the best place to start. Ashtor's broad conclusion that the Black Death was devastating to Egypt has never been seriously challenged, and he is still the most cited source for the specifics of economic decline in this period. In 1970, Abraham Udovitch (together with Robert Lopez and Harry Miskimin) summed up what was known about the economic trajectory of Egypt in the late Middle Ages (Lopez, Miskimin, and Udovitch 1970). Udovitch concluded that economic decline was quite severe during the 1350 to 1500 interval. Around the same time, studies of monetary transformation by Jere Bacharach (1971 and 1983) drew deserved attention to the problems posed by the adoption of copper currency in Egypt during the late fourteenth and early fifteenth centuries. The formal study of the Black Death in Egypt began with Michael Dols (1977). In his book, Dols included a section on the economic impact of the Black Death. As was the case with Ashtor and Udovitch, his conclusions about the economic impact of plague depopulation were altogether negative. Later work by Dols (1979, 1981) focused primarily on the plague outbreak of 1430. As the data that we have for this outbreak is much more extensive than that for the Black Death itself, Dols made a case study of Cairo and concluded that overall mortality in that city was on the order of 90,000.[1]

After Dols's work, there were no studies dedicated specifically to the Black Death in Egypt—or the Middle East—until my own comparative monograph (Borsch 2005). However, there were a number of studies in the economic history of Egypt that examined the problem indirectly. The work of Boaz Shoshan (1983) on grain prices, from which he considerably expanded the data on prices and exchange rates for late medieval Egypt, focused on the role of monetary factors in the economic turbulence of the 1400s. Shoshan was one of a series of scholars—Giles Hennequin (1974), Adel Allouche (1994), Warren Schultz (1998, 2011), and John Meloy (2001)—who studied various aspects of the monetary system in the wake of the Black Death. Among this group there seems to have been a quiet consensus that the monetary woes of the 1400s were in many ways bound up with falling economic production. Carl Petry (1994) devoted a chapter of his work to the economic trajectory of Egypt in the post-Black Death period, painting a bleak picture of economic events, especially when it came to the political economy of corruption and its impact on the economy as a whole. From a very different perspective, Sato Tsugitaka (1977) was really the first scholar who studied the Egyptian irrigation system during the Mamluk period, and his work is indispensable for anyone studying economic changes in the rural economy in the interval between 1347 and 1517.

Adam Sabra's work (2000) indirectly addresses the subject of plague depopulation via an examination of famine relief in the Mamluk period of rule (1250–1517). His detailed analysis of Egypt's inflationary cycles is an indispensable guide to the economic trajectory of Egypt at this time. At roughly the same time, two Egyptian historians produced detailed and innovative studies of Egyptian economic life that included a great deal of detail about the rural economy of Egypt after the Black Death. 'Imād Abū Ghāzī (2000), a historian who produced what was effectively the first archive-based monograph dedicated to the rural economy of Egypt, explored the changes in the agrarian economy that arose because of land sales conducted by the cash-strapped Circassian Mamluk regime.

1 Dols (1977: 204–12) initially examined the outbreak of 1430 and provided a table that attributed 91,845 deaths to plague for that year, a figure in close proximity to that given by the fifteenth-century chronicler Ibn Taghrībirdī, who had estimated 100,000 deaths (Popper 1954–63, 4: 72, 181). Dols's later analysis of this epidemic (1981) included a thorough re-examination of population levels for Cairo.

The work of ʿĀmr Najīb Mūsā Nasir (2003) addresses a host of hitherto overlooked aspects of the rural economy, breaking ground in terms of the depth and detail given to rural economic change in the wake of plague depopulation. In terms of archival work on the rural economy, it should also be noted that the Japanese scholar Daisuke Igarashi (2006, 2008, 2010, and forthcoming) has extensively investigated archival collections of *waqf* documents (created by formal institutions established by charitable donation) in order to study agrarian developments; his forthcoming monograph on the political economy of *waqf* foundations deals with the economic change related to plague depopulation.

Meanwhile, Sevket Pamuk (2007) has taken up the subject of east-west divergence and its relationship to plague depopulation. Since then, he has (with Maya Shatzmiller) published analyses that study wage trajectories following plague outbreaks (Shatzmiller 2012; Pamuk and Shatzmiller 2014). Two other recent contributors to this area of economic history are the Malaysian scholar Wan Kamal Mujani (2008 and 2011), who studies economic developments at the very end of the Mamluk period, and the Swedish economist Johan Söderberg (2006), who has produced a new and novel examination of prices, an examination that employs methodological tools new to the study of the Black Death in the Middle East.

Another recent work in Arabic, indispensable for anyone studying the economic impact of plague depopulation in Egypt, is that of Muhammad al-Zāmil (2008). This book is full of insightful observations and detailed analysis of economic developments—particularly developments in the rural sphere. Perhaps the most innovative recent study is by Julien Louiseau (2011). In *Reconstruire la maison du sultan, 1350–1450: ruine et recomposition de l'ordre urban au Caire*, Louiseau conducts a detailed mapping of Cairo that examines the areas of the city most affected by the *khirāb*, or economic decline of Egypt. Using a broad archeological reconstruction of fifteenth-century Cairo, this massive two-volume work studies the aftermath of the Black Death and its effects on the built environment, including graves as well as ruined palaces, mosques, and housing structures.

Finally, looking at the subject of plague in the longer term, there is new work by Alan Mikhail (2008, 2011, 2013) and Sam White (2010) on Ottoman Egypt. Mikhail, whose work studies the trail of plague mortality stretching all the way to the nineteenth century, focuses attention on the environmental history of plague, and his innovative use of archival court records gives him a unique perspective on the disease's long-term tenure in the eastern Mediterranean. Long after plague had been banished from Europe it endured in the Middle East, and it continued to haunt Egypt, with outbreaks recurring approximately every nine years for over half a millennium, from 1347 to 1894 (see also Varlık 2014, in this issue).

Measuring Rural Depopulation

The Black Death was thus the first of many blows that struck the Egyptian population; cycles of plague outbreaks continued into the 1400s and well beyond—and some of these outbreaks were nearly as bad as the Black Death itself (Dols 1977: 305–14).[2] The many outbreaks of the fifteenth century carried away enough victims that they left deep scars in the collective memory. An account narrated by al-Maqrīzī (*al-Sulūk*, 4: 227) describes the outbreak of 1412 in the following terms:

> خربت الإسكندرية و بلاد البحيرة و أكثر الشرقية و معظم الغربية و الجيزة و تدمرت بلاد
> الفيوم و عم الخراب بلاد الصعيد بحيث بطل منها زيادة على أربعين خطبة كانت تقام في يوم
> الجمعة. و دثر ثغر أسوان – و كان من أعظم ثغور المسلمين. فلم يبق به أمير و لا كبير و
> لا سوق و لا بيت. و تلاشت مدائن الصعيد كلها. و خرب من القاهرة و ظواهرها زيادة على
> النصف من أملاكها. و مات من أهل إقليم مصر بالجوع و الوباء نحو ثلثي الناس.

> (Alexandria was laid waste [by these troubles] and so was [the Nile Delta province of] al-Buḥayra. The greater part of [the province of] al-Sharqīya was ruined, and the majority of [the two provinces] al-Gharbīya and Giza were desolated. The [province of] the Fayyum was devastated. Destruction was widespread in Upper Egypt as well – so much so that more than forty sermons that were held on Fridays were abrogated. *[The intent here is to convey that more than forty villages/towns large enough to have a congregational mosque were abandoned.]* The port city of Aswan was destroyed, and it was once one of the greatest of Muslim port cities; now nothing remains in it of amirs, influential people, marketplaces, or houses. Most of the cities of Upper Egypt have been obliterated. Cairo and its outskirts have lost half their wealth. And two-thirds of the population of Egypt has been wiped out by famine and plague.)

Al-Maqrīzī is trying to describe the scale and scope of economic and demographic devastation, though a mortality of two-thirds was probably only witnessed at times and in places where plague outbreaks were at their most intense. The plague cycles of 1430 and 1460 were two such outbreaks: they were the worst to follow the Black Death. Both lasted for about four and a half months. In Cairo, the plague of 1430 claimed about 90,000 lives and the 1460 outbreak some 70,000 lives.[3]

---

2 Dols provides a fairly detailed appendix of the outbreaks that followed the Black Death, to the end of the Mamluk period (1517 CE). He concludes (1977: 223–24) that there were some twenty-eight outbreaks in Egypt in the interval 1349–1517 CE, with cycles of recurrence every five and a half years.

3 Quantitative primary evidence (including figures for daily death tolls) supports this conclusion. For the 1430 plague, see al-Maqrīzī (*al-Sulūk*, 4: 822–26), Ibn Ḥajar

What we know about these plague outbreaks—qualitatively and quantitatively—are details provided by eye-witness observers, like Ibn Ḥajar al-ʿAsqalānī and al-Maqrīzī for the 1430 plague and Ibn Taghrībirdī for the 1460 plague. These three men (among other witnesses) were members of the elite class of urban scholars. What they record are the number of plague deaths per day (and sometimes the totals for certain periods of time). These numbers were conveyed to them by high-ranking members of the Circassian (Mamluk) military regime and its civilian bureaucracy. The bureaucrats themselves obtained the figures for the number of plague deaths per day by one of two methods. The first was derived from an account of deaths listed by name and registered by the Department of Inheritances. But this was only a partial record, perhaps one-third of all urban deaths, because the vast number of anonymous and propertyless poor were not counted. The second method was more comprehensive and consisted of counting corpses that were brought to a *muṣallā*, which might best be translated as "prayer site" or "oratory."

The *muṣallā* was an open place with a more limited ceremonial scope than a mosque. It was often located at a city's gates, with a designated wall for the prayer niche (*mihrab*). The *muṣallā* most often referenced in the course of these two outbreaks was that of the Bab al-Nasr at the northern end of Fatimid Cairo. Here, bodies were brought for the brief "funeral prayer" (*janāza*) that preceded actual burial. In 1430, however, these funeral prayers were performed with great haste over long lines of bodies. This mass blessing was then followed, in 1430, by burial en masse, with graves dug out for forty or more corpses at a time (Ibn Taghrībirdī, *Ḥawādith*, 14: 341). From these *muṣallā*, of which Cairo had about fourteen in 1430 and seventeen in 1460, the total number of deaths per day were recorded by civilian bureaucrats—sometimes under the direction of leaders (*amirs*) of the regime. These tallies were apparently detailed and conducted with as many as three independent witnesses. Sometimes rounded and sometimes not, the numbers present a complex picture of different urban sectors in which there were mosques, markets, and gates that served as *muṣallā*.

---

al-ʿAsqalānī (*Inbā'*, 9: 200), Ibn Iyās (*Badā'i'*, 2: 113), and Ibn Taghrībirdī (*Ḥawādith*, 14: 339–43). The primary sources for the 1460 plague are Ibn Taghrībirdī (*Ḥawādith*, 16: 130–47; see the translation by Popper (1954–63, 4: 90–100). See also Ibn Iyās (*Badā'i'*, 2: 357). On the 1430 plague, see also Dols (1981: 404–11), who had clearly intended to study the 1460 plague as well (1981: 409).

Analyzing the Data for Rural Plague Mortality

Thanks to these contemporary records, urban death tolls (numbers of deaths per day) from different sources can be compared with one another, and the resulting ratios indicate the data's probable validity. Once a confirmable ratio is established, one can calculate total deaths per day by extrapolating from a single data point (such as a datum from one of the *muṣallā*). From these ratios, final death counts can then be posited and graphed, to represent the number of deaths per day over time.

The graphs for rural mortality from plague outbreaks (**Graphs 1–3**, on pp. 134–5, below) are based on this method of calculation. However, it should be noted that compiling rural depopulation statistics presents more of a challenge. The same sources available for Cairo can also be mined for data on rural plague outbreaks in 1430 and 1460, as well as for one in 1403–04 and another in 1407 (al-Maqrīzī, *al-Sulūk*, 3: 1126 and 4: 43). But the mortality figures that we have for towns and villages outside of Cairo are much less systematic, so we must assess the scale of rural depopulation by adapting and applying the plague curves determined for Cairo. Moreover, we do not know precisely how these rural figures were compiled, but it seems logical that the *muṣallā* funeral rite (and associated body count), as a generalized Islamic practice, worked in roughly the same manner in a village as in a city.

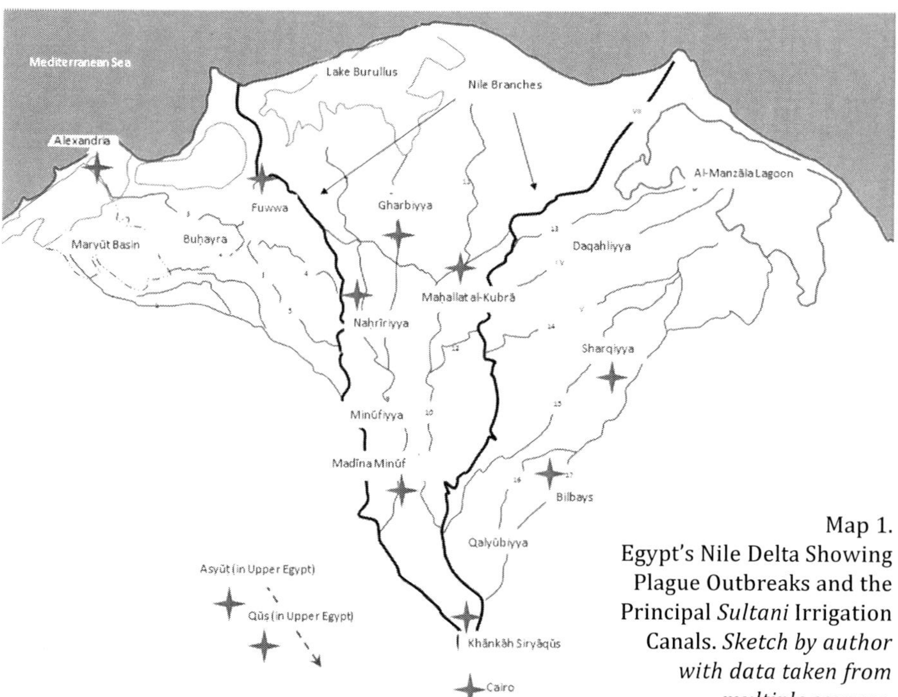

Map 1.
Egypt's Nile Delta Showing Plague Outbreaks and the Principal *Sultani* Irrigation Canals. *Sketch by author with data taken from multiple sources.*

Map 1 on the previous page shows the distribution of rural outbreaks that have so far been documented. **Tables 1–3** opposite display data collected from the available sources for the three outbreaks (1403, 1430, and 1460). These figures are rough estimates, as attested by the urban witnesses who recorded them. Hence, the goal here is to convey a sense of *scale and scope*: did hundreds die in large towns like al-Maḥallat al-Kubrā (below)—or was the total mortality in the thousands—or even tens of thousands?

For estimating mortality in these rural locations, Cairo's peak death rates for 1430 and 1460 were scaled down to the two death rates that we have for al-Maḥallat al-Kubrā in 1460 (**Table 3**: 250 per day in February and 300 per day in March): see **Graph 1**. These two curves, which align closely with that of the scaled-down curve for Cairo, can then be averaged and combined into one curve: see **Graph 2**.

Summing up the interpolated areas suggested by this amalgamated curve yields an estimated total number of deaths: approximately 10,000 for the plague outbreak of 1460 in al-Maḥallat al-Kubrā alone. This total mortality can then be tested against the total deaths of the 1430 outbreak in the same locale, for which we have a figure of some 5,000 deaths by January of 1430, some sixty days into the epidemic (Table 3). The sixty-day mark in the 1460 graph above (Graph 2) reads as 4,000 total deaths. The fact that the two figures are comparable suggests that the scale is correct—even if the figures themselves are rounded estimates.

We also have estimated death tolls for the Nile Delta town of Minūf al-ʻUlyā (see Madīna Minūf on Map 1, above) in 1407 CE: a peak death rate of 140 per day and a total death count of 4,400. The same method of adapting the Cairo plague curve (see **Graph 3**), takes a peak death rate of 140 and generates an estimated total deaths of 4,652. The closeness of the estimated total deaths (4,652) and the reputed actual total deaths (4,400) could be a coincidence, but it more likely suggests, again, that the *scale* of the toll reported in our sources is correct—and that for Minuf al-ʻUlya, a total mortality between 4,000 and 5,000 for this epidemic is a realistic estimate.

In sum, Minūf al-ʻUlya was subjected to a series of major outbreaks in 1403, 1407, 1430, and 1460, each claiming several thousand lives. If this method of estimating rural depopulation is effective, then some other towns and villages—like al-Naḥririyya and al-Maḥallat al-Kubrā—must have suffered a similar fate. Prior to this unfolding catastrophe, populations for these provincial centers were likely in the range of 20,000 to 40,000. Al-Qalqashandī describes Minūf al-ʻUlyā as "medium" (*mutawassiṭa*) and al-Maḥallat al-Kubrā as "large" (*ʻaẓīma*). The loss of 5,000 to 10,000 inhabitants in successive blows suggests depopulation

Table 1. Plague Outbreak of 1403

Locale	Daily rate of plague deaths	Sum of plague deaths to date	Month	Sources
Qūṣ		17,000		al-Maqrīzī (*al-Sulūk*, 3: 1126) for 806/1403
Asyūṭ		11,000		al-Maqrīzī (*al-Sulūk*, 3: 1126) for 806/1403

Table 2. Plague Outbreak of 1430

Locale	Daily rate of plague deaths	Sum of plague deaths to date	Month	Sources
Delta (Damanhur, Nahririyya)			December 1429	al-Maqrīzī (*al-Sulūk*, 4: 821)
Maḥallat al-Kubrā		5000	January 1430	Ibn Taghrībirdī (*al-Nujūm*, 14: 337–39); al-Maqrīzī (*al-Sulūk*, 4: 821)
Alexandria	100		February 1430	al-Maqrīzī (*al-Sulūk*, 4: 824); Ibn Taghrībirdī (*al-Nujūm*, 14: 338)
Naḥrīriyya		9000	February 1430	Ibn Taghrībirdī (*al-Nujūm*, 14: 338)
Minufiyya, Qalyubiyya	600		March 1430	al-Maqrīzī (*al-Sulūk*, 4: 825)
Fuwwa, Bilbays			March 1430	al-Maqrīzī (*al-Sulūk*, 4: 827)
Siryaqus	200		March 1430	Ibn Iyas (*Badā'i'*, 2: 138)
Upper Egypt			April 1430	al-Maqrīzī (*al-Sulūk* 4: 829); Popper (1954–63, 4: 93)

Table 3. Plague Outbreak of 1460

Locale	Daily rate of plague deaths	Sum of plague deaths to date	Month	Sources
Sharyqiyya, Gharbiyya			January	Ibn Iyās (*Badā'i'*, 2: 357); Ibn Taghrībirdī (*al-Nujūm*, 16: 139); Popper (1954–63, 4: 93)
Maḥallat al- Kubrā	250		February	Ibn Taghrībirdī (*al-Nujūm*, 16: 140); Popper (1954–63, 4: 93)
Siryaqus	400		March	Ibn Taghrībirdī (*al-Nujūm*, 16: 140); Popper (1954–63, 4: 93)
Maḥallat al-Kubrā	300		March	Ibn Taghrībirdī (*al-Nujūm*, 16: 140); Popper (1954–63, 4: 93)
Madinat Minuf	200		March	Ibn Taghrībirdī (*al-Nujūm*, 16: 140); Popper (1954–63, 4: 93)

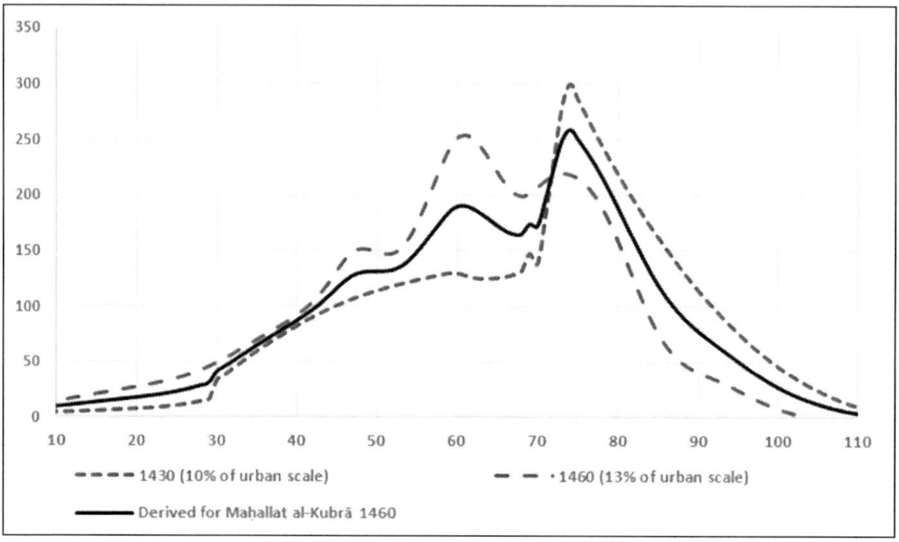

Graph 1. Al-Maḥallat al-Kubrā in 1460 CE: Graph of Plague Deaths over Time as Measured against a Scaled Curve for Cairo

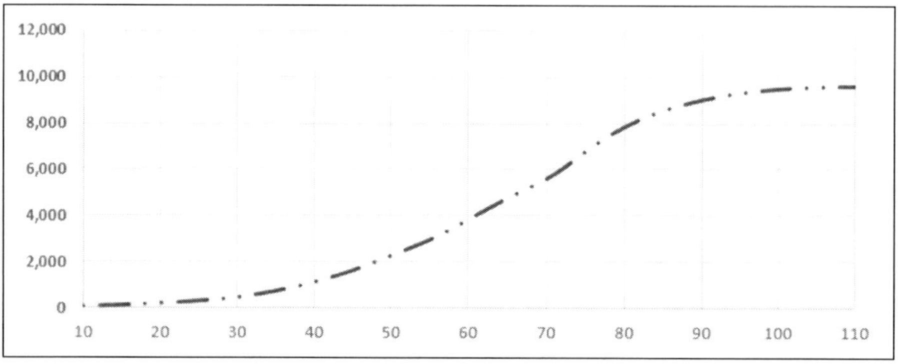

Graph 2. Al-Maḥallat al-Kubrā in 1460 CE: Graph of Rising Death Toll over Time

substantially higher than the one-third estimated by Dols (1977) for Egypt as a whole. The Egyptian historian ʻImād Abū Ghāzī (2000: 65–66), who closely examined rural Egypt via archival documents, suggests that rural Egypt lost more than 40% of its population from 1347 to 1517.

The numbers derived above suggest that Abū Ghāzī's estimate is realistic. Geography argues for it as well: the layout of Egypt's rural areas suggests that it facilitated the spread of plague. Egypt's Nile Valley is a thin strip of arable land, bounded by desert, hugging the Nile River at all points, while Egypt's Delta is crisscrossed with canals and inland waterways that were used for transporting grain on small ships. These spatial

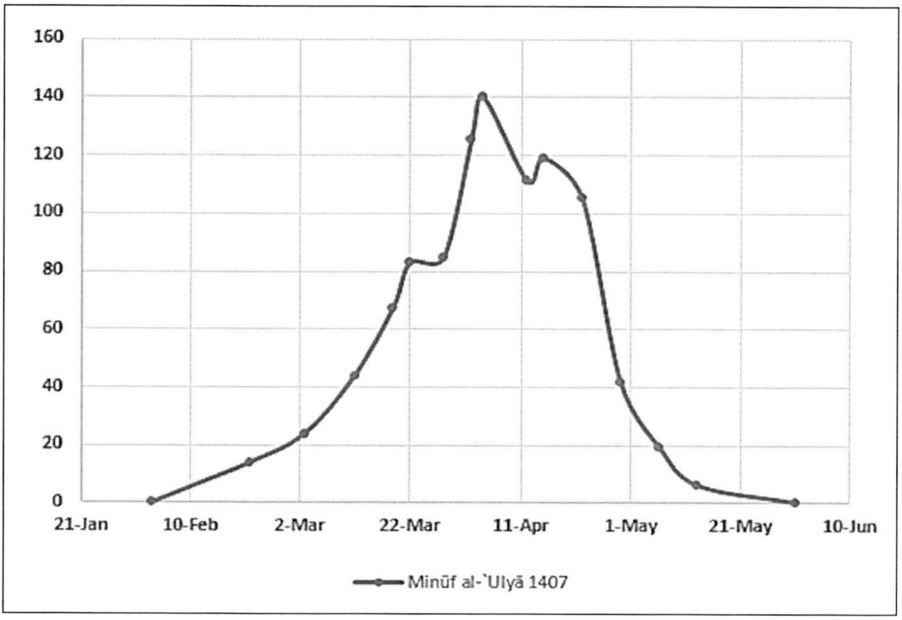

Graph 3. Minuf ʿUlyā in 1407 CE: Graph of Estimated Plague Deaths over Time (as Measured against Cairo Curve)

configurations are ideal for the dissemination of plague-bearing rats and fleas. The annual Nile flood would then have abetted plague mortality by drowning the fields surrounding the villages, forcing rats to seek shelter in human habitations located on higher ground (Conrad 1981). The fact that plague outbreaks continued to strike Egypt with substantial force well into to the nineteenth century may itself be largely attributable to geography (Mikhail 2011: 214–21).

The Irrigation System and the Rural Economy

If rural depopulation was severe, what did it spell out for Egypt's economy? This is where the subject of irrigation plays a major role: to study Egypt's medieval irrigation system is, essentially, to study the economy of preindustrial Egypt. No other aspect or foundation of Egyptian economic activity had a larger impact on its overall economic output.

A few words on the system itself and how it functioned are in order here. Medieval Egypt's irrigation system relied on the spring monsoon over the western Indian Ocean: the monsoon, which fell on the highlands of Ethiopia in June, caused the Nile to flood in the early autumn. As the Nile rose some seven meters up from its low-water level, floodwater was channeled to flood canals (called variously: *khalīj*, *tura*, and *baḥr*) that

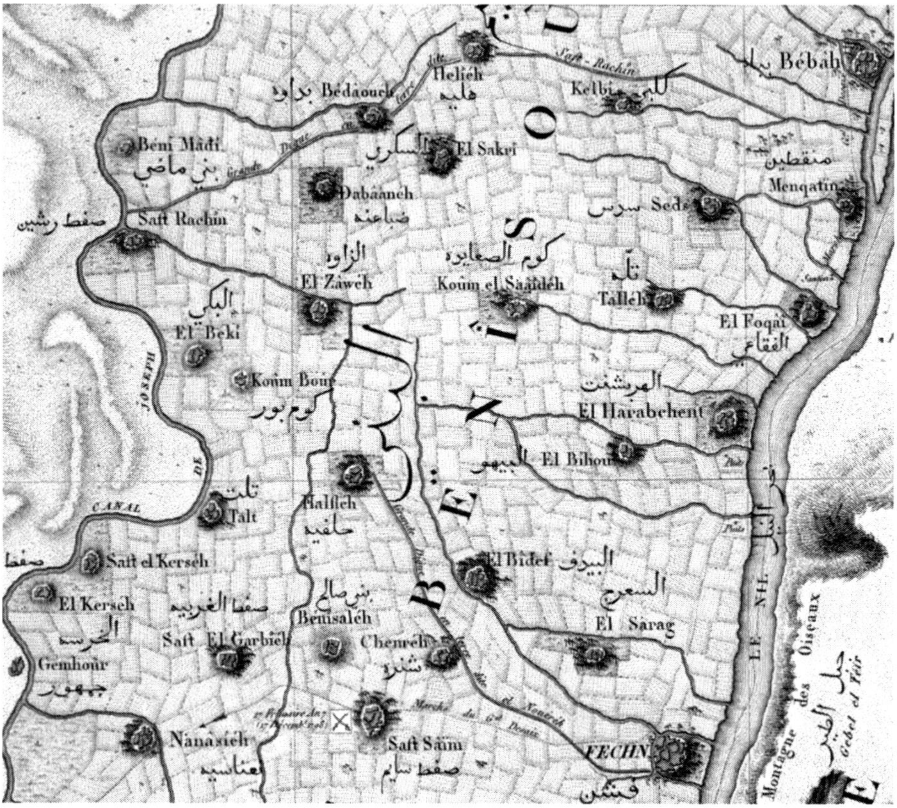

Map 2. Flood Canals in Upper Egypt, *c.* 1800 (Nile River at Right, Baḥr Yūsuf at Left)[4]

led water from the Nile River and collected it in enormous basins (Arabic: *ḥawḍ* or *aḥwād*) (**see Map 2**).

The walls containing the water in these basins were enormous dikes (Arabic: *jisr* or *jusūr*), and they held the water in the basin, allowing it to soak into the soil over a period of about a month and a half. Alluvial sediment that washed down from the Ethiopian highlands with the floodwater also settled into the soil, which accounted for Egypt's rich agricultural fertility.[5] When this period of soaking the soil was complete, the remain-

4 Map by M. Schouani, printed in Pierre Jacotin's *Déscription de l'Égypte* (1826); reproduced by kind permission of the David Rumsey Map Collection, no. 3964022.

5 The British colonial hydraulic engineer William Willcocks (1913, 1: 302) analyzed the floodwater's sediment and determined that it contained nitrogen, phosphoric acid, and other nutrients. There were 1.5 kilograms of suspended alluvial matter per cubic meter of floodwater and two-thirds of this came out of solution and was deposited, one millimeter a year, as a layer on Egypt's soil. The deposition of alluvium,

ing floodwater was allowed to flow back into the Nile and sowing of seed for the winter crop would commence. So Egyptian agriculture was fundamentally dependent upon its irrigation system—and damage to the irrigation system meant severe damage to Egypt's agrarian sector.

Canals themselves were classified as either perennial canals (*ṣayfī*) or flood canals (*nīlī*). The former were deep enough, and/or had gated weirs, that they were able to provide water year-round, while the latter were only filled during the flood season. These irrigation components, the canals, the dikes, the dams, and the weirs, were controlled by and maintained by the provincial *walī* (governor) and his *mubāshirūn* (roughly, staff or bureaucrats) in the respective provincial capital. From there the governor and his staff acted as authority and liaison for the irrigation system. In their interactions with village elders (*shaykh*, *mashāyīkh*) and village experts (among them the *khawlī*), the provincial authority played a role as both coordinator and coercer.

While much of the agricultural work in medieval Egypt was comparatively light, this was not so for the irrigation system. Enormous labor was required to keep the system going. The village irrigation system itself demanded a heavy toll of labor, but so did the large-scale sultani system that connected the villages to one another—and to the Nile.

During the Mamluk period, Egypt's irrigation system fell into two neat categories. The first of these, the *baladi* system, was the local, village-level system. The village community was supposed to take care of it, without the help of any broader (communal) or higher (coercive) authority, even if the irrigation bureaucracy still played a prominent role in that process. The *sultani* system, by contrast, was everything the *baladi* system was not: it was outside the boundary of the village; it was a non-local system; it was a regional system; it was controlled from a remote center; it linked larger parts of the system together; it linked one part of the *baladi* system to other parts of the *baladi* system; and it connected the *baladi* system, at most points, to the Nile River.

---

dating some 10,000 years back to the last Ice Age, formed a layer roughly ten meters thick in Egypt's Nile Delta. See also Beaumont (1993: 25–29), Ward (1993: 229 and 231), Bowman and Rogan, (1999: 2), Stanley and Warne (1998: 797–804), and Barois (2010: 25). The rich muddy water, the "red water," was highly prized by Egyptian farmers. The scholarly elite of Mamluk Egypt were well aware of the cause of the flood, the source of the alluvial matter, and its properties. Ibn Iyās, writing at the end of the fifteenth century, discusses the crucial difference between the barren prospects of spring water and the enriching quality of the Nile mud. His testimony is one of many in a long tradition of Islamic natural philosophers who examined the various aspects of Egypt's Nile flood (*Nuzhat*: 101–04, 108–12).

The numbers of irrigation laborers that were needed to maintain the *sultani* system, according to three different fifteenth-century authors, are 50,000 for Upper Egypt and 70,000 for Lower Egypt (al-Suyūṭī, *Ḥusn*, 2: 320; al-Maqrīzī, *Khiṭaṭ*, 1: 60; Ibn Iyās, *Nuzhat*: 137). There are also references to the total cost of irrigation maintenance, estimated at 25% of the annual revenue income of the non-hereditary *iqṭā'* landholdings, which would add up to several million gold dinars. It is not clear, however, how the expenditures were supposed to break down. If one takes labor-to-population ratios as a guide, 120,000 irrigation laborers out of a rural population in the millions—where the ratio of labor to total population was in all likelihood on the order of 70%—would seem a rather paltry workforce for a country with such a large and rich arable terrain. However, this figure of 120,000 clearly applied only to the larger-scale interconnecting *sultani* system, and not to the thousands of village systems that fed into the sultani system.[6]

As it turns out, these numbers are quite realistic. If we compare them to nineteenth-century statistics, they match quite closely (see **Table 4**), which means that contemporary reporters were probably talking to someone close to the source, in a *diwan* of the central regime, who understood the system well. For example, after the British occupation of Egypt in 1882, the colonial irrigation engineer William Willcocks (1913, 2: 815) reported that some 400 adult males per village, that is all males between fifteen and fifty years of age, were liable for seasonal corvée work. Willcocks's estimate may have been on the high side; the real figure might have been less than 350, given a likely adult male labor pool (aged fifteen to fifty) consisting of perhaps 25% to 30% of a total village population hovering between 1000 and 1500.

What was the exact nature of this labor, and why did it carry a heavy toll? It seems clear from both modern and medieval sources that the bulk of the work was composed of the annual "reconstruction" of the system in the spring, starting in the Coptic month of Ṭūba. This annual spring work, which was needed to undo the damage wreaked by the Nile flood itself, was (in the Mamluk period) directed by the *kāshif al-jusūr* (provincial *sultani* system inspector) of which there was one for each province, rotating in appointment on a year-to-year basis. The provincial governor (*wālī*) also played an important role here, and his mandate often intersected with that of the *kāshif al-jusūr* (Baḥr 1999, 38–52).

6 See al-Qalqashandī (*Subḥ*, 3: 515–16); Ibn Shahīn al-Ẓāhirī (*Zubdat*: 129); and al-Maqrīzī (*Khiṭaṭ*, 1: 101). See also Cooper (1973: 77), Tsugitaka (1977: 183–84), and Nāṣir (2003: 172, 177).

Table 4. Fifteenth-Century Data on Number of Workers Compared to Nineteenth-Century Data

Year	Laborers	Days Labor	Earthwork (m^3)	Source
1400s	120,000			al-Suyūṭī (*Ḥusn*, 2: 320; *Khiṭaṭ*, 1: 60); Ibn Iyās (*Nuzhat*: 137)
1879	120,000	152	29,000,000	Barois (2010: 68)
	165,000	100		Willcocks (1913, 2: 815)
	125,000	100		Willcocks (1913, 2: 815)
	95,093	100		Willcocks (1913, 2: 815)
1884	125,000	150	29,000,000	Willcocks (1913, 2: 815)
1885	91,000	117	21,000,000	Barois (2010: 69)

There were two principal tasks that took up the lion's share of the spring labor requirements: dredging canals and rebuilding dikes.[7] The dredging of canals meant, for the larger canals, the use of a kind of shoveling device called a *jarrāfa*, which was a large box-like scraper for the bottoms of canals, triangular and measuring eighty centimeters to the side. One or two men would sit on this box to weight it down and dig into the accumulated silt, and when full it would be emptied at the side of the canal (Ibn Shahīn al-Ẓāhirī, *Zubdat*: 128; see also Shaw 1962: 227–28). The dredging of smaller canals usually involved peasants using shovels, and there was a "shovel levy" (a reference to equipment of various kinds) that seems to have been measured for each individual village (Tsugitaka 1997: 230). There was a levy of oxen as well (Abū Zayd 1987: 62).[8] Dredging the

7 Julien Barois (2010: 37), writing in the nineteenth century, makes it clear that the dikes and canals occupied the time of repair crews about equally. In Upper Egypt, he counted 3,550,000 cubic meters of earthwork on the dikes and 4,650,000 in the canals; in all, 8,200,000 cubic meters. He also provided an estimate of the volume of earthwork per hectare for dikes (5.5 cubic meters) and canals (8.7 cubic meters), for a total of 14.30 cubic meters of earthwork per hectare.

8 The shovel levy was assigned in units called *qiṭa'*, perhaps one apparatus per *qiṭa'*, but I suspect it came to have some other standardized meaning that was becoming disassociated with the actual equipment, and may eventually have referred to money payments—or levies of manpower in corvée. See "Rural Society in Medieval Islam," a website maintained by the College of Queen Mary, University of London: <http://www2.history.qmul.ac.uk/ruralsocietyislam/index.html> [accessed October 11, 2014]. It includes a very useful quantitative tool which documents al-Nābulusī's financial information for the Fayyum in the thirteenth century, and the spreadsheet of "Demographic Information" includes the shovel levy, which researchers Rappaport and Shahar suggest using as a relative indicator of population. The levies, in number

siltation buildup in the irrigation supply (*sawq*) and drainage (*maṣraf*) canals, whether they were flood canals (*nīlī*) or perennial canals (*ṣayfī*), took up a huge amount of time and heavy labor. Rates of siltation varied widely, and were often anywhere between 0.5 to 1.5 meters per year (Willcocks 1913, 1: 320). Considering that there were probably well over a hundred *sultani* canals for Lower Egypt, and at least half as many for Upper Egypt, it is easy to see how the dredging of all of this silt made for a very heavy manpower requirement (Willcocks 1913, 1: 329).[9] The second task, equally daunting, was to repair the dikes (*jusūr*) that had been cut/broken (*qaṭa'*) to let water in and out in the flood season. This process, the *shāqq*, involved rebuilding the dikes, usually with a material known as *labsh* (approximately, a mixture of mud and straw) (Abū Zayd 1987: 64). The places where cuts and breaches in the dikes had been made and then mended were known as *quṭū'* and formed irregular joints that gave these dikes a zig-zag pattern. The dikes, like the canals, amounted to a very substantial volume of earthwork, and some of them could be as much as 20 kilometers in length (see **Table 5**).

These tasks ate up a lot of man-days (irrigation laborers were all male). One medieval source estimates that the shoring up of dike breaches (*maqāṭi*: made to let water into the basins)—and presumably repairs to flood damage elsewhere along the dike—required the labor of about a hundred men and fifty oxen with *jarārīf* (shovels) and *miḥārīth* (plows) for five months (Baḥr 1999: 50–51). Medieval records also indicate that the number of *sultani* dikes in the Delta numbered in the several hundreds. From these sources, we can estimate something on the order of 350 *sultani* dikes in the Delta. This (350 × 100 laborers) would account

---

of *qiṭa'*, vary from a low of .083 for one village to a high of 9 for a particularly large village. The average for the Fayyum is 1.16 and the sum total 104.66. Al-Nābulusī also discusses an instance where a hundred *jarrāfa* (*qiṭa'*) were levied from the Fayyum as a whole, with ninety-five being the number actually collected. Other totals are found in numerous sources. One example is two hundred *qiṭa'* levied for the construction of the Jisr Shībīn in Qalyūbiyya in the early 1300s, a job that cost about 60,000 gold dinars, employed 12,000 in labor, and lasted three months. So 1 *qiṭa'* of *jarrāfa* was presumably a fairly substantial amount by itself. For detail on the Jisr Shībīn, see al-Maqrīzī (*al-Sulūk*, 2: 466–67).

9 Even with half of Upper Egypt's arable given over to perennial irrigation, there were still forty-five major flood canals in use, and presumably all of these would have been classified as *sultani* in the medieval period, as they each seemed to have served more than one village. Given that, one should double the figure to forty-two for Upper Egypt. And then, given that Lower Egypt had a much higher density of irrigation components, it is easy to see why something well in excess of a hundred would be reasonable.

Table 5. Dike Lengths and Volume of Earthwork[10]

Locale	Name of Dike	Length (m)	Total Volume of Earthwork (m^3)
Al-Minyā	Ṭahnashāwī	23,450	592,196
Mallawi	Kudyah	14,000	1,376,000
Asyūṭ	Donhea	8750	175,000
Manfalūt	Banī Kalb	17,500	551,638
Manfalūt	Maharriq	17,500	551,638
Girgā	Manshīyah	15,750	1,935,000
Upper Egypt	Annual	183,390	11,999,208

for half of the 70,000 men required for work in the Delta, with canal-dredging probably requiring another 35,000 men. Again, these estimates are not intended to be exact, but rather to approximate the scale and scope of manpower. The nineteenth-century data provides a very important cross-reference, with figures ranging from 95,000 to 150,000 men at work for 100 to 150 days, suggesting the validity of these medieval numbers. Egyptian flood dikes were enormous, and the data on dikes from the 1800s (**Table 5**) give a good idea of the volume of earthwork that medieval Egyptians accomplished every spring. The figures in the table are a guide to the dimensions of spring reconstruction.

When the manpower capacity, the volume moved per man-day (which averaged about 1 to 1.5 meters cubed), is applied to these figures, we see again that the total labor requirements were imposing and would easily add up to the 120,000 estimated by the medieval sources. Medieval accounts also match these dike figures in terms of length, total volume of earthwork, and man-days employed.

What this means, for our purposes, is that the decay of this labor-intensive system was a very likely result of the scarcity of rural labor caused by plague mortality. There were, moreover, a number of contributing factors that greatly intensified the irrigation system collapse, and these appear to have been maladaptive responses to the economic shock of depopulation. Egypt's military elite played a role here: these elites, essentially synonymous with the urban landholding caste at this time, added to the crisis by forcing rents upward, coercing corvée in the place of wages, redirecting irrigation-system taxes to their own coffers, and in essence looting the rural economy (Borsch 2005: 42–60). These things added to the direct damage of depopulation and irrigation labor scarcity, making for a

10 Sources: Clot-Bey (1840: 473–74) and Rivlin (1961: 285).

poisonous combination of factors whose effects on the irrigation system became quite apparent by the early fifteenth century. Many witnesses of this period testify to these problems.[11] The encyclopedist al-Qalqashandī, writing in the early fifteenth century, notes that "in our times, the maintenance of the *baladi* (local village) systems are being neglected, and upkeep of the *sultani* (interconnecting) system has been limited to the most trivial repairs that have little impact on production." Furthermore, he continues, "the level of the Nile has, at many times, been as high as 19 or even 20 cubits, and despite this, the irrigation system does not provide adequate floodwater and agrarian production is weakened" (*Subḥ*, 3: 516).

Al-Qalqashandī's intention, in emphasizing the height of the annual Nile flood, is quite clear, and his meaning is echoed by several other contemporary chroniclers. The subject of flood heights was a source of endless anxiety for Egyptians whose prosperity rose and fell with the outcomes of the annual flood. The ideal flood level at this time was between 17 and 18 cubits (a cubit was a linear measure of .462 meters) on the upper end of the scale on the Nilometer: a stone pillar used to measure the Nile flood. The level celebrated by old tradition was 16 cubits, at which mark the flood was said to have reached fulfillment—or completion (*wafā'*)—at a point in the flood season, usually in August, when there was a public ceremony and the main canal (Khalīj Amīr al-Mu'minīn) was opened.[12] Above that, 17 to 18 cubits was regarded as a sufficient level for providing floodwater to the majority of the agricultural areas, whereas a level lower than 17 cubits might risk leaving areas under-watered and dry.[13] On the other hand, a level higher than 18 cubits, somewhere in the range of 19 to 20 cubits, was considered potentially dangerous: an overly high flood could wreak a lot of damage—to the irrigation system, and to villages and homes; an over-inundation could also drown a significant portion of the cultivable region (Ibn Iyās, *Nuzhat al-umam*, 88–89; al-Maqrīzī, *Khiṭaṭ*, 1: 60; Barois 2010: 24).

Clearly, then, al-Qalqashandī's narrative suggests that these quantitative rules have been changed: that a level of 19 to 20 cubits, far from

---

11 See al-Maqrīzī (*al-Sulūk*, 4: 564, 618, 646, 678, 709–10, 750–53, 806–09, 834, 863, 874, 903–04, 931, 950); Ibn Iyās (*Nuzhat*, 182); Ibn Taghrībirdī (*Ḥawādith*, 4:573); Ibn Iyās (*Badā'i'*, 5: 114–15); Suyuti (Husn, 2: 302). See also Petry (1994: 114–15 and 124–25).

12 Al-Maqrīzī (Khiṭaṭ, 1: 55); see also Abū Zayd (1987: 18) and Nāṣir (2003: 173). Traditionally, the flood was said to begin its rise on the night of the Feast of Saint Michael ('Īd Mīkā'īl), on the twelfth day of the Coptic Month of Ba'una (June 20).

13 Specifically, 12 to 13 cubits was considered dangerously low (Said 1993: 98).

providing too much water, was in fact not providing enough; despite high flood levels, much of the agricultural land was going dry. The Nile itself was not to blame, nor even the sediment that built up on the river bed, sediment that caused its natural crest level to rise every year. It was, in fact, the irrigation system itself that was causing the problem. When canals became silted up and blocked, floodwater was prevented from reaching the irrigation basins, even when the Nile level was far more than adequate (al-Maqrīzī, *al-Sulūk*, 4: 903). And when dams and weirs were in disrepair, floodwater was no longer being provided according to schedule. And of greatest importance was the role of the dikes. The Nile reached its peak in the Coptic month of Tūt (approximately September). When the flood was at or near peak, water was led into the flood basins.[14] The floodwater was then held in these enormous basins for forty to fifty days.[15] Any shortening of this time period would mean that the basins were insufficiently full for watering the winter crop. When the Nile began to descend in the Coptic month of Bābih (roughly October, in the fifteenth century), it was essential that the dikes held the water in as the flood went down (Willcocks 1913, 1: 307, 311). Any failure in the dike system (cuts in the dikes, holes in the dikes, breaches in the dikes) meant a failure to check this flow.[16] It meant that water would leak from the system before the proper time, and therefore meant a failure to irrigate the flood basins and a failure to provide adequate watering for the critically important winter crop.[17]

14 The schedule called for specific, targeted openings at different times, such as at Nawrūz (New Year's Day), on the first day of the Coptic month of Tūt (corresponding to September 12) and on the 'Īd al-Ṣalīb (the Festival of the Cross) on the seventeenth day of the Coptic month of Tūt (corresponding to September 29). See Abū Zayd (1993: 18–19) and Willcocks (1913, 1: 304).

15 The reported average time is forty-five days (Willcocks 1913, 1: 301). Other durations are also given (Barois, 2010: 25).

16 The management of the *sultani* system included provisions for watchmen who were assigned to monitor the canals and dikes carefully, to watch for any breaks in the dikes or problems with canals. See the roles of the *khufarā'* and *ḥurrās* in Ibn Mammātī (*Qawānīn*: 229). See also Cooper (1993: 229), Tsugitaka (1977: 333), and Abū Zayd, (1983: 13).

17 When flood was to be let into a confined area, the dikes were broken open. The places where they were broken open were called *quṭū'*. From the same Arabic root, we get the word for open ruptures in the dikes (*maqāṭi'*) that were repaired in the early spring. In the Coptic months of Ṭubih (January 10 to February 8) and Amshīr (February 9 to March 9), dikes that had been broken open in the early autumn, to let water in, were sealed up again using harrows (*jarārīf*) and mud mixed with straw (*labsh*). See Ibn Mammātī (*Qawānīn*: 244–45); see also Abu Zayd (1987: 17, 64–65) and Cooper (1973: 103).

In this instance, al-Qalqashandī indicates that this delicate process was not being observed. Damage to the system, failure to maintain and repair dams, dikes, and canals, was causing it to malfunction. The failure of the canals to supply the water, along with the failure of the dikes to hold the water in, was causing the basins to go dry. Hence, damage to the system was causing a very high flood level (19 to 20 cubits) to look like a very low flood level, leaving much of the agricultural land dry.[18] So in this sense, damage to the irrigation structure was not only wreaking havoc with the operation of the system, but also with the level indicators that allowed for proper control of the system.[19] Managers of the system, depending upon a traditional corpus of knowledge, thus might anticipate flood damage and respond accordingly, when in actual fact, the level of the flood was barely adequate. It is clear from this account that serious harm had come to the irrigation system.

By the early fifteenth century, irrigation system decay was apparent to all observers. Plague depopulation, coming in cycles for the last half-century, had been taking its toll, denuding the rural labor force of its numbers. The notes taken by Ibn Iyās in the late fifteenth century, coupled with those of other witnesses, suggest that the irrigation system in Upper Egypt had been gravely impaired by that time, and that the Lower Egyptian system had been affected in a similar manner (Borsch 2000: 137–39). Furthermore, the changes in the indicators—this confusion by which flood levels could no longer be read—is also palpable in the sources for this time. To know that serious maintenance was needed was one thing, but to realize that a traditional timetable, developed over centuries, was malfunctioning, was another thing altogether (Nāṣir 2000: 170). It was recognized that the time-tested ways of controlling the flood were now failing. There was also a sense that the traditional system of flood prediction had gone awry. During the flood of 1468, Nile officials were reputedly stunned when their predictions based on patterns of alluvial deposit failed for the first time since the Islamic conquest of Egypt in 640

18 If, for whatever reason, flood levels were too low, the impact of abandoned land could affect the afflicted rural areas for years. 'Abd al-Laṭīf al-Baghdādī' furnishes us with an account of the two years that followed a disastrously low flood in the year 1200, when the flood waters, "receded without the country having been sufficiently watered, and before the convenient time, because there was no one to arrest the waters and keep them on the land" (al-Baghdādī, *Kitāb al-'ifāda*: 253–54).

19 Openings and closings of the canals and dikes followed a very complicated and precise schedule set down in the *qawānīn al-riyy* (the rules, also called "logs" or "registers" for irrigation). See Ibn Mammātī (*Qawānīn*: 205–32) and al-Maqrīzī (*al-Sulūk*, 1: 61, 171). See also Cooper (1973: 397) and Thayer (1993: 123).

CE. Other events, such as the highly unusual crest of the river in 1479—arriving half a month early on the twenty-ninth day of the Coptic month, Abīb (August 6)—added to the general level of anxiety (Petry 1994: 123). For the year 1508, we are told that the flood surged "fifty fingers" (1.125 meters)[20] in a single day—and this apparently had happened only twice since the Arab conquest (Petry 1994: 123).

The magnitude of the crisis and the uncertainty it was causing thus loomed very large in the eyes of these contemporaries. It seemed to them that the Nile, as well as the irrigation system, could no longer be trusted. But as bad as the psychological impact may have been, the physical effects were of course more immediate—and bone-dry flood basins were not the only concern here, as level indicators went awry. It seems clear that episodes of destructive flooding made at least as much of an impression as did episodes of drought, involving, as these episodes did, the destruction of dikes that were caught in the flood's wake. One record from the year 1432 CE notes that "dikes were ruined and many lands drowned, and water rushed into many of the villages before the proper time (for filling the basins). Summer crops such as cucumbers, sesame, and indigo were all ruined—to the loss of thousands of dīnārs" (al-Maqrīzī, *al-Sulūk*, 4: 874). Just as broken dikes could allow floodwater to leak from basins before the watering was done, so too could they fail to hold back high levels of water, as they were designed to do. Hence, just as a high crest could still leave many lands dry, a normal crest could swamp low-lying villages with a torrent of water.[21] More distressing were times when these two curses were compounded, and a flood too high was also a flood too low. In the same year that a destructive flood was sweeping through and ruining villages in many areas, the opposite was occurring in other parts of the country: areas were being left dry by the absence of this same flood. Floodwater was surging in places where dikes failed to protect low-lying lands, and pouring out of areas where dikes were failing to retain water (al-Maqrīzī, *al-Sulūk*, 4: 874). The combination of the twin evils added to the sense of confusion and dismay.[22]

---

20 One finger on the Nilometer was 2.25 centimeters or 1/24th of a .541 cubit (*dhirā'*) (Allouche 1994: 88).

21 Ibn Iyās (*Nuzhat*, 88–89), al-'Asqalānī (*Taysīr*: 171), al-Qalqashandī (*Subḥ*, 3: 515), and al-Maqrīzī (*al-Sulūk*, 4: 806–09, 874). See also Barois (2010: 36), Abū Zayd (1987: 61), and Nāṣir (2003: 171–72).

22 Under these conditions, it seems likely that there were problems with salinity as well. The land category of *sibākh* was designated for areas that could not be cultivated due to high salt content: see Ibn Mammātī (*Qawānīn*: 204); al-Maqrīzī (*al-Sulūk*, 2:

Most witnesses seem to have been aware that these twin disasters of drowning and parching were connected to the underlying irrigation system decay. For the years 1432 and 1435, al-Maqrīzī (*al-Sulūk*, 4: 874) makes a clear connection between these problems and system damage and notes that the decay of the system was compounding and multiplying the natural vulnerability of Egypt's inundation agriculture. Chronicles of the fifteenth century are, in fact, replete with very specific examples of what went wrong with the system as it fell apart (Borsch 2005: 44). And system failure, when it occurred, could happen on a very large scale. Problems with the larger, interconnecting (*sultani*) system could have a profound effect not only on downstream villages, but on the local, village (*baladi*) systems, too. In the year 1428, for example, there was an enormous toll of damage. Disaster struck the villages of Zifta, Shubra, and their outlying areas and was blamed upon the neglect of the irrigation system maintenance. In 1477, the chronicler al-Ṣayrafī tells how major parts of Cairo were badly damaged by floods because of dike failure in the area (cited by Nāṣir 2003: 173). Separate reports from Ibn Ḥajar al-'Asqalānī and Ibn Iyās inform us that a major disaster occurred when the enormous *sultani* dike of the Baḥr Abī al-Manajjā failed and numerous downstream villages were drowned by floodwater. And violent flood surges, intimidating during times when the system was functioning well, became catastrophic as the system fell apart.[23] Frequently, large sections of the *baladi* system were taken down as parts of the *sultani* system failed. This is hardly surprising, bearing in mind that the *sultani* dikes and canals were just as important for protecting the *baladi* system from water as they were for supplying it. The vulnerability of the *baladi* system meant that

130, 166); see also Tsugitaka (1977: 230) and Cooper (1973: 33, 37). Willcocks (1913, 1: 308) says that "If the distribution is bad [...] some basins receive little but sand, others have far more than their share of rich mud, and the greater part have nothing but the finest particles of mud with a large proportion of salts; especially is this the case where white water has stood for any length of time without any perceptible flow."

23 It is important that one visualize the flow dynamics of the system. A flood which might only be 2 meters above the ground can wreak major havoc when a large volume of the water is penned back by a major dike. Julien Barois (2010: 33), observing the system in the nineteenth century, noted that "when one of these dikes becomes broken by the pressure of the water, great havoc may result, because in general the level of the flood much exceeds that of the riparian lands, and especially in certain parts of the Delta the high water reaches normally 2 meters above the soil of the valley." Some *sultani* dikes were of huge proportions. One dike in the suburbs of Cairo was 16 meters high and built to a depth of 32 meters. See Tsugitaka (1977: 229–30). So too would depressions created by ruined canals pen up water, where it could apply stress to already weakened dikes.

Table 6. Estimated Agrarian Production over Time

Year (CE)	Agrarian Output (1315 = 1)	Source
1315	1.00	Borsch (2005: 77)
1400	0.50	Extrapolated from treasury figures (Ibin Shahīn, *Zubdat*: 107)
1410	0.45	Mujani (2008: 1113)
1517	0.42	Borsch (2005: 80–88)
1528	0.36	Michel (2002 : 197–251)
1597	0.45	Borsch (2005: 80–88)

sections would go down like dominos, the failure of one set of basin dikes meaning that the entire chain, as many as eight basins in length, would be threatened with collapse (Borsch 2000: 459–60).

Problems appeared at intervals. Calm could prevail for decades only to be suddenly followed by catastrophic and unpredictable crashes of whole segments of the system.[24] This cycle seems to have continued through to the end of the fifteenth century, and it had a number of effects on the wider economy, and not just the rural sector. It was in this context, we can say, that Egypt's irrigation system collapsed via a process of punctuated equilibrium (Borsch 2004: 461). Egypt's fifteenth-century irrigation system seems to have persisted in a state of slow change/slow neglect until sudden and dramatic episodes of regional collapse occurred. Each time the system's functioning was punctuated by an episodic crash, repair costs escalated and the task of restoring the system became significantly more daunting. By the end of the Mamluk period (1517 CE), Egypt's irrigation infrastructure had been largely ruined by the direct and indirect impact of plague depopulation. In addition to the evidence that we have from the fifteenth century chroniclers—and the data for irrigation labor—estimates of total agrarian production (**Table 6** and **Graph 4**) lead to the same conclusion.

Here, data points gleaned from sources composed in the course of the fifteenth century are supplemented by data from the early Ottoman era, which also recorded irrigation system decay. For example, the Ottoman land survey, conducted in 1528, offers data for the northwest Delta province of al-Buḥayra (**Map 3**), which allow us to compare the irrigation system's performance in that year with that of the 1315 land survey con-

24 Ibn Taghrībirdī (*Ḥawādith*, 4: 67), al-ʻAsādī (*al-Taysīr*: 92–93), and Ibn Iyās (*Badāʾiʿ*, 5: 114–15; *Nuzhat*: 182). See also Borsch (2000: 461).

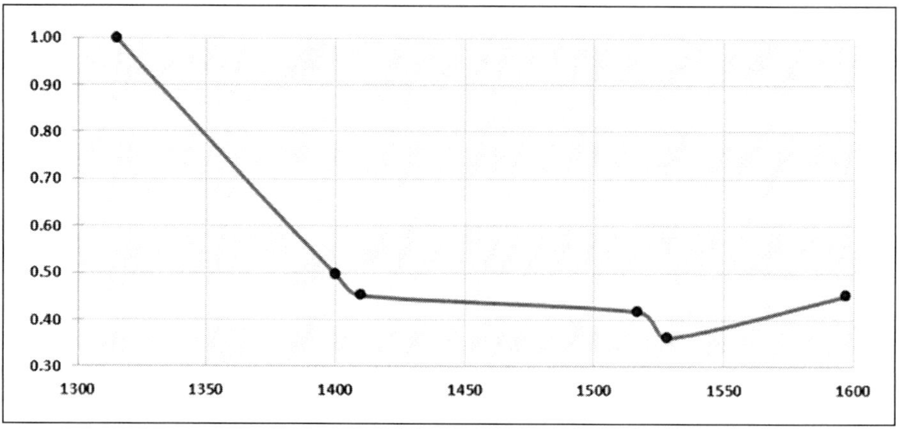

Graph 4. Estimated Agrarian Output of Egypt (1.0 = Land Survey of 1315 CE)

ducted when the Mamluk Sultanate was at its economic peak. The spatial patterns of decay (villages with little or no output on the downstream ends of the provinces' *sultani* canals) indicate system decay in excess of 60% (Michel 2002). If we look much further ahead, we find a scene of mortality and economic disruption that seems to resemble that of the fifteenth century. The death toll of the plague outbreak in Cairo, in 1791 CE, was one of the worst of the Ottoman period; it is evocative of the terrible 1430 and 1460 outbreaks, with peak mortalities of 1,500 and 2,000 deaths per day (Mikhail 2011: 221–23). Given the analysis above for the fifteenth-century outbreaks, it seems unlikely that these peak mortality rates were exaggerated; total death tolls for Cairo, reported as well over 50,000, are realistic. The city of Alexandria can serve as a special example of demographic catastrophe over this long term, its population dropping from an estimated 100,000 in the Mamluk era to some 6,000 to 8,000 by the early nineteenth century (Le Père 1818: 10; Panzac 1978: 85; Panzac 1987: 86-87).[25]

25 We do not have any reliable population data for the medieval population of Alexandria, but Mamluk-era figures for the number of silk weavers in the city give us a rough sense of the scale of population at this time, and two separate accounts provide estimates that are close to one another. If there were over 10,000 silk weavers in the late thirteenth and early fourteenth centuries (one report lists some 14,000 for 1380, another some 12,000 for 1295) one might guess that a very *minimum* population level might be reasonably close to 100,000, which would assume that a very high percentage of the adult (presumably male) population was engaged in silk weaving. But given the plethora of trades in Alexandria and other cities of the Mamluk Sultanate at this time, it seems unlikely that silk weaving comprised so high a share of the total working (again presumably male) population. 100,000 would be a minimum.

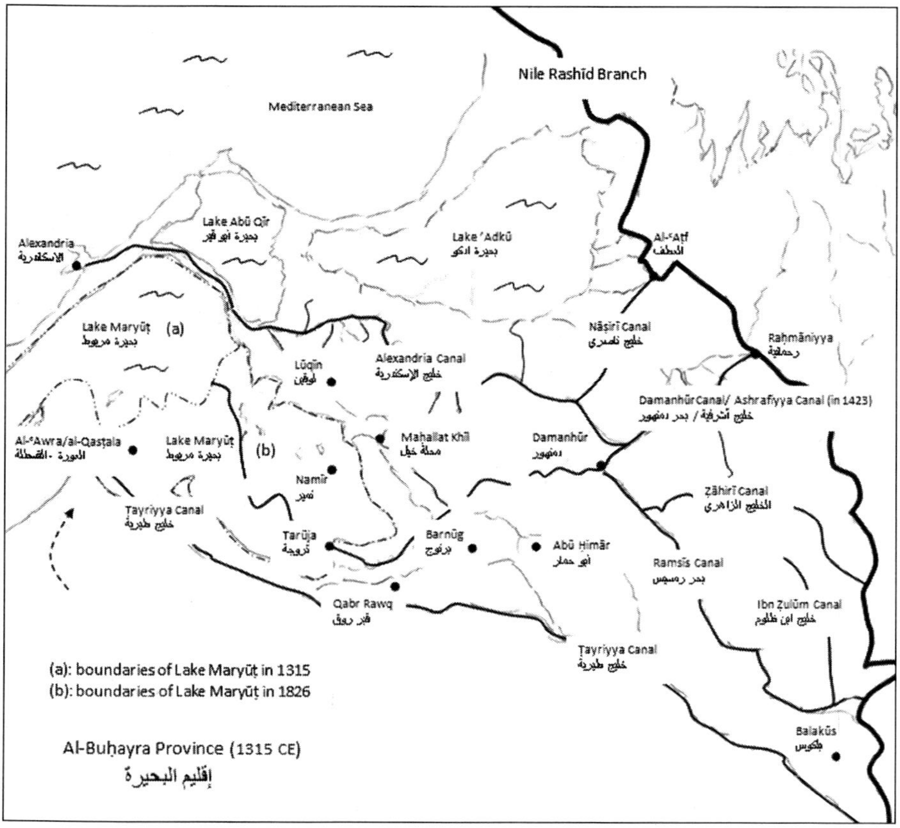

Map 3. The Province of Buḥayra Showing Sultani Canals.
Sketch by author after maps in Jacotin (1828).

An Agenda for Future Studies of Plague's Impact in Egypt and Elsewhere

The case of medieval Egypt calls for further examination of the irrigation system in a long-term perspective that includes the Ottoman period as well as the Mamluk era considered here; study of the early nineteenth century would provide a valuable comparison based on population figures as well as on land survey data. It also goes without saying that the impact of plague in the Middle East as a whole calls for much more attention, especially given its role in shaping the long-term divergence between the economies of this region and that of Europe. Indeed, this article's analysis of Egypt's demographic and economic response to plague outbreaks suggests that other irrigation systems might have been similarly affected. An agenda for future research would therefore include analogous systems like that of Mamluk Syria, Iran's network of underground canals (*qanats*), and the irrigation system of Iraq. Comparisons of irrigation systems could also extend to case studies of plague depopulation and its potential economic impact in South Asia (e.g., Sri Lanka) and East Asia as well. In addition to China's irrigation system, the flood recession economy of Cambodia's Angkor Kingdom is an especially interesting candidate for future research, precisely because Angkor's sophisticated irrigation network fell apart in the fifteenth century: an event suspect in its timing. This collapse has hitherto been attributed to its extreme complexity, but the study of population levels could suggest other causes.[26] Paying attention to changing irrigation economies, more broadly, could therefore help us to trace the impact of plague depopulation in world history.

Egypt's long-term response to plague-induced demographic decline proves that outcomes differed drastically from place to place, contingent upon dependent variables like social structure and environment. But there are other important lessons to be learned from future studies of plague in this area. For example, Egypt has the potential to teach us something new about plague's biology. After all, its experience with plague lasted for a very long time: it was still tormented by the disease in the eighteenth and nineteenth centuries. As Nükhet Varlık observes (2014, in this issue), a truly global approach to the study of this pandemic complicates the neat Eurocentric periodization of plague's history and must be factored into new narratives and future scholarly approaches. So what made Egypt's disease trajectory (and perhaps that of the Middle East as well) so different? My tentative answer would be that Nile flood geography and its influence upon insect and rodent vectors played a substantial role, and I propose this as another agenda item for future research (see Carmichael 2014, in this issue). Furthermore, it is worth considering how Egypt's mass graves, which we suspect were as plentiful there as in Europe, might supply bioarcheological data comparable to that derived from the East Smithfield cemetery of medieval London (see DeWitte 2014, in this issue). Egypt's famous aridity, and the process of desiccation that has yielded so many well-preserved bodies from antiquity, is an important factor here. Consider the multitude of sandy graves amid the two huge cemeteries (the *Qarafatayn*, they were called) ringing the eastern edge of Cairo. We might find a rich if grim treasure trove of evidence in some of these graves, soft tissue residue as well as skeletal remains worthy of careful study.

---

26 Theories range from war to environment to irrigation system complexity: Moore 1989; James 1995; Higham 2002; Penny et al. 2005; Stone 2006 and 2009; Chandler 2007; Evans et al. 2007; Fletcher et al. 2008; Kummu 2009; Buckley et al. 2010; Diamond 2011.

Bibliography

Medieval Sources

al-'Asādī, Muḥammad ibn Muḥammad. *al-Taysīr wa-al-i'tibār wa-al-taḥrīr wa-al-ikhtibār fīmā yajibu min ḥusn al-tadbīr wa-al-taṣarruf wa-al-ikhtiyār*, ed. 'Abd al-Qādir Aḥmad Ṭulaymāt (Cairo: Dār al-Fikr al-'Arabī, 1968)

Badr al-Dīn al-'Aynī, Maḥmūd. *'Iqd al-jumān fī tārīkh ahl al-zamān*, ed. Muhammad Muhammad Amīn, 4 vols. (Cairo: al-Hay'ah al-Miṣrīyah al-'Āmmah lil-Kitāb, 1987)

al-Baghdādī, 'Abd al-Laṭīf. *Kitāb al-'ifādah wa-al-i'tibār*, ed. and trans. John A. and Ivy E. Videan (London: Allen and Unwin, [1965])

Ibn 'Abd al-Wahhāb Nuwayrī, Aḥmad. *Nihāyat al-'arab fī funūn al-'adab*, ed. Saīd 'Abd al-Fattāḥ 'Āshūr, 33 vols (Cairo: al-Mu'assaa al-Miṣrīya al-'Āmma lil-Ta'līf wa al-Tarjama wa al-Ṭabā'a wa al-Nashr, 1964)

Ibn Ḥajar al-'Asqalānī, Aḥmad ibn 'Alī. *Inbā' al-ghumr bi abnā' al-'umr*, ed. Ḥasan Ḥabashī, 9 vols. (Beirut: Dār al-Kutub al-'Ilmiyya, 1969)

Ibn Iyās. *Badā'i' al-zuhūr fi-waqā'i' al-duhūr*, ed. Muṣṭstafá Muhammad, 5 vols. (Cairo: al-Hay'ah al-Miṣrīyah al-'Āmmah lil-Kitāb, 1982)

Ibn Iyās. *Nuzhat al-umam fī-l-'ajā'ib wa'l-ḥikam*, ed. Muḥammad Zaynham Muḥammad 'Azab (Cairo: Maktaba Madbūlī, 1995)

Ibn al-Jī'ān, Yaḥyā ibn al-Maqarr. *Kitāb al-Tuḥfa al-sanīya bi-asmā' al-bilād al-Miṣrīya*, ed. Bernhard Moritz (Cairo: Imprimerie nationale, 1898)

Ibn Mammātī, Al-As'ad. *Kitāb al-qawānīn al-dawānīn*, ed. A. S. Atiya (Cairo: al-Jam'īya al-Zirā'iya al-Malakīya, 1943)

Ibn Shahīn al-Ẓāhirī, Khalīl. *Kitāb zubdat kashif al-mamālik wa-bayan al-ṭuruq wa-al-masālik*, ed. Paul Ravaisse (Paris: Imprimerie nationale, 1894)

Ibn Taghrībirdī, Yūsuf. *Ḥawādith al-duhūr fī madá al-ayyām wa-l-shuhūr*, ed. William Popper, 4 vols. (Berkeley: University of California Publications in Semitic Philology, 1930–42)

Ibn Taghrībirdī, Yusūf. *al-Nujūm al-zāhira fī mulūk Miṣr wa'l-Qāhira*, ed. Fahīm Muhammad Shaltūt and Jamāl al-Dīn Shayyāl, 16 vols. (Cairo: al-Hay'ah al-Miṣrīyah al-'Āmmah lil-Kitāb, 1972)

al-Maqrīzī, Aḥmad Ibn 'Alī. *Kitāb al-mawā 'iẓ wa-l-i 'tibār bi-dhikr al-khiṭaṭ wa-l-āthār*, 2 vols. (Cairo: [printer unknown], 1853–54)

al-Maqrīzī, Aḥmad Ibn 'Alī. *Kitāb al-Sulūk li-Ma'rifat Duwal al-Mulūk*, ed. Muḥammad Muṣṭafā Ziyāda, 12 vols. (Cairo: Lajnat al-Ta'līf wa al-Tarjama wa al-Nashr, 1956–73)

al-Qalqashandī, Aḥmad ibn 'Alī. *Subḥ al-a'shā fī sinā'at al-inshā*, ed. Muḥammad Ḥusayn Shams, 15 vols. (Beirut: Dār al-Kutub al-'Ilmiyya, 1987)

al-Suyūṭī, Khalīl Manṣūr. *Husn al-muḥāḍarah fī tārīkh Miṣr wa-al-Qāhirah*, 2 vols. (Beirut: al-Maktabah al-'Aṣrīyah, 2009)

Modern Sources and Secondary Scholarship

Abū Ghāzī, 'Imād Badr al-Dīn. 2000. *Taṭawwur al-ḥiyāzah al-zirā'īyah fī Miṣr: zaman al-Mamālīk al-Zharākisah: dirāsah fī bay 'amlāk Bayt al-Māl.* al-Haram (Giza: 'Ayn lil-Dirāsāt wa-al-Buhūth al-Insānīyah wa-al-Ijtimā'īyah)

Abū Zayd, Muhammad Mahmūd 'Ali. 1987. *al-Nīl wa-Miṣr: dirāsah li-athar al-Nīl fī al-ḥayāh al-iqtiṣādīyah wa-al-ijtimā'īyah fī Miṣr min al-fatḥ al-Islāmī ḥattá muntaṣaf al-qarn al-rābi' al-Hijrī* (Cairo: Dār al-Hidāyah)

Allouche, Adel. 1994. *Mamluk Economics: A Study and Translation of al-Maqrīzī's "Ighāthah"* (Salt Lake City: University of Utah Press)

Ashtor, Eliyahu. 1949. "Prix et salaires à l'époque mamlouke: une étude sur l'état économique de l'Égypte et de la Syrie à la fin du Moyen Âge," *Revue des études islamiques* 17: 49–94

Ashtor, Eliyahu. 1969. *Histoire des prix et des salaries dans l'Orient médiéval* (Paris: S.E.V.P.E.N)

Ashtor, Eliyahu. 1976. *A Social and Economic History of the Near East in the Middle Ages* (Berkeley: University of California Press)

Ashtor, Eliyahu. 1977. "Levantine Sugar Industry in the Later Middle Ages—An Example of Technological Decline," *Israel Oriental Studies* 7: 226–80

Bacharach, Jere. 1971. "Circassian Monetary Policy: Silver," *Numismatic Chronicle* 11: 267–81

Bacharach, Jere. 1976. "Circassian Monetary Policy: Copper," *Journal of the Economic and Social History of the Orient* 19: 32–47

Bacharach, Jere. 1983. "Monetary Movements in Medieval Egypt, 1171–1517," in *Precious Metals in the Later Medieval and Early Modern Worlds*, ed. J. F. Richards, 159–81 (Durham, NC: Carolina Academic Press)

Baḥr, Majdī 'Abd al-Rashīd. 1999. *al-Qaryah al-Miṣrīyah fī 'aṣr salāṭīn al-Mamālīk, 648–923 H/1250–1517 M* (Cairo: al-Hay'ah al-Miṣrīyah al-'Āmmah lil-Kitāb, Far 'al-Ṣiḥāfah)

Barois, Julien. 2010. *Irrigation in Egypt*, trans. A. M. Miller (Washington, DC: Government Printing Office)

Bavel, Bas van. 2006. "Rural Wage Labour in the Sixteenth-Century Low Countries: An Assessment of the Importance and Nature of Wage Labour in the Countryside of Holland, Guelders and Flanders," *Continuity and Change* 21: 37–72

Beaumont, P. 1993. "Climate and Hydrology," in *The Agriculture of Egypt*, ed. C. M. Craig, 16–38 (Oxford: Oxford University Press)

Borsch, Stuart. 2000. "Nile Floods and the Irrigation System in Fifteenth-Century Egypt," *Mamluk Studies Review* 4: 131–45

Borsch, Stuart. 2004. "Environment and Population: The Collapse of Large Irrigation Systems Reconsidered," *Comparative Studies in Society and History* 46: 451–68

Borsch, Stuart. 2005. *The Black Death in England and Egypt: A Comparative Study* (Cairo: American University Press)

Bowman, Alan K., and Eugene Rogan (eds.). 1999. *Agriculture in Egypt from Pharonic to Modern Times* (Oxford: Oxford University Press)

Buckley, B. M., K. J. Anchukaitis, D. Penny, R. Fletcher, et al. 2010. "Climate as a Contributing Factor in the Demise of Angkor, Cambodia," *Proceedings of the National Academy of Sciences* 107, no. 15: 6748–52

Carmichael, Ann G. 2014. "Plague Persistence in Western Europe: A Hypothesis," *The Medieval Globe* 1: 157–191

Chandler, David. 2007. *A History of Cambodia*, 4th ed. (Boulder, CO: Westview Press)

Clot-Bey, Antoine Barthélemy. 1840. *Aperçu général sur l'Égypte* (Paris: Fortin, Masson)

Conrad, Lawrence. 1981. "The Plague in the Early Medieval Near East" (PhD dissertation, Princeton University)

Cooper, R. S. 1973. *Ibn Mammati's Rules for the Ministries: Translation with Commentary of the "Qawānin al-Dawāwīn"* (PhD dissertation, University of California, Berkeley)

Description de l'Égypte ou recueil des observations et des recherches qui ont été faites en Egypte pendant l'expédition de l'armée française. Atlas géographique. 1828. 2nd ed., France, Commission des monuments d'Égypte (Paris: Imprimerie de C. L. F. Panckoucke)

DeWitte, Sharon N. 2014. "The Anthropology of Plague: Insights from Bioarcheological Analyses of Epidemic Cemeteries," *The Medieval Globe* 1: 97–123

Diamond, Jared. 2011. *Collapse: How Societies Choose to Fail or Succeed* (London: Penguin)

Dols, Michael. 1977. *The Black Death in the Middle East* (Princeton, NJ: Princeton University Press)

Dols, Michael. 1979. "The Second Plague Pandemic and its Recurrences in the Middle East: 1347–1894," *Journal of the Economic and Social History of the Orient* 22: 162–89

Dols, Michael. 1981. "The General Mortality of the Black Death in the Mamluk Empire," in *The Islamic Middle East, 700-1900: Studies in Social and Economic History*, ed. Abraham Udovitch, 397–428 (Princeton, NJ: Darwin Press)

Evans, D., C. Pottier, R. Fletcher, S. Hensley, et al. 2007. "A Comprehensive Archaeological Map of the World's Largest Preindustrial Settlement Complex at Angkor, Cambodia," *Proceedings of the National Academy of Sciences* 104, no. 36: 14277–82

Fletcher, R., D. Perry, D. Evans, C. Pottier, et al. 2008. "The Water Management Network of Angkor, Cambodia," *Antiquity* 82: 658–70

Hennequin, Gilles. 1974. "Points de vue sur l'histoire monétaire de l'Égypt musulmane au moyen-âge," *Annales islamologiques* 12: 1–36

Hennequin, Gilles . 1977. "Nouveaux aperçus sur l'histoire monétaire de l'Égypt à la fin du moyen-âge," *Annales islamologiques* 13: 179–215

Higham, Charles. 2002. *The Civilization of Angkor* (Berkeley: University of California Press)

Igarashi, Daisuke. 2006. "The Establishment and Development of al-Diwan al-Mufrad: Its Background and Implications," *Mamluk Studies Review* 10: 117–40

Igarashi, Daisuke. 2008. "The Private Property and Awqaf of the Circassian Mamluk Sultans: The Case of Barquq," *Society for Near Eastern Studies in Japan* 63: 167–93

Igarashi, Daisuke. 2010. "The Evolution of the Sultanic Fisc and *al-Dhakhira* during the Circassian Mamluk Period," *Mamluk Studies Review* 14: 85–108

Igarashi, Daisuke. Forthcoming. *Land Tenure, Fiscal Policy, and Imperial Power in Medieval Syro-Egypt* (Chicago: Middle East Documentation Center)

Jacotin, Pierre. 1826. *Description de l'Égypte, ou Recueil des observations et des recherches qui ont été faites en Égypte pendant l'expedition de l'armée française. Atlas géographique dédiée au Roi*, 2nd ed. (Paris: Imprimerie de C. L. F. Panckoucke)

James, J. 1995. "Shuttle Radar Maps Ancient Angkor," *Science*, n.s., 267, no. 5200: 965

Kummu, M. 2009. "Water Management in Angkor: Human Impacts on Hydrology and Sediment Transportation," *Journal of Environmental Management* 90, no. 3: 1413–21

Le Père, Gratien. 1818. *Mémoire sur la ville d'Alexandrie* (Paris: Imprimerie royale)

Lopez, Robert, Harry Miskimin, and Abraham Udovitch. 1970. "England to Egypt, 1350-1500: Long Term Trends and Long Distance Trade," in *Studies in the Economic History of the Middle East*, ed. Michael Cook, 93–128 (London: Oxford University Press)

Louiseau, Julien. 2011. *Reconstruire la maison du sultan, 1350–1450: ruine et recomposition de l'ordre urban au Caire* (Cairo: Institut français d'archéologie orientale)

Meloy, John. 2001. "Copper Money in Late Mamluk Cairo: Chaos or Control?," *Journal of the Economic and Social History of the Orient* 44: 293–321

Michel, Nicolas. 2002 "Villages désertés, terres en friche et reconstruction rurale en Égypte au début de l'époque ottomane," *Annales islamologiques* 36: 197–251

Mikhail, A. 2008. "The Nature of Plague in Late Eighteenth-Century Egypt," *Bulletin of the History of Medicine* 82, no. 2: 249–75

Mikhail, A. 2011. *Nature and Empire in Ottoman Egypt* (Cambridge: Cambridge University Press)

Mikhail, A. 2013. "Plague and Environment in Late Ottoman Egypt", in *Water on Sand: Environmental Histories of the Middle East and North Africa*, ed. A. Mikhail, 111–32 (Oxford: Oxford University Press)

Moore, E. 1989. "Water Management in Early Cambodia: Evidence from Aerial Photography," *Geographical Journal* 155, no. 2: 204–14

Morberg, A. 1915. "Regierungs Promemoria eines egyptischens Sultans," in *Festschrift Eduard Sachau zum siebzigsten Geburtstage*, ed. Gotthold Weil, 406–21 (Berlin: Reimer)

Mujani, W. K. 2008. "Sources for the Economic Decline of the Circassian Mamluks in Egypt (872–922AH/1468–1517CE): Are They There?," *Islamic Quarterly* 52: 161–77

Mujani, W. K. 2011. "The Nile and Irrigation during the Mamluk Period (1468–1517)," *Australian Journal of Basic and Applied Sciences* 5, no. 9: 2264–68

Naṣir, ʿĀmr Najīb Mūsā. 2003. *al-Ḥayāt al-iqtiṣādiya fī Miṣr al "Asr al-Mamlūkī"* (Ammān: al-Shurūq)

Pamuk, Sevket. 2007. "The Black Death and the Origins of the "Great Divergence" across Europe, 1300–1600," *European Review of Economic History* 11: 289–317

Pamuk, Sevket, and Maya Shatzmiller. 2014. "Plagues, Wages, and Economic Change in the Islamic Middle East 700–1500," *Journal of Economic History* 74: 196–229

Panzac, Daniel. 1978. "Alexandrie: évolution d'une ville cosmopolite au XIXe siècle," *Annales islamologiques* 14: 195–215

Panzac, Daniel. 1987. "Alexandrie, peste et croissance urbaine (XVIIe-XIXe siècles)," *Revue de l'Occident musulman et de la Méditerranée* 46: 81–90

Penny, D., C. Pottier, M. Kummu, R. Fletcher, et al. 2005. "Hydrological History of West Baray, Angkor, Revealed through Palynological Analysis of Sediments from the West Mebon," *Bulletin de l'École française d'Extrême Orient* 92: 497–521

Petry, Carl. 1994. *Protectors or Praetorians? The Last Mamluk Sultans and Egypt's Waning as a Great Power* (Albany: State University of New York Press)

Popper, William. 1954–63. *History of Egypt, 1382–1469 A.D.*, 4 vols. (Berkeley: University of California Press)

Rappaport, Yosef, and Ido Shahar. "Rural Society in Medieval Islam: 'History of the Fayyum'" <http://www2.history.qmul.ac.uk/ruralsocietyislam/index.html>

Rivlin, Helen. 1961. *Agricultural Policy of Muhammad 'Ali in Egypt* (Cambridge, MA: Harvard University Press)

Sabra, Adam. 2000. *Poverty and Charity in Medieval Islam* (Cambridge: Cambridge University Press)

Said, R. 1993. *The River Nile: Geology, Hydration, and Utilization* (Oxford: Pergamon)

Schultz, Warren. 1995. "Mamluk Money from Baybars to Barquq: A Study Based on the Literary Evidence and the Numismatic Evidence" (PhD dissertation, University of Chicago)

Schultz, Warren 1998. "The Monetary History of Egypt, 642-1517," in *The Cambridge History of Egypt, Volume I: Islamic Egypt, 640–1517*, ed. Carl Petry, 318–38 (Cambridge: Cambridge University Press)

Schultz, Warren. 2011. "Recent Developments in Islamic Monetary History," *History Compass* 9: 71–83

Shatzmiller, Maya. 2012. "The Economic History of the Medieval Middle East: Strengths, Weaknesses, and the Challenges Ahead," *International Journal of Middle East Studies* 44: 529–31

Shaw, Stanford J. 1962. *The Financial and Administrative Organization and Development of Ottoman Egypt* (Princeton, NJ: Princeton University Press)

Shoshan, Boaz. 1983. "Money Supply and Grain Prices in Fifteenth Century Egypt," *Economic History Review* 36: 47–67

Silverstein, Adam J. 2007. *Postal Systems in the Pre-Modern Islamic World* (Cambridge: Cambridge University Press)

Söderberg, Johan. 2006. "Grain Prices in Cairo and Europe in the Middle Ages," *Research in Economic History* 24: 189–216

Stanley, D. J., and A. G. Warne. 1998. "Nile Delta in its Destruction phase," *Journal of Coastal Research* 14, no. 3: 794–825

Stone, R. 2006. "The End of Angkor," *Science* 311, no. 5766: 1364–68

Stone, R. 2009. "Tree Rings Tell of Angkor's Dying Days," *Science* 323, no. 5917: 999

Thayer, Jennifer M. 1993. "Politics and Power Networks in Ancient Egypt" (PhD dissertation, New York University)

Tsugitaka, Sato. 1977. *State and Rural Society in Medieval Islam: Sultans, Muqta's, and Fallahun* (Leiden: Brill)

Varlık, Nükhet. 2014. "New Science and Old Sources: Why the Ottoman Experience of Plague Matters," *The Medieval Globe* 1: 193–227

Ward, P. N. 1993. "Systems of Agricultural Production in the Delta," in *The Agriculture of Egypt*, ed. G. M. Craig, 229–64 (Oxford: Oxford University Press)

White, Sam. 2010. "Rethinking Disease in Ottoman History," *International Journal of Middle East Studies* 42: 549–67

Willcocks, William. 1913. *Egyptian Irrigation*, 3rd ed., 2 vols. (London: Spon and Chamberlain)

al-Zāmil, Muhammad Fathī. 2008. *al-Taḥawwulāt al-'iqtiṣ ādīyah fī Miṣr 'awākhir al-'Uṣūr al-Wusṭá* (Cairo: al-Majlis al-A'lá lil-Thaqāfah)

Stuart Borsch (sborsch@assumption.edu) is an associate professor of history at Assumption College in Worcester, Massachusetts. His primary field of research is the economic history of the medieval Islamic world. Among his previous works is *The Black Death in Egypt and England* (2005), a study aimed at explaining how plague depopulation produced different economic outcomes for two countries, Egypt and England. Whereas England was able to recover from the Black Death, it is clear that Egypt did not, and the root cause was the difference in social structure and landholding practices. Borsch now works on projects related to the Egyptian irrigation system. Most recently, he finished a piece on the history of the Alexandria canal during the medieval and early modern periods. He is also studying long-term changes in the irrigation system of the province of al-Buḥayra. Other recent work focuses on historical changes in the rural markets of Egypt and monetary disruption following the Black Death.

Abstract Starting with the Black Death, and continuing over the century and a half that followed, plague depopulation brought about the ruin of Egypt's irrigation system, the motor of its economy. For many generations, the Egyptians who survived the plague therefore faced a tragic new reality: a transformed landscape and way of life significantly worsened by plague, a situation very different from that of plague survivors in Europe. This article looks at the ways in which this transformation took place. It measures the scale and scope of rural depopulation and explains why it had such a significant impact on the agricultural infrastructure and economy.

Keywords Medieval Egypt, irrigation, plague, depopulation, economic decline, agrarian economy.

PLAGUE PERSISTENCE IN WESTERN EUROPE: A HYPOTHESIS

ANN G. CARMICHAEL

HUMAN PLAGUE OUTBREAKS occur after fleas infected with *Yersinia pestis* can find no other preferred hosts. Thus, plague is similar to the vector-borne infectious diseases that have been described as "spillovers," because humans are not directly involved in the primary ecological processes that govern pathogen persistence (McMichael 2010; Ostfeld 2011; Quammen 2012). Plague persists via transmissions within a population of reservoir hosts, such as Eurasian great gerbils and marmots. This hidden, silent stage of plague transmission is now called "maintenance phase" plague,[1] and involves only burrowing rodents and their fleas. Burrows provide protected microenvironments for temporary survival of both bacteria and flea larvae (Anisimov, Lindler, and Pier 2014; Wimsatt and Biggens 2009). The precise mechanisms and ecological triggers that cause a wider, explosive "amplification phase" of plague, when highly susceptible animals begin to die, are not yet fully understood (Gage 2012). Intensive laboratory and field research projects focus on events early in a "transmission shift": from ongoing flea-borne transmission within a maintenance host population to rapidly widening rodent die-offs, spread by many flea species (Buhnerkempe et al. 2011).

Today, several low-tech, early-alert surveillance systems teach people living near plague hotspots how to notice deaths among the rodents involved in plague amplification. Should the warning signs escape notice, laboratory and/or autopsy investigation of sudden human deaths in a plague-endemic region become the next-best alert that it is time to inter-

I owe an incalculable debt to Monica Green and Carol Symes, for their editorial interventions; to Fabian Crespo, Nükhet Varlık, and Michelle Ziegler for detailed feedback on various points of my argument; and to George Sussman for his very helpful suggestions and edits. During the earliest formulations of this paper, my colleague Ellen Dwyer provided critique crucial to my eventual argument; her comments at that inchoate stage proved invaluable.

1 The terms "sylvatic" or "enzootic" are still used to refer to plague transmission exclusively among animals. More uncommonly, maintenance phase plague is called "primary plague," and amplification (the spread to highly susceptible animal hosts), "secondary plague." On the shifting scientific terminology, see Gage and Kosoy (2005).

rupt plague's spread. The remedy in both cases is the same: using pesticides to kill the fleas and flea larvae in areas near human habitation or worksites (Dennis and Staples 2009; Duplantier 2012; Stenseth et al. 2008). *Yersinia pestis* persists because it can infect a wide range of fleas, many of which do not feed on humans (Hinnebusch 2010).

Environmental conditions that favor flea activity and replication are linked to plague amplification (Wimsatt and Biggins 2009; Adjemian et al. 2007; Davis, Calvet, and Leirs 2005; Keeling and Gilligan 2000). Indeed, *Yersinia pestis* evolved from its ancestor, *Yersinia pseudotuberculosis*, through the acquisition of DNA permitting the infection of fleas. Because *Y. pseudotuberculosis* is able to live and replicate freely, typically in water, it needs genes that allow it to utilize environmental resources as nutrients. The new species *Yersinia pestis* lacks such capacity: it is an obligate pathogen. Instead, flea-borne transmission permits *Y. pestis*'s survival, as well as its capacity to survive at the body temperature of fleas (26°C/79°F), a capacity which is conferred by two unique plasmids (i.e., DNA molecules within the bacterium, but separate from the DNA chromosome of the organism). Even though slightly over 90% of the DNA is the same in both organisms, the "extra-chromosomal" or plasmid DNA is essential to the extraordinary virulence of *Yersinia pestis* (Hinnebusch 2005; Keim and Wagner 2009; Eisen and Gage 2009).[2] Because most fleas are able to clear *Y. pestis* infection from their gastrointestinal system relatively quickly, evolutionary pressure selects for strains of plague that overwhelm mammalian immune defenses, ensuring high concentrations of bacteria in the bloodstream. When fleas feed on an infected mammal, most of these insects can become transiently infected, able to transmit the organism to a new mammalian host (Perry and Fetherston 1997; Stenseth et al. 2008; Suntsov 2012). In sum, knowing that the evolution and survival of *Yersinia pestis* depends upon conditions favoring flea replication and dispersal changes how we historians can approach the problem of plague's four-hundred-year persistence in Western Europe.

---

2 Many of the genes which *Y. pestis* shares with *Y. pseudotuberculosis* became "pseudogenes" serving no known purpose. Some of the novel virulence genes that *Y. pestis* develops after the flea bite are genes that block many of the systemic immune defenses that warm-blooded mammals deploy. These genes are turned on ("upregulated") at a temperature of 37°C/98.6°F. Similar to other emergent pathogens, *Y. pestis* lost or scrambled key components of the chromosomal DNA of the ancestor organism, and it acquired the two additional plasmids unique to the killer bacterium, possibly in separate stages (Hinnebusch 2005). Many of the functions new to *Y. pestis* related to flea-borne transmission, but some included virulence factors in mammals, particularly the ability to cause an overwhelming pulmonary infection (Price, Jin, and Goldman 2012).

Bio-historical interest in European plagues typically concentrates on the origins and nature of the disease that appeared in 1347. Secondarily, interdisciplinary interest once centered on the possible reasons for plague's eventual disappearance from Western Europe: a region that, for the purposes of this historical study, I will limit to medieval Christendom. Nicely summarized a generation ago by Stephen Ell (1984), plague's disappearance subsequently became a relatively less interesting locus of interdisciplinary debate. The best-supported arguments for plague's disappearance pointed to historical factors (such as modernization, change in interregional trade patterns, targeted public health measures) rather than specific identifiable biological or environmental changes in eighteenth-century Europe.

Until very recently, biologically oriented analysis of the cause, spread, and decline of plague outbreaks in Europe also focused on the habitats and habits of the genus *Rattus*, the species of rodents assumed to be fundamental to understanding medieval and early modern plague. Those who strongly supported the view that the Black Death was caused by *Yersinia pestis* (e.g., Benedictow 2004; Audoin-Rouzeau 2003), as well as those who equally vigorously opposed that view (Twigg 1984; Cohn 2002; Christakos et al. 2005), assumed that black rats and two anthropophilic fleas (*Xenopsylla cheopis* and *Pulex irritans*) were required for the spread of plague across Europe. The constraints imposed by the rat/flea model made the rapid temporal and spatial diffusion of human mortality in the Black Death epidemic of 1347–53 a site of intense historical debate. Benedictow (2004) concluded that plague could spread very quickly, "metastasizing" to settlements along rivers and roads, gradually diffusing into the agrarian spaces that surrounded towns: an argument consistent with some earlier work on British India. That is, passive redistribution of infected fleas and rats could infect sizeable populations of black rats (*Rattus rattus*) in cities, towns, and market centers.

My analysis assumes that many more mammalian and flea species were involved in plague maintenance and amplification in late medieval Europe, just as is the case today.[3] Now that we are sure that the excess mortality of the great mid-fourteenth century epidemic was caused by

3 Bolton's helpful, very recent (2013) essay appeared too late to fully inform my present research. I agree with his shift in emphasis to non-*Rattus* plague host species, and will not here repeat his important summary of plague transmission by fleas that do not become "blocked," a classic mechanism for plague described in Bacot and Martin (1914). Their work led to a long-standing assumption that one flea species, *Xenopsylla cheopis*, was the primary insect vector in plague epidemics.

Yersinia pestis, it is vitally important to understand the ecological features of areas where high levels of human mortality are discernible. Ecology is the study of interrelationships among all living organisms, as well as with their physical surroundings. This means that the anthropocentrism of familiar contagion-based diffusion analyses hinder our full understanding of the initial catastrophe. Contagion-based understanding of Black Death plague mortality tends to elide evidentiary lacunae, in order to claim that the epidemic was uniform, sparing only a few cities, towns, and regions. But given that *Y. pestis* has been identified as the primary cause of the overall pandemic, this molecular-archeological finding redraws the ecological and historical questions that we must now confront.

For example, the apparent speed of plague's spread across different European regions and within human populations has traditionally been calculated by mapping accounts that offer very little more than a brief allusion to an epidemic: these have been staple findings of the contagion-driven model of Black Death diffusion. Retheorizing and problematizing maps of Black Death mortality is therefore an important next step, as David Mengel (2011) has shown. Meanwhile, it is now evident that the initial mid-fourteenth century epidemic cannot be explained by appealing to a uniquely virulent emergent strain of *Y. pestis* at the time of the Black Death. The archaic *Y. pestis* DNA recovered from Black Death plague pits shows no significant genetic differences from bacterial strains of plague still extant today. Further study of the plague genome in its ecological contexts is consequently another important next step, as we try to understand "the genetic changes involved in [plague's] transformation from a sylvatic pathogen to one capable of pandemic human infection on the scale of the Black Death" (Bos et al. 2011: 506; and see Green 2014, in this issue).

But genomic and molecular-archeological studies cannot account for the initial demographic collapse and the lingering population stagnation that characterizes many areas of Western Europe in the century following the Black Death. We must look to other historical factors to explain mortality patterns, indeed, bringing to the foreground many that have long been a part of more complex understandings of the late medieval period. For example, DeWitte's analysis of Black Death victims buried in East Smithfield, London (2009, 2010, and 2014, in this issue), provides strong evidence that poor prior health status increased an individual's risk of dying during a plague epidemic. Recent syntheses of economic and demographic evidence suggest that the surviving population was *not* a more privileged one that escaped a Malthusian trap; epidemics and famines recurred, exacerbated by warfare in many regions. Borsch (2014, in this issue), meanwhile, analyzes the processes of social and economic collapse, undermining the stability of crucial infrastructures supporting urban populations. I find the global framework provided by Bruce Campbell's recent synthesis of northern hemisphere climate change to be most promising (Campbell 2010, 2011, 2013). Overall, I was inspired to focus on plague outside urban centers by Campbell's suggestion that the long secular decline in population numbers and overall population health during the period 1300–1800 CE are best situated in a wider ecological and climatic context.

With the knowledge that *Yersinia pestis* accounts for the dramatic mortality levels seen in the Black Death, we should expect that different localities would have experienced mortality crises of quite different dimensions. Yet historians of European plagues have shown a strong tendency to connect only the bigger data-rich dots, remaining unimpressed by patchy and problem-ridden evidence from rural hinterlands. As a consequence, a common claim is that plague became almost exclusively an urban phenomenon in Europe by the fifteenth century. (e.g., Alfani 2013). Renewed, detailed study of the paths and timing of recurrent waves of plague in Western Europe is necessary, given what we now know of the ecology of *Y. pestis.* Plague first spills over around a limited number of maintenance reservoirs, which are "heterogeneous at global, regional, and local scales" (Eisen and Gage 2012: 63). How, then, does it travel between rural areas, small market centers, and larger cities?[4] The papers by Nükhet Varlık (2014) and Michelle Ziegler (2014, both in this issue) offer detailed observations on amplifying rodent host species (Varlık) and the circumstances and locations in which flea "super-production" would have amplified flea-borne transmissions to susceptible mammals, including humans (Ziegler). Here I will direct attention to a remote region serving as habitat for a possible plague maintenance host.

Plague today is found on most, but not all, continents. It was eradicated from Australia by the mid-1920s but persists in both North and South America, in many regions of Africa, and across Eurasia east of the Black Sea. On continents where plague is found, reservoirs are heterogeneously arrayed: thus, transmission hotspots are discontinuous. Were there simi-

4 Not all waves of plague in Europe would have been generated by spillovers from remote maintenance foci. In an extraordinarily valuable case study of endemic plague in London, *c.* 1550–1665, Cummins, Kelly, and Ó Gráda (2013), show that plague persisted for up to a century in London, without requiring reintroduction of the pathogen from rural hinterlands or maritime commerce. A city the size of London (population *c.* 60,000 in 1550) would have supported a heterogenous population of *Rattus rattus* rodents, some surviving and resistant, others susceptible. When fleas could not find a nearby rodent host, however, humans would serve.

lar zones in Europe where plague could have been maintained in a reservoir host, readily amplified by fleas to involve susceptible wild rodents and lagomorphs (e.g., squirrels, voles, rabbits), and eventually extending to the infamous black rat (*Rattus rattus*) and/or human fleas (*Pulex irritans*) to cause a dramatic plague outbreak? My restudy of plague persistence in Western Europe begins with archival sources indicating that plague could have persisted in the southern Alpine region, in just such natural reservoirs. Europe's alpine zones are not often discussed in historical work on the Black Death and its recurrences, because research understandably centers on devastating late-stage zoonotic spillovers, the epidemics. Evidence nonetheless exists for plague in Europe's alpine uplands, suggesting a new approach to the larger story.

A Few Plague Deaths along High Mountain Roads, 1567

Milan's public health office, an impressive and extensive bureaucracy since the 1400s, systematically monitored plague cases on the state's northern frontier. Traditional Milanese plague surveillance evolved by concentrating on principal trade routes and nodes linked to the military boundaries of Lombardy, including those roads leading toward various Alpine passes (Pracchi 1971: 5–14 and 165–72). But surveillance over upper Lombardy collapsed during the half-century of horrors attending the "Italian Wars" (1499–1559), which subjected all of northern Italy to recurring food shortages, plagues, and pestilences (Mallet and Shaw 2012; Alfani 2013). Foreign troops repeatedly crossed the mountains into northern Italy, and often it seemed that plague came with them.

By the late winter and early spring of 1567, after hostilities had ended, public health officials in Milan resumed aggressive plague surveillance. According to a well-placed Dominican, Gasparo Bugati, they assumed that the city of Lyon presented the greatest danger of plague this particular year. Italian princes had fled Lyon after paying homage to the new Holy Roman Emperor in 1565. The following year, plague spread eastward over the Savoyard-controlled western Alps, ravaging areas involved in most transalpine commercial and communications networks. When Bugati published his massive history of Milan up to the year 1569, he believed that these heightened precautions proceeded from a constant fear of another catastrophic plague like that of 1524, the worst in living memory.[5] In that

5 "[. . .] partì di lungo pel timor della peste gia per queste parti principiata, e incrudelità poi per l'Alpi, che traversano la Savoia ne gli Suizzeri, & ne' Grigioni: tanto che in Chiavena, & per quei suo contorni morirono gi huomini de' dieci gli otto: cagione

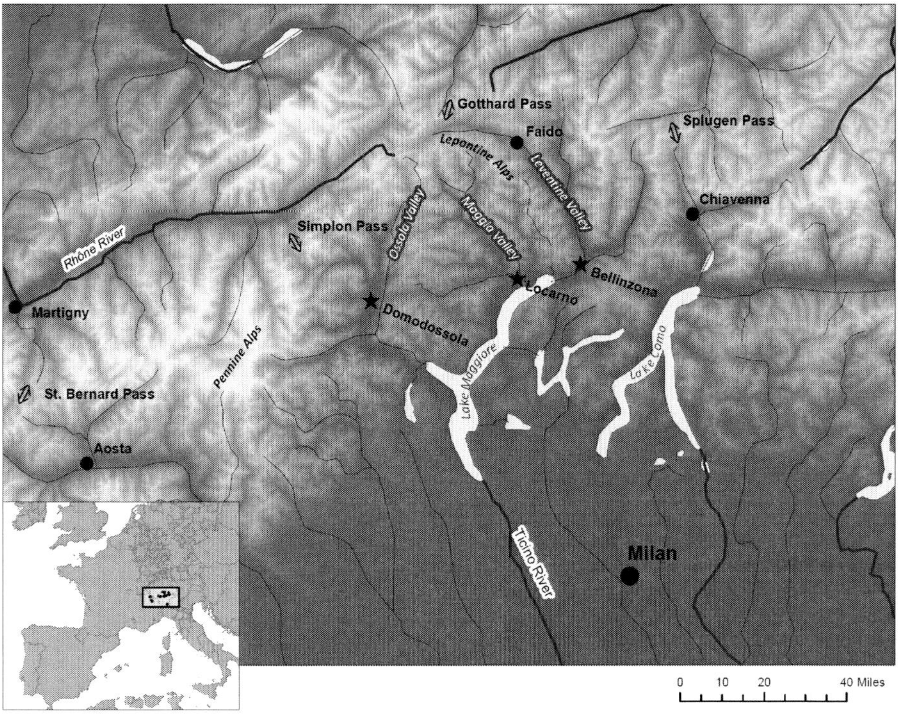

Map 4. Locales in the Southern Alps Reporting Plague Outbreaks to Milan (Spring 1567). *Map created by Theresa Quill for Indiana University Libraries, 2013.*

year, almost 50,000 had died, out of a population fewer than 100,000, and economic recovery was fitful, crippled further by protracted regional warfare (Bugati 1570: 1047; d'Amico 2012: 11–13, 33; Zanetti 1977).

From more specific surviving archival documents in the health office, we know that the Milanese expected that plague would funnel through the mountains. In 1567, letters sent in early spring from local officials in three southern Alpine market towns reported recent plague cases in hamlets to their north.[6] Although many of these Italian-speaking settlements can no

che à Milano si fecero strettissime guardie, come quello che ricordavasi della infinita strage dell'anno del 1524. passato, & si per questa diligenza, come principalmente per la pieta d'Iddio conservossi intatta."

6 All of the letters referenced here come from records of the Conservatori alla Sanità in the Archivio di Stato of Milan, p.a. [parte antiqua], n. 279: a box containing a bundle labeled *peste*. Unnumbered letters are cited by date. For example, a letter from Bellinzona, dated March 30, 1567, notes new plague cases in three settlements in the Leventina valley, one place named Tortengho (two deaths, two ill), another named Calpiogno (a woman died), and a third called Mairengho, where "some little children" had fallen ill.

longer be found on modern maps, the reporting centers are still important today. Domodossola, Locarno, and Bellinzona all had centuries-long ties to Milan, and informants in each town provided some details about each suspected plague case. The map locates principal places either named in these letters or relevant to itineraries by which travelers from Lyon would have reached Milan. These three mountain towns were vital to Milan's strategic and economic interests because they were situated on Ticino River tributaries that emptied into Lake Maggiore near Locarno, thirty miles west of Bellinzona. The Ticino reforms south of the lake, crossing the plains to meet the Po River.

Control of the Ticino River, which often served as a geographical boundary between Lombardy and the Italian Piedmont, was a vital economic interest to Milan during the Middle Ages. Milan's rise to power and prominence as a regional state capital was due to novel water-management strategies: because no great river ran through the city, its economic expansion depended on sustained innovative, hydrological projects, binding all these areas into a network of cities and regions with different local resources (Boucheron 2001). By the late thirteenth century, Milan became one of the richest cities in Europe, able to exploit the Alpine river tributaries within an already vast canal system. The famous *vie dei marmi*—the marble routes—brought great marble and granite stones, and the men who carved them, from the mountains to the cities (Soldi Rondinini 1989). Canals transported building supplies, meat, pelts and a steady infusion of immigrants from the Alpine regions (Grillo 1994). In the sixteenth century, migrants from the southern Alps still found work as porters and domestic servants in Milan; other hill-town people, including skilled artisans (e.g., stone masons), followed patterns established for centuries, resettling in the metropolis or living half of each year in each location (d'Amico 2012: 55). Alpine furs lined some of the Milanese gloves, bonnets, and caps which were sought after around Europe.

In 1567, plague appeared in different mountain valleys that were separated east to west by formidable peaks.[7] Not only would it have been nearly impossible, given the season and the distances, for these sporadic cases to be transmitted by human contact, the cases of plague show no

7 Many of the tiny places named in these letters had connections to Milan stretching back many centuries. Initially, the tie was to the distinctive Ambrosian Church of the earlier Middle Ages; much of today's Swiss Canton Ticino, still Italian-speaking, was once called the *vallate ambrosiane* (Ambrosian valleys). With the Visconti and Sforza *signorie*, they each independently established pacts and agreements tying them to the regional state of the fourteenth and fifteenth centuries: see Chittolini 1985.

straightforward movement of infection along one or another route from Lyon which humans could have used. To appreciate the significance of the archival evidence, some preliminary historical and geographical background is useful.

Bellinzona and Domodossola were (and still are) Italian-speaking centers that served travelers connecting to mountain passes, but the routes northward diverged significantly. The Gotthard Pass, 45 miles northeast of Bellinzona moving up into the Leventina Valley, was more frequently used by German-speaking merchants and migrants (Racine 2004). It led into the Uri Canton and the Reuss Valley, at the headwaters of the Rhine River. Domodossola (so named because it is at the head of the Italian Ossola Valley) instead connected Lombard travelers to the French-speaking Valais Canton, through the Great St. Bernard Pass. Heavily used since the early Middle Ages, the Great St. Bernard route linked Mediterranean Italy to the Low Countries and British Isles via the Rhineland. Many of the travelers (and armies) moving through the St. Bernard Pass and the Mont Cenis Pass (further to the west and thus not on the map provided) would more easily proceed south through Ivrea and Aosta, and to Turin and Genoa. In the mid-sixteenth century these cities and lands, today part of Italy's Piedmont province, were controlled by the counts of Savoy, and were not areas the Milanese could monitor easily.

A third major Alpine pass essential to Milanese trade was the Simplon Pass, just 41 km (25 miles) away from Domodossola. While closer to the town than was the route to the Great St. Bernard Pass, reaching the Simplon involved a steep climb into the Lepontine Alps. This was the most direct route if plague were spreading between Lyon and Milan by a series of contacts. Access to the Simplon route had been created by medieval Milanese merchants eager to circumvent tolls exacted by agents of the count of Savoy, in control of the western French Alps (Bergier 1997). The Simplon route followed the upper Rhône River as it passed by Martigny. From that important medieval hub, one would continue toward Geneva and alternate routes north through the Jura Mountains, toward Burgundy, Champagne, and Paris. By comparison, it was the longer, and in several ways more rigorous journey—especially as it presented various seasonal challenges—but the Simplon route did not necessarily entail higher transport costs. The Romans had not used the Simplon, and the Gotthard Pass and the St. Bernard Pass were also used more in the medieval centuries than in antiquity. (The Romans had instead cleared and exploited passes in the far western Cottian and Graian Alps, for the conquest and administration of Gaul.) During the later Middle Ages, Milanese trade thus steadily pulled the axis of transalpine communications eastward to the Central Alps (Frangioni 1983: 18–22; Ugolini 1985; and Bergier 1997).

The salience of these complex geographical features to the Milanese plague surveillance of 1567 is their connection with routes and passes along Ticino River tributaries. However, long before this time, larger ecological and political changes to the region had affected the entire southern Alpine zone during this period: changes that (as I argue) facilitated the establishment of plague maintenance foci. An historical ecology of Alpine-region plague cannot respect the political, linguistic, and social boundaries that have hitherto shaped most historical study of the past. Essentially, we should first understand that different Alpine passes threaded north-south traffic through different Alpine valleys, thereby passing towns and hamlets that may look close to one another on some maps, but were not actually in easy trading distance one from the other.

At the beginning of February 1567, health deputies in Locarno (situated between Domodossola and Bellinzona) relayed news of suspicious deaths in the Val Maggia. Two women had died suddenly, one of them with a *bugnone* (bubo) behind one ear. The officials wrote to say that they had implemented plague controls, but did not describe their actions further. In mid-February, a frustrated health commissioner in Domodossola independently complained of costly trade and travel restrictions, claiming that he had been on the lookout for plague for the previous three years, guarding the roads day and night. He expected that travelers from Lyon or Savoy would bring plague, but had no knowledge of events in Locarno. Two months later, a more detailed letter from Bellinzona, dated April 25, reported cases near a larger settlement in the Leventina valley, halfway to the Gotthard pass:

> The day before yesterday we wrote to you about some cases occurring in Faido in which we suspected plague. To be certain, we sent out one of our deputies and he provided a written report certifying that in this place of Faido a little boy died of plague, [and that he had also] discovered a man who had the disease in one armpit.[8]

Reassuring Milan's health office that they (officials in Bellinzona) had implemented appropriate procedures, they volunteered details of uncon-

8 Milano, Archivio di Stato, Conservatori alla Sanità , p.a., n. 279: "L'altro ieri una l[ette]ra. scrivessemo[...]le certi casi occorsi in Faido dubiosi di peste, et per sapper sicuramenti come era il fatto haveramo man[dat]ti uno de n[ost]ri Deputati al ritorno del quale fatta la sua rellatione che subito ne haressemo scritto la verità a quelle. Cosi è gionto detto n[ost]ro Deputato certificandone ch fa esso luogho di Faido è morto uno putto di peste, et uno huomo essergli scoperto tal morbo sotto una sella. ¶ Dipui che nelle Montagne d'esso luogho di Faido à quelli luoghi dove già muolt' giorni fa la peste anchor regnava fa progresso. Il tutto si fa per reguardarsi v[ostri] s[ignori]. . ."

nected cases in three tiny settlements where they found other presumptive plague cases; they verified oral reports by undertaking direct bodily inspection of the victims; then they prepared to receive district officials, dispatched by orders from Milan, to investigate the full extent of the infected zone.

From other reports this same year, the Milanese knew that the geographical scope of the plague threat was not limited to the Canton Ticino. During the spring and early summer months, the health office and even well-informed citizens received a steady stream of similar alerts from officials in Bergamo and mountain areas as far to the east as Trent. Plague menaced the Grigioni (Grisons), a German-speaking Swiss canton much further east, in a region connecting Milan to the Splugen Pass by way of Chiavenna.[9] Still other cases popped up along the roads that doubled back eastward into the Venetian Trentino. Plague reports coming to Milan from these areas further east included similar postmortem descriptions of confirmed plague deaths, but (with practiced facility) they blamed plague's spread preemptively on travelers or undesirable migrants, or on infractions to good order by smugglers, tax evaders, and delinquent watchers.

Thus in 1567, plague menaced Milan's Alpine fringe: west, east, and center. Yet specific trade and travel connections to the known plague in Lyon were elusive. Despite consistent and worrisome news, cities and towns of the northern Italian plains did not confront an epidemic later that year. From the end of winter into the summer, the Milanese authorities received and responded to plague reports. Spared the worst, they eventually filed away letters that required no further action. There is no evidence (at least in the box of papers now containing these letters) concerning how Milan's health office ultimately assessed these mountain-region plague threats. Considering the letters strictly as historical evidence, we know that the Milanese had mostly well-established routines of remote, rural-area surveillance in place by the mid-sixteenth century. The control that Milan could exert was impaired during the decades of war, but economic integration of upper Lombardy and the southern Alps had not been fractured either by warfare or the shift in political boundaries when the Canton Ticino became part of the Swiss Confederation. Officials

---

9 Bugati (1570: 1047): ". . . partì di lungo pel timor della peste gia per queste parti principiata, e incrudelità poi per l'Alpi, che traversano la Savoia ne gli Suizzeri, & ne' Grigioni: tanto che in Chiavena, & per quei suo contorni morirono gi huomini de' dieci gli otto: cagione che à Milano si fecero strettissime guardie, come quello che ricordavasi della infinita strage dell'anno del 1524. passato, & si per questa diligenza, come principalmente per la pieta d'Iddio conservossi intatta."

in the hinterlands were in the habit of reporting plague to the office in Milan, regardless of their transient political allegiances.

More detail about the diffusion of sporadic plague outbreaks through the southern Alps might lead us to a better understanding of the beginnings of the great epidemic that pummeled northern Italy later, in the 1570s. The point of this preliminary excursion is, instead, to show that early spring cases could not have been connected to one another by normal channels of human communication and interaction. All these routes, through high mountains and treacherous late winter Alpine climes, seem labyrinthine paths for plague to travel from one known-infected city, Lyon, to another large and vulnerable city, Milan.

Endemic Plague in Alpine Europe during the 1560s

Sporadic Alpine plague cases in the Canton Ticino illustrate that contagion-based transmission scenarios for the spread of plague do not map onto the evidence from 1567. The zone at risk was too wide, the known cases disconnected, the terrain too difficult, the season uncooperative. Contemporary with these Milanese records, archival evidence of endemic plague in other areas of Alpine Europe actually suggests plague *persistence* in this general region during the mid-sixteenth century and for at least a century before that. In the Haute-Maurienne, this evidence is illuminated by some extraordinary dramatic and artistic artifacts.[10] In 1567, a village near the northern outlet of the Mont Cenis Pass, Lanslevillard, orchestrated the performance of a traditional mystery play, the *Mystère de Saint Sébastian*, in honor of the saint frequently invoked in times of plague. This two-day dramatic event was probably based on a much older template (Symes 2011) scripted in the early fifteenth century, before the painting of the murals in Lanslevillard's chapel of Saint-Sébastien (1446–1518), which also document this village's long experience of recurrent plague outbreaks (see **Plate 2** on page 230). Other performances of plays dedicated to that saint were mounted elsewhere in the Maurienne in the mid-1560s, as they had been a generation earlier, when the plague last circulated there. Indeed, there is widespread evidence of many other artistic and theatrical responses to plague in this region (Leandri-Morin 1997). In a few instances, we have specific archival evidence to show that such performances fulfilled a community's prophylactic vow (made at a time when

10 The Maurienne follows the Arc river valley and connects Lyon to Turin across the Mont Cenis Pass, by way of Susa and the Susa Valley. Outbreaks here are typically explained by its proximity to trade.

plague raged) to honor the saint (Chocheyras 1971; Lebègue 1975). All of this evidence points to the plague's wide diffusion into the transverse Maurienne valley, as well as along the longitudinal ones of Canton Ticino.

Study of plague in an ecological zone such as the Alpine region is difficult. Historians tend to search for plague within a specific archive, a political domain, or urban setting. Many different kinds of boundaries—political, linguistic, religious, social, economic—frustrate attempts to gather and evaluate evidence from ecologically similar regions of Europe that sprawl across these boundaries. Thus, the rather limited evidence presented here can be usefully compared to that uncovered by William Naphy, mostly from Genevan archives, and by Edward Eckert, using principally south German parish records.

Naphy's research found that 1567–72 was the single worst plague interval in Geneva's history (Naphy 2002: 13–16, 18–19, 108–19, and 163). He initially wanted to understand why, from 1470 to 1530, records from the western Alps provided dramatically increasing reports of plague deliberately spread by "greasers" (*engraisseurs*). This accusation was a manifestation of the popular notion that plague could be transferred by oily substances, carried by persons who themselves did not contract plague (see also Preto 1987). Though similar fears of plague spreaders had emerged in the western Alps at the time of the Black Death (Guerchberg 1948; Arrizabalaga 1994; Cohn 2007), later medieval fear of plague-carriers in the western Alps coincided with a surge in witchcraft persecutions. Prior to Naphy's research, scholars had argued that witches and "greasers" were variant expressions of general popular anxiety during an age of rapid social and economic change to the countryside. After all, Geneva was still a small city (less than 20,000) that served as a refuge for displaced country people during the late fifteenth and early sixteenth centuries. Situated along the dangerous confessional fault lines of the Protestant Reformation, Geneva and its leaders had to discern heresy from superstition, even in plague times.

But contrary to his expectation, Naphy found that the fear of persons spreading plague was fueled by a gradual recognition that plague was endemic. Between 1470 and 1530, local plague epidemics increased, but Geneva's governing elite treated each outbreak as a new external threat. Accordingly, they applied costly reactive measures to each newly discovered case of plague. When their *de facto* approaches failed, they made little effort to stanch rumors that plague workers (nurses, launderers, gravediggers, barber-surgeons, and so on) were seeding new cases in order to hang onto their high, hazard-pay wages. By 1567–72, frustrated city managers finally adopted the more proactive, remote surveillance approach Milan had long taken. They began to treat plague as something flowing from the countryside all around them, not something deliberately spread in the city by persons hoping to sustain the plague. Accordingly, they spent money during quiescent intervals. They funded the retention of pest-house staff over winter months and required medical certification of cause of death. They applied sustained attention to the identification of new plague cases and put brakes on commercial ties between these people and places and the general urban community. After 1572, "greasers" finally became harder to find, and the plague seemed to release its century-long grip.

In a study focused on a region just north of the Alps, epidemiologist Edward Eckert (1996) analyzed parish death records that covered an eighty-year span, from 1560 to 1640. Mapping intervals of crisis mortality at the local level, he found two distinctive pathways implicated in plague outbreaks within the region. He argued that larger-scale trade corridors transmitted plague from maritime areas to southern, German-speaking European towns and villages. But once plague reached the interior, outbreaks moved around the entire region in pathways defining a "closed system": that is, without a new plague wave coming from the maritime epicenters. These internal cycles repeated every five to ten years. Thus, Eckert emphasized different spatial and temporal differences between local crisis mortality in the German-speaking regions north of the Alps (stretching from the Rhine river to today's Czech Republic) and the patterns of plagues that originated in European maritime cities. He argued that we should look at regional clusters of plague rather than study only focal epidemic outbreaks, and see that plague moved by "traveling waves" from one cluster to another contiguous cluster.[11]

Eckert parsed evidence from hundreds of parish registers, spanning a century and covering a generous portion of Central Europe, but focused entirely on Protestant records that provided no evidence of similar events in the Alps, Catholic Bavaria, or Slavic-speaking regions further east. His mapping of temporal plague patterns within larger regions is nevertheless quite valuable, because it helps us to see that plague outbreaks were neither random nor sporadic. (Lacuna-ridden documentation and uncertainties about the historical diagnosis of plague deaths can otherwise lend

11 The characterization of "traveling waves" comes from Adjemian et al. (2007): a historically interesting spatio-temporal review of the eastward expansion of plague from western coastal cities of the United States in 1900, from which it spread across the Rocky Mountains, and then extended as far east as Kansas. Within forty years, plague traversed 2250 km (nearly 1400 miles).

the impression that plagues followed no clear pattern.) Although Eckert's evidence is consistent with my hypothesis that Alpine plague foci existed, I question his assumption that plague had to be repeatedly reintroduced to the coastal cities of Western Europe in order to set these regional plague cycles in motion. In a subsequent evaluation of the factors leading to bubonic plague's retreat from Central Europe over the long eighteenth century, Eckert accordingly emphasized the decline of exogenous plague introductions to the maritime coasts in order to explain plague's eventual disappearance (Eckert 2000). Here, Nükhet Varlık's recent work on plague in the Ottoman empire makes untenable Eckert's backdated assumption that trade with Anatolia could have been the proximate origin of late medieval European plagues.[12] The path of plague spread in the fifteenth and sixteenth centuries instead moved the other way, from Venice and its hinterlands eastward into the Balkans and Black Sea littoral (Varlık 2012 and 2014, in this issue).

The Western Alps and Black Death Mortality

Interdisciplinary application of recent plague ecology to historical investigations of the Black Death requires a regional focus in addition to research at the global and local levels.[13] The southeastern region of what is now France is happily an ideal place to begin such inquiry. Those familiar with narrative histories of the Black Death—in particular, with Rosemary Horrox's collection of sources—know that striking accounts of the Black Death in Marseille and Avignon illustrate different aspects of the catastrophe than the accounts that we have from Tuscan and English sources. The magnitude of the demographic catastrophe and social disruption in Marseille has been well studied (Smail 1996; Michaud 1999). Similarly, a range of texts generated in and around the court of Pope Clement VI include staple Black Death accounts by the natural philosopher Conrad von Megenberg (Gotschall 2003); the physician Guy de Chauliac (1363/1997: 2, 119); and the musician Ludwig van Kempen, a close friend of Francesco Petrarca, writing in Avignon (trans. in Horrox 1994: 41–45). Petrarca himself had fled Avignon, taking refuge from the pestilence in the Vaucluse,

12 I am especially grateful to Nükhet Varlık for correspondence with me on this point, and her ideas on how altitude and Mediterranean ecology, as environmental determinants, might support possible Alpine plague foci. See her essay (2014) in this issue.

13 Here, as elsewhere throughout this essay, I use "Black Death" with temporal specificity, to refer to the singular epidemic wave 1347–53.

right at ground zero of plague's spread into the French Alps.[14] From the Provençal region broadly, including also southwestern France and northern Iberia, we possess the notorious written accounts of the early, widespread riots and massacres of Jewish communities (Cohn 2007; Foa 1992: 7–23; Nirenberg 1998: 231–49; Shatzmiller 1974; and Biraben 1975: 54–71), now further substantiated by the work of Colet and colleagues (2014, in this issue).

Plague seeped into these temperate alpine regions from early-infected Mediterranean port cities, moving toward Europe's upland interiors, high plains, and Massif Central. Alpine regions included the Pyrenees (linked to eastern Iberian ports), the Julian Alps (in Venice's hinterlands), and, above all, the maritime and western (French) Alps, where we have disproportionately more urban archival evidence of the plague's spread and social effects than elsewhere. The Apennine chain in Italy is also an alpine zone, but one characterized by a Mediterranean climate regime (Nagy, Grabherr, and Thompson 2003). I am limiting discussion here to the alpine region where we have substantial and diverse documentation about the Black Death, but Tàrrega (Colet et al. 2014, in this issue) and many other market centers in upland Iberia could illustrate a similar pattern of severe Black Death mortality in regional market centers connected to alpine zones (Emery 1967; Phillips 1998).

Historical evidence and contexts are as fundamental to the new interdisciplinary study of past plague as are the ecological and environmental determinants of regional plague amplification. Biraben's monumental plague history (1975) argued that plague's effects during the Black Death were not uniform, but instead varied according to the season during which the plague first arrived. Evidence subsequently wrested from the Savoyard archives confirms his observation. Such geographical variation in mortality experience is far more characteristic of the previous diffusion of *Yersinia pestis* than it is of human infection spread by contagion. Evidence of plague's incursions into Alpine Savoy is, for this time period, abundant, permitting some demographic study of Black Death mortality in rural hinterlands (Carrier and Mouthon 2002). At the same time, many different important social and political changes overlap the Black Death's

---

14 We do not know precisely when Petrarca was at his villa in Vaucluse. He was in Avignon until November 1347, when he left for Parma and Verona. He learned of the death (in Avignon) of the woman whom his love poems made famous (Laura) while he was in Verona, and was likely in the Vaucluse to finish his *Secretum* in 1349–50. That year, he went to Rome for the Jubilee and returned to the Vaucluse for the last time, 1351–53, before moving to Milan. See Kirkham and Maggi (2009: xix–xx).

diffusion through the western Alps: for example, the most brutal phase of the Hundred Years' War (Sumption 1990: 6–13) and the rising political and military career of the extraordinary young duke of Savoy, Amadeus VI, who created a transalpine feudal state (Cox 1967). From the late 1340s through the 1360s, the entire region was subjected to new stresses on local resources, primarily caused by demobilized soldiers coalescing into mercenary companies.

Given the number and variety of potential mammalian hosts for *Yersinia pestis* in these human-churned landscapes, it is reasonable to postulate the establishment of enzootic plague foci, although not with geographical precision. Thankfully, unusually detailed accounts of Savoyard district administrators allow historical reconstruction of the multi-century processes of the region's occupation, cultivation, and late medieval abandonment (Carrier and Mouthon 2010: 11–30 and 171–205). For example, we know from Savoyard archival sources that high mortality during the Black Death epidemic occurred in the *bailliages* of Chambéry, Chablais, Bugey, Bresse, the Viennois, the Maurienne, the Tarentaise, and in the Italian Piedmont, the Val d'Aosta, and the marquisate of Susa. Two especially useful social and demographic studies of localized Black Death mortality in Savoy show that plague mortality was greater in the surrounding countryside than in the towns, that the season at which the plague arrived affected the severity and duration of the epidemic interval, and that the Alpine population steadily declined in the fourteenth and fifteenth centuries. Gelting (1991) establishes that Martigny, an important market town connecting travel from either the Mont Cenis Pass or the Simplon Pass to Geneva, suffered rural population losses up to 45% during the Black Death. Andenmatten and Morerod (1987) likewise show that Black Death losses in hinterlands of larger centers—in their case, Lausanne and Geneva—were greater than within urbanized settlements. As I have already suggested, evidence from remote villages in the Maurienne indicates that these communities continued to struggle with recurrent plague outbreaks throughout the fifteenth and well into the sixteenth centuries.

A regionally integrated analysis of economic and ecological changes within the western Alps following the Black Death would be most welcome, since the many extant surveys concentrate instead on individual French *départements* or Swiss cantons. Even histories of the duchy of Savoy, which Amadeus VI transformed over the central decades of the fourteenth century into a transalpine state, are similarly fragmented along modern national divides (Vester 2013). For now, the storied version of some of the events commonly described in political and military histories of the region suggests that the Black Death accelerated a profound reversal and deterioration of human occupation of Savoy's mountain regions, with the disappearance of cultivation and settlements fundamental to Savoy's rise as a regional power during the twelfth and thirteenth centuries. We know so much about these rural areas because the young Amadeus's advisors moved quickly to stabilize his tax base and central administration, documenting revenue collections from both autonomous and comital landholdings in each castellany. The Count himself was busy exerting military power to keep the dynastic holdings intact. During the seven years between 1348 and 1356, when he had reached twenty-two years of age and made his first important diplomatic treaty, Count Amadeus traveled tirelessly with huge entourages, entailing all the horses and all the grain required to keep these large mammals well provisioned. Meanwhile, throughout the 1350s, mountain people in his domain had to forage for survival. Neither the stranded and hungry English and French soldiers from the Provençal wars, nor Amadeus and his retinue, would have confronted the protracted subsistence crises that locals endured.

Even where the plague did not strike directly, tax burdens multiplied and local environmental conditions deteriorated in the upland communities. In both Lombardy and Savoy, the most destabilizing reflection of larger climate change was the recurrence of crippling spring flooding (Tropeano and Turconi 2004; Bravard 1989).[15] Spring floods amplified the foliage of semi-arid Alpine valleys, thus feeding small rodents and providing abundant humidity for the replication and activity of their various fleas. In plague ecological field studies, this sequence is referred to as a "trophic cascade" (e.g., Salkeld et al. 2010, on changing vacillations of prairie dog populations).[16] The preconditions for a rural plague epizootic were amply supplied in the years surrounding the Black Death.

The Black Death did not affect all regions of Europe equally; even neighboring, or similarly situated, towns experienced quite disparate overall mortality. In analyzing the spread of the Black Death via spotty mentions of high mortality, some scholars have inferred equally catastrophic losses from comparable places where we have no documentation. We should

15 Important recent historical studies of multi-decadal climate change includes those of McCormick et al. (2012), for late antiquity, or Campbell (2011 and 2013), for the late medieval period; but neither focuses on the Alpine regions nor the great rivers that originate there. This is surprising, because climatologists today see global alpine regions as sentinel areas of large ecological change: see Allainé and Yoccoz (2003). Squatriti (2010) usefully couples written documentation of northern Italian flooding to climate changes of late antiquity.

16 One of the earliest mentions of Alpine marmots is in 1339, by a Benedictine prior imposing restrictions on peasants' hunting (Carrier and Mouthon 2010: 141).

resist this temptation. Filling in the map between localities where some evidence of plague exists is not without foundation when estimating the true costs of the Black Death pandemic in Europe, but we do need to exercise considerable caution when drawing conclusions about the in-between areas of these maps (Mengel 2011). Not unreasonably, tracing the path of plague in 1347–53 typically inspires careful researchers to follow waterborne and overland routes of human communications. Indeed, historians must usually follow human-generated sources, as I did in describing sinuous mountain back roads where the plague cases of early 1567 were located. But diffusion of *Yersinia pestis,* spreading via rodents and their fleas, does not replicate human itineraries.

The "Second Pestilence" of 1359–63

The lack of evidence for some places, such as Bohemia (which Mengel 2011 has studied), may not be evidence for the absence of plague during the 1347–53 epidemic. However, the dearth of Black Death evidence from urbanized Lombardy and especially from Milan, its capital, is differently problematic. We know from the famous account of Gabriel dei Mussis (trans. in Horrox 1994: 14–26) that Piacenza was severely infected, most likely as plague spread inland along the Po River. Piacenza was fewer than 42 miles south of Milan, a city of nearly 100,000 people. And yet secure contemporary evidence of the Black Death in Lombardy is almost nonexistent (Albini 1982: 14–17). Why would Milan and many other towns and cities to the north of the Po River, all of which were larger than most rural market centers anywhere in Europe and Britain, be spared a disease supposedly spread by contagion? Oddly, many historians accept the claim by a Florentine plague survivor, Matteo Villani, that Milan escaped catastrophic mortality in 1348–49 because its ruler took cruel and aggressive isolationist measures to board up infected houses when the first cases of the new disease appeared (e.g., Benedictow 2004: 95; Christakos et al. 2005: 215). While a few places in Milanese suburban districts reported epidemic outbreaks in 1350, during the high traffic caused by pilgrims to Rome this Jubilee year, no evidence of these outbreaks is unambiguously plague-related (Albini 1982: 15–16; Michaud 1998).

Instead, the first devastating plague in Milan and the major cities of Lombardy occurred in 1361–63 (Del Panta 1982: 118). Francesco Petrarca fled Milan in the late spring of 1361, as the city faced its initial experience with the catastrophic new epidemic. His son remained behind. Long disappointed by the young man's adolescent choices and limited achievements, Petrarca consigned his nuanced remorse to pages of a precious manuscript copy of Virgil which his own father had given him:

> Our Giovanni, born to my toiling and my sorrow, brought me heavy and constant cares while he lived, and bitter grief when he died. He had known few happy days. He died in the year of our Lord 1361, in the 25th year of his age, in the night between Friday and Saturday the 9th and 10th of July. The news of his death reached me in Padua late on the afternoon of the 14th. He died in Milan in the unexampled general devastation wrought by the plague, which hitherto had left that city immune from such evils, but now has found it and has invaded it. (Kirkham 2009: 5).

The other deaths Petrarca recorded in this manuscript are of those he loved most: Laura (in Avignon, April 1348, of plague); his closest friend, Ludwig van Kempen, also called Louis Heiligan (in Avignon, 1361, of plague), and his grandson Francesco, aged 2 years, 4 months (in Pavia, 1363, toward the end of a plague). Writing to Francesco Nelli, a favorite correspondent and a former tutor of his son, while he was still grieving for Ludwig, Petrarca dedicated his *Letters of Old Age* to his friend's memory:

> [T]his year [1361/62] has not only equaled but even surpassed the earlier one in many regions, especially here in Cisalpine Gaul, and has almost completely emptied along with many other cities the most flourishing and populous Milan, untouched until now by these disasters. (Petrarca 1361–73/1992: 1).

Many of Petrarca's other correspondents survived the initial wave of plague, only to die in the next epidemic. Francesco Nelli subsequently died of plague, in Avignon, in 1363.

Seen from the perspective of England or Florence, this "second plague" is often called the "plague of children," likely because a very large baby-boom generation dominated the population at risk a decade after the first epidemic, in those places where it had caused substantial mortality.[17] Otherwise, occurrences of the "second plague," and the places where it was severe, have received the muted acclaim consonant with its "second" sobriquet. Glénisson long ago observed that some areas in France's Massif Central were far more devastated during the 1360s plague than they had been at the time of the Black Death. Moreover, he traced the north-to-south overland itinerary of the second epidemic's spread, noting the substantially different pattern from the Black Death (Glénisson 1968; see also Albini 1982: 14–18 and 82). Plague's initial spread from the alpine and high upland communities of the western Alps, down to great metropolitan

17 New perspectives on population immunity, as discussed by Crespo and Lawrenz (2014, in this issue), are likely to change our understanding of how human populations adapt when living near plague enzootic foci.

centers such as Milan, seems most likely to have occurred during the second wave of plague, not the first, and this anomalous temporal-geographical evidence led me to locate persisting plague foci in a way consistent with modern plague ecology. This second wave of plague in Europe, as well as the even more neglected later European plague recurrences over the following centuries, may claim a greater importance in plague history generally if we reposition plague within larger ecological and environmental contexts.

The Alpine Marmot: A Potential Host for Persisting Plague in Europe

The western Eurasian alpine system is vast, and its temperate-zone mountains include the Pyrenees, the alpine groups variously referred to as maritime, western, south-central (or Italian), Julian, Dinaric and Carpathian, and the Apennines (Nagy, Grabherr, and Thompson 2003). All these mountain regions are connected to the Mediterranean climate zone, where undershrubs are prominent and winters are mild and wet. Undershrub vegetation survives better than forests in these fire-prone regions, and provides habitats for many nesting and burrowing rodents. Mild, wet winters support year-round flea activity, and all the way up to the high mountain pastures the fleas would have found a great variety of indigenous rodent and lagomorph hosts for plague.[18] The French Alps have a now-dwindling variety of likely plague-susceptible species, including lagomorphs (hares), sciuridae (squirrels), mice, dormouse species, voles, and both *Rattus rattus* and *Rattus norvegicus* (Ariagno 1976). Many other mammalian genera and species implicated in maintaining plague elsewhere also inhabit, or once inhabited, the southern and western European Alps (Armitage 2013).

Alpine regions linked to Mediterranean plague ports were therefore, I contend, ecologically ideal homes for the introduction and propagation of the plague bacillus. At the time of the Black Death, moreover, all these upland zones were under considerable ecological stress, both chronically (following centuries of intensive development of the uplands and alpine pastures) and acutely (due to destabilizing flooding events). The longer-

18 Generally, I rely here on a model for the spatial diffusion of plague epizootics offered by Davis et al. (2008). Full elaboration of the hypothesized movement of plague from coastal regions into the Mediterranean and western alpine hinterlands would require a separate study. Varlık (2014, in this issue) provides illustrative detail of the rodents inhabiting zones from the mountains to the great city of Istanbul.

term anthropogenic changes to land use and settlement are important to fold into our understanding of medieval history (Hoffmann 2014). Nicholas Carrier and Fabrice Mouthon (2010) have summarized ecological transformations in the French and Italian Alps during the medieval era, describing how these different, contiguous ecological regions became fundamentally connected through human activities. Beginning in the eleventh century, communities of monks vied with local lords and autonomous civilian communities for control of the use and access to high alpine pastures. Alpine meadows were given over to pastoral farming, not only to exploitation by transhumance, but (by the mid- to late thirteenth century) to the multiplication of permanent settlements in the high pastures and more extensive forest-clearing on slopes leading up to these pastures. Where pastoral activity was not easy, the peaks attracted new mining investments. Mountain peoples who once farmed lived much of the year very close to famine, scratching their meals from the ground.

Once these alpine communities were linked to the grain-rich plains, the extraction of mountain resources intensified; even more uplands were exploited for products which the plainsmen wanted in return. As beneficiaries of economic trade integration, people in the mountainous areas of Europe became ecologically bound to urban regions outside these zones, and cereals were staple imports to the region during the seasons when travel was easier. Over the colder months, the hunting of larger rodents and carnivore competitors (both for food and pelts or fur) had been common across the region since early Neolithic times, but remodeling the flora and fauna of the entire European Alpine region occurred only during the last millennium. Medieval monastic documents occasionally mention marmots (von Tschudi 1870: 750–69; Shopkow 2010: 242), which is significant (see below). As early as the 1330s, edicts indirectly refer to pressure on larger fauna of the region, when great feudal lords feared that the peasants could compromise their sport hunting (Blache 1922). Even more spectacular changes to the Alpine region's ecology and human settlement patterns occurred over the fourteenth through seventeenth centuries (Carrier and Mouthon 2010; Viazzo 1989).

In sum, diverse regional stressors and the creation of vital economic ties and new demands on high mountain pastures made an easier entry for *Yersinia pestis* at the time of the Black Death. The upland landscapes were fragmented by human occupation and early commercialized livestock rearing, here and there connecting commensal rodents to the fleas of a great many other plague-susceptible mammals. The precise mechanisms for a very rapid wave of epizootic die-offs during the Black Death epidemic remain elusive, requiring further research if the primary hypothesis presented in this paper—the existence of a suitable reservoir host for plague—offers a plausible model for plague persistence in Continental Western Europe more generally. If plague were well established in Europe's southern alpine region, the circumstances under which occasional early spring plague cases would occur—such as those suggested in the letters to the Milanese health office in 1567—can be readily imagined. Tilling and/or living in Alpine valleys might have brought the occasional subsistence farmer into contact with burrowing rodents, and if those hosts maintained plague infection, sporadic human plague outbreaks would have occurred (Ariagno 1976).

One candidate species for plague maintenance in the uplands would be the Alpine marmot (*Marmota marmota*), a highly social, burrowing, hibernating species that is a favorite of tourists in Switzerland today (Tomé and Chaix 2003). The species is closely related to rodent hosts of plague elsewhere in Eurasia (Allainé and Yoccoz 2003). For example, *M. marmota* is morphologically similar to the *M. bobac* species common in Kazakhstan, and to the Manchurian marmots (*M. sibirica*) made famous by Wu Lien-Teh's investigations of plague in Manchuria during 1910–11 (Summers 2011: 107–29). Marmot popoulations expanded during the last glaciation across the temperate Alpine zone (Zimina and Gerasimov 1973), but did not survive unmolested thereafter. Between 10,000 and 7000 BCE, early hunters rid the upper Rhone area of the western Alps (e.g., the Jura mountains) of marmots, ibex, and chamois. At the same time, intensified pasturage and resource extraction during the medieval era created new habitats for marmots within higher elevation forest clearings. Because the roots of trees make burrow-formation quite difficult, potential new marmot habitats were created when trees were felled or burned for increasing pasturage (Armitage 2013). Surviving alpine marmot colonies today inhabit the region above the treeline (altitude varies by Alpine location) along with two species of voles, but their steady disappearance is a much more recent process, further threatened today by global warming and by competition for the highest alpine pastures and slopes.

Human uses of Alpine marmots can only be documented over the last half-millennium. Beginning with the sixteenth-century naturalists, we have direct testimony of marmots being captured and kept as pets. Felix Platter, the famous Protestant Swiss printer of the early sixteenth century, briefly had a captive Valais marmot in his collections, as we learn from his daybook entries of the early 1560s (Katritzky 2012: 20). Tourists and travelers encountered marmot pelts, used for luxury bedding in nineteenth-century chalets (Raverat 1872: 14–20; Gayot 1889). Outside the mountain region, the rodent had already become a familiar performer in French cities. During the eighteenth and nineteenth centuries, mountain people from the one-time kingdom of Savoy migrated seasonally to France's cities and towns, desperately poor and eking out a winter living by offering services that lowlanders found either necessary or amusing—for example, sweeping chimneys, killing rats, or begging for pittances by entertaining passersby with trained ferrets and marmots, memorialized as the "marmotte en vie."[19] Because these economic migrants returned to the high meadows come spring, they were not seen as intrinsically dangerous, in contrast to feared, rootless vagabonds of the pre-Revolutionary period. Poster illustrations captured the quaint dress and humble activities of the Savoyards (Hufton 1972). European naturalists of the nineteenth century became fascinated with marmots as a hibernating species, reporting local knowledge of their habitats and the ease of extracting animals from their burrows soon after the first snowfall. Species-targeted exploitation accelerated on the eve of the so-called "Third Pandemic" of plague.

Epilogue: Global and Historical Perspectives on Ecological Change and Plague Persistence in Europe

The Alpine marmot was not necessarily uniquely responsible for plague maintenance in that region, as seems to have been the case with the Siberian marmot during the pneumonic plague catastrophe of 1910–11 in Manchuria. In most of today's permanent plague foci, *Yersinia pestis* can infect a local array of small mammals and their fleas. Although Suntsov (2012) argues that Eurasian marmot species, generally, were the original maintenance host for plague's evolution as a species, the burrow structure of great gerbils (*Rhombomys opimus*) has also made them candidates (Randall et al. 2005; Wilschut et al., 2013). As in regions of the globe where plague was newly introduced during the "Third Pandemic," a variety of amplifying hosts and their fleas would have promoted plague persistence in the Mediterranean and temperate Alpine zones during the second pandemic. Rather than focusing entirely on *M. marmota*, we should note the general characteristics of Alpine zones and the high meadowlands that marmots favor. Thus equally important would be the wide range of potential amplifying hosts common throughout the Alpine foothills and high massif regions of Western Eurasia, species that Varlık details in her dis-

19 For an eighteenth-century image of a young man with a trained marmot and what appears to be a street organ, see Claude-Louis Desrais, designer, "Petits métiers, cris de Paris," available online at <http://catalogue.bnf.fr/ark:/12148/cb40312379s> [accessed September 18, 2014].

cussion of rural plague transmissions (Varlık 2014, in this issue; specifically for the western Alps, see Allainé and Yoccoz 2003). In particular, the southern face of the Eurasian Alpine system, linked to Mediterranean climates and ecology, bears important ecological similarities to modern areas where newly introduced plague persisted. Grove and Rackham (2001: 11–65) emphasize common characteristics of "mediterraneoid" zones across the globe: a mosaic of landscapes, predominant undershrubs and savanna, steppes with more grasses than woody plants, warm wet winters, hot dry summers. Almost all of California, Chile, and, to a lesser extent, South Africa have regions comparable to Mediterranean uplands, and all became areas where plague established new, permanent maintenance foci during the late nineteenth and early twentieth century.

Temperate-climate alpine rodents better survive occasional bitter winters because snowfall is heavy, protecting the ground from sheet ice that impairs their survival. But whether many colonies could have survived the aggressive and prolonged winters during the Little Ice Age (roughly 1550–1830; see Parker 2013) is difficult to say. Early and late snowfalls could have shortened the reproductive season of most burrowing rodents, especially marmots, but the species could have survived and thrived if it were not targeted by hunters and hungry mountain dwellers. The historical evidence at present offers greater support for sustained habitat destruction and/or human-driven landscape alteration, profound since 1700 throughout Europe.

With or without northern hemispheric cooling during the Little Ice Age, the fauna and flora biodiversity of the Alpine and Mediterranean upland regions steadily declined, processes that continue today. By the time French and English investigators rushed to East, West, and South Asia to investigate outbreaks of plague in the 1890s, a world of plants and animals once commonly known in earlier centuries had disappeared. Europeans, including scientists, found the natural and human environments of the strikingly "other" colonial metropoles utterly foreign spaces a century ago. Was it also difficult for them to imagine that the humble black house rat—much less the ibex, chamois, badger, and bear of the western Alps—had once been fairly ubiquitous around European human settlements? In Britain, the aggressive use of rat poisons, from the 1680s on, may have cleared the way for the rat species dominant there today, *Rattus norvegicus* (Konkola 1992). At least as early as 1800, a few British zoologists had noted the disappearance of the "old English rat," which we now know was *Rattus rattus* (Burt 2006). But most plague observers in British India had no knowledge that the Indian or "tropical plague rat" was once a domestic species back home. A flea that renowned entomologist N. Charles Rothschild named *Pulex cheopis* in 1903, for the great Egyptian pyramids where he found it, became *Xenopsylla cheopis* within five years, its Greek- derived prefix (*xeno*) capturing its "foreign" status as an "Indian rat flea" ([U.S.] *Public Health Reports* 1907). But both *R. rattus* and *X. cheopis* once had a cosmopolitan distribution across Eurasia (McCormick 2003).

Today, the single most active plague maintenance focus causing human deaths is in the uplands of subtropical Madagascar, where a different flea genus (*Synopsyllus*) spreads plague continually among highland rodents (800 meters or more above sea level). *R. rattus* is the dominant species there, "found everywhere: in houses, villages, fields, and also in the forests," but hedgehogs, insectivores, and small mammals such as shrews and tenrecs help to amplify plague (Andrianaivoriamana et al. 2013: quotation at e2382; see also Rahelinirina et al. 2010, and Vogler et al. 2013). High degrees of poverty, the difficulty of recognizing atypical human plague infection, and insufficient governmental resources to apply to surveillance lead to high and persisting plague in Madagascar today: the consequences of which Michelle Ziegler's (2014) contribution to this issue makes clear. In other words, the famous British Commission for the Investigation of Plague in India (1906/07), used by many different historians of the Black Death (e.g., Cohn 2002; Benedictow 2004) might better reflect its imperial (European) historical context than the ecology of plague in the early twentieth century (e.g., Chandavarkar 1992; for French Indochina, see Latour 1988: 59–110; and recently Au 2011: 29–49).[20] Katherine Royer (2014) has shown how the observations of colonial physicians and surgeons (who had long lived and served in British India) were rejected or discarded by Bombay-based scientists from London. Hence, actual plague experience throughout the northern Indian subcontinent may need to be reconstructed historically, based on her work.

The historical moment of the Black Death introduced a highly virulent flea-borne pathogen to densely settled regions crippled by multiple economic and ecological stressors. A wide variety of potential plague hosts and vectors intrinsic to the Alpine regions faced a combination of climate-driven and anthropogenic destabilization in the years surrounding the beginnings of the great plague: massive spring flooding events, intermittent droughts, and high traffic of demobilized soldiers and camp supporters after the English victory at Crécy (1346). All were likely factors in the

20 Mathematician Nicolas Bacaër (2012) has even shown how the plague data generated by the 1906/07 Commission provides a misleading picture of the magnitude and temporal progression of the human epidemic on Bombay Island.

devastating and uncharacteristically rapid spread of plague between 1347 and 1349. Now that we know that mortality in this great, catastrophic epidemic was at least partly caused by *Yersinia pestis*, the study of plague history is not at an end; only a narrow and protracted debate about the presence of the plague pathogen has been resolved. An altogether different set of historical questions, prompted by the findings of modern plague ecology, must begin to bridge the local, the regional, and the global. Interdisciplinary historical study of evidence for prior global climate change, exemplified by Campbell (2010, 2011, 2013) and McCormick et al. (2012), seems to point a way forward.

Bibliography

Adjemian, J. Z., P. Foley, K. L. Gage, and J. Foley. 2007. "Initiation and Spread of Traveling Waves of Plague, *Yersinia pestis*, in the Western United States," *American Journal of Tropical Medicine and Hygiene* 76, no. 2: 365–75

Albini, Giuliana. 1982. *Guerra, fame, peste: crisi di mortalità e sistema sanitario nella Lombardia tardomedioevale* (Bologna: Cappelli)

Alfani, Guido. 2013. *Calamities and the Economy in Renaissance Italy: The Grand Tour of the Horsemen of the Apocalypse* (New York: Palgrave Macmillan)

Allainé, D., and N. G. Yoccoz. 2003. "Rodents in the European Alps: Population Ecology and Potential Impacts on Ecosystems," in *Alpine Biodiversity in Europe*, ed. L. Nagy, G. Grabherr, C. Körner, and D. B. A. Thompson, 339–50 (Berlin: Springer)

Andenmatten, Bernard, and Jean-Daniel Morerod. 1987. "La peste à Lausanne au XIVe siècle (1348/49, 1360)," *Étude de Lettres* 2–3: 19–49

Andrianaivoarimanana, V., K. Kreppel, N. Elissa, J.-M. Duplantier, et al. 2013. "Understanding the Persistence of Plague Foci in Madagascar," *PLoS Neglected Tropical Diseases* 7, no. 11: e2382

Anisimov, A. P., L. E. Lindler, and G. B. Pier. 2004. "Intraspecific diversity of *Yersinia pestis*," *Clinical Microbiology Review* 17, no. 2: 434–64

Ariagno, D. 1976. "Essai de synthèse sur les mammifères sauvages de la region Rhône-Alpes," *Mammalia* 40: 125–60

Armitage, K. B. 2013. "Climate Change and the Conservation of Marmots," *Natural Science* 5, no. 5A: 36–43

Arrizabalaga, J. 1994. "Facing the Black Death: Perceptions and Reactions of University Medical Practitioners," in *Practical Medicine from Salerno to the Black Death*, ed. L. García Ballester et al., 237–88 (Cambridge: Cambridge University Press)

Au, S. 2011. *Mixed Medicines: Health and Culture in French Colonial Cambodia* (Chicago: University of Chicago Press)

Audoin-Rouzeau, F.. 2003. *Les Chemins de la peste: le rat, la puce et l'homme* (Rennes: Presses universitaires de Rennes)

Bacaër, N. 2012. "The Model of Kermack and McKendrick for the Plague Epidemic in Bombay and the Type Reproduction Number with Seasonality," *Journal of Mathematical Biology* 64, no. 3: 403–22

Bacot, A. W., and C. J. Martin. 1914. "Observations on the Mechanism of the Transmission of Plague by Fleas," *Journal of Hygiene*, Plague Supplement, 3: 423–39

Benedictow Ole J. 2004. *The Black Death, 1346–1353: The Complete History* (Woodbridge: Boydell)

Bergier, Jean-François. 1988. "Territorio, economia e società nella storia delle Alpi," in *Le Alpi per l'Europa: una proposta politica*, ed. Edoardo Martinengo, 25–54 (Lugano: Jaca)

Bergier, Jean-François. 1997. "Le traffic à travers les Alpes et les liasons transalpine," in *Pour une histoire des Alpes: Moyen Age et temps modernes*, section II, 1–72 (Aldershot: Ashgate)

Biraben, Jean-Noël. 1975. *Les hommes et la peste en France et dans les pays européens et méditerranéens*, vol. 1 (Paris: Mouton)

Blache, Jules. 1922. "Les trappeurs du Vercors au Moyen-Âge," *Revue de géographie Alpine* 10, no. 2: 305–10

Bolton, J. L. 2013. "Looking for *Yersinia pestis:* Scientists, Historians and the Black Death," in *The Fifteenth Century, XII: Society in an Age of Plague*, ed. C. Rawcliffe, 15–38 (Woodbridge: Boydell)

Borsch, Stuart. 2014. "Plague Depopulation and Irrigation Decay in Medieval Egypt," *The Medieval Globe* 1: 125–156

Boucheron, Patrick. 2001. "Water and Power in Milan, *c.* 1200–1500," *Urban History* 28: 180–93

Bouquet, Jean-Jacques. 1963. "Quelques remarques sur la population du comté de Savoie au XIVe siècle d'après les comptes de subsides," *Revue historique vaudoise* 71: 49–80

Bravard, J. P. 1989. "La Metamorphose des rivières des Alpes françaises à la fin du Moyen Âge et a l'epoque moderne," *Bulletin de la Société Géographie de Liège* 25: 145–57

Bugati, Gasparo. 1570. *Historia universale [...] dal principio del mondo fino all'anno 1569* (Venice: Gabriel Giolito)

Buhnerkempe, M. G., R. J. Eisen, B. Goodell, K. L. Gage, et al. 2011. "Transmission Shifts Underlie Variability in Population Responses to *Yersinia pestis* Infection," *PLoS One* 6, no. 7: e22498

Burt, Jonathan. 2006. *Rat* (London: Reaktion)

Campbell, Bruce M.S. 2010. "Physical Shocks, Biological Hazards, and Human Impacts: The Crisis of the Fourteenth Century Revisited," in *Economic and Biological Interactions in Pre-Industrial Europe, from the 13th to the 18th Centuries*, ed. S. Cavaciocchi, 13–32 (Florence: Firenze University Press)

Campbell, Bruce M.S. 2011. "Panzootics, Pandemics and Climate Anomalies in the Fourteenth Century," in *Beiträge zum Göttinger Umwelthistorischen Kolloquium, 2010–2011*, ed. B. Hermann, 177–216 (Göttingen: Universitätsverlag)

Campbell, Bruce M. S. 2013. "The Great Transition: Climate, Disease and Society in the 13th and 14th Centuries," The Ellen McArthur Lectures, University of Cambridge <http://www.econsoc.hist.cam.ac.uk/podcast-campbell.html> [accessed January 9, 2014]

Carrier, Nicolas, and Fabrice Mouthon. 2002. "Extentes et reconnaissance de la principauté savoyarde: une source sur les structures agraires des Alpes de la Nord (fin XIIIe–fin XVe siècle)," in *Terriers et plans-terriers du XIIIe au XVIIIe siècle*, ed. Ghislan Brunel, Olivier Guyotjeannin and Jean-Marc Monceau, 217–40 (Rennes: Association d'histoire des sciences rurales)

Carrier, Nicolas, and Fabrice Mouthon. 2010. *Paysans des Alpes: les communautés montagnardes au Moyen Âge* (Rennes: Presses universitaires de Rennes)

Castelnuovo, Guido. 2000. "Centri urbani, organizzazione del territorio e vie di traffico nell'area alpina occidentale: Chambéry, Torino e le loro montagne (X–XV secolo)," *Histoire des Alpes* 5: 109–23

Chandavarkar, R.. 1992. "Plague, Panic and Epidemic Politics in India, 1896–1914," in *Epidemics and Ideas: Essays on the Historical Perception of Pestilence*, ed. Paul Slack, 203–40 (Cambridge: Cambridge University Press)

Chevé, D., and G. Boëtsch, 2007. "Image-source: un préalable iconographique à l'étude de toute représentation de la peste à l'époque moderne," in *Peste entre épidemies et sociétés*, ed. M. Signoli, 331–44 (Florence: Firenze University Press)

Chittolini, Giorgio. 1985. "Principe e comunità alpine in area lombarda alla fine del medio evo," in *Le Alpi per l'Europa: una proposta politica*, ed. Edoardo Martinengo, 219–36 (Lugano: Jaca)

Christakos, G., et al. 2005. *Interdiscipinary Public Health Reasoning and Epidemic Modelling: The Case of Black Death* (New York: Springer)

Chocheyras, Jacques. 1971. *Le théâtre religieux en Savoie au XVIe siècle: avec des fragments inédits* (Geneva: Droz)

Cohn, Samuel Kline, Jr. 2002. *The Black Death Transformed: Disease and Culture in Early Renaissance Europe* (London: Arnold)

Cohn, Samuel Kline, Jr. 2007. "Black Death and the Burning of Jews," *Past and Present* 196: 3–36

Cohn, Samuel Kline, Jr., and Guido Alfani. 2007. "Households and Plague in Early Modern Italy," *Journal of Interdisciplinary History* 38: 177–205

Colet, Anna, Josep Xavier Muntané i Santiveri, Jordi Ruíz Ventura, Oriol Saula, et al. 2014. "The Black Death and its Consequences for the Jewish Community in Tàrrega: Lessons from History and Archeology," *The Medieval Globe* 1: 63–96

Cox, Eugene L. 1967. *The Green Count of Savoy: Amadeus VI and Transalpine Savoy in the Fourteenth Century* (Princeton, NJ: Princeton University Press)

Crespo, Fabian, and Matthew B. Lawrenz. 2014. "Heterogeneous Immunological Landscape and Medieval Plague: An Invitation to a New Dialogue between Historians and Immunologists," *The Medieval Globe* 1: 229–257

Cummins, N., M. Kelly, and C. Ó Gráda. 2013. "Living Standards and Plague in London, 1560–1665," *Social Science Research Network* <http://ssrn.com/abstract=2289094> [accessed September 10, 2014]

d'Amico, Stefano. 2012. *Spanish Milan: A City within the Empire, 1535–1706* (New York: Palgrave Macmillan)

Davis, S., E. Calvet, and H. Leirs. 2005. "Fluctuating Rodent Populations and Risks to Humans from Rodent-Borne Zoonoses," *Vector-Borne and Zoonotic Diseases* 5, no. 4: 305–14

Davis, S., et al. 2007. "Plague Metapopulation Dynamics in a Natural Reservoir: The Burrow System as the Unit of Study," *Epidemiology and Infection* 135, no. 5: 740–48

Davis, S., et al. 2008. "The Abundance Threshold for Plague as a Critical Percolation Phenomenon," *Nature* 454, no. 7204: 634–37

Del Panta, Lorenzo. 1982. *Le epidemie nella storia demografica italiana (secoli XIV–XIX)* (Turino: Loescher)

Dennis, D. T., and J. E. Staples. 2009. "Plague," in *Bacterial Infections of Humans: Epidemiology and Control*, ed. Philip S. Brachman and Elias Abrutyn, 597–612 (New York: Springer)

DeWitte, Sharon N. 2009. "The Effect of Sex on Risk of Mortality during the Black Death in London, A.D. 1349-1350," *American Journal of Physical Anthropology* 139, no. 2: 222–34

DeWitte, Sharon N. 2010. "Age Patterns of Mortality during the Black Death in London, A.D. 1349–1350," *Journal of Archaeological Science* 37, no. 12: 3394–3400

DeWitte, Sharon N. 2014. "The Anthropology of Plague: Insights from Bioarcheological Analyses of Epidemic Cemeteries," *The Medieval Globe* 1: 97–123

Duplantier, J.-M. 2012. "Surveillance and Control of Plague," in *Yersinia: Systems Biology and Control*, ed. Elisabeth Carniel and B. Joseph Hinnebusch, 183–200 (Norfolk, UK: Caister Academic Press)

Eckert, Edward A. 1996. *The Structure of Plagues and Pestilences in Early Modern Europe: Central Europe, 1560–1640* (Basel: Karger)

Eckert, E. A. 2000. "The Retreat of Plague from Central Europe, 1640–1720: A Geomedical Approach," *Bulletin of the History of Medicine* 74, no. 1: 1–28

Eisen, R. J., et al. 2008. "Persistence of *Yersinia pestis* in Soil under Natural Conditions," *Emerging Infectious Diseases* 14, no. 6: 941–43

Eisen, R. J., and K. L. Gage. 2009. "Adaptive Strategies of *Yersinia pestis* to Persist during Inter-Epizootic and Epizootic Periods," *Veterinary Research* 4: 14

Eisen, R. J., and K. L. Gage. 2012. "Transmission of Flea-Borne Zoonotic Agents," *Annual Review of Entomology* 57, no. 1: 61–82

Ell, S. R. 1984. "Immunity as a Factor in the Epidemiology of Medieval Plague," *Reviews of Infectious Diseases* 6, no. 6: 866–79

Emery, Richard W. 1967. "The Black Death of 1348 in Perpignan," *Speculum* 42: 611–23

Foa, Anna. 1992. *The Jews of Europe after the Black Death* (Berkeley: University of California Press)

Frangioni, Luciana. 1983. *Milano e le sue strade: costi di trasporto e vie di commercio dei prodotti milanesi alla fine del Trecento* (Capelli: Bologna)

Gage, K. L. 2012. "Factors Affecting the Spread and Maintenance of Plague," in *Advances in Yersinia Research*, ed. Alzira Maria Paiva de Almeida and Nilma Cintra Leal, special issue, *Advances in Experimental Medicine and Biology* 954, no. 1: 79–94

Gage, K. L., and M. Y. Koysoy. 2005. "Natural History of Plague: Perspectives from More than a Century of Research," *Annual Review of Entomology* 50: 505–28

Gayot, Eugène. 1889. *La marmotte* (Paris: Firmin-Didot)

Gelting, M. H. 1991. "The Mountains and the Plague: Maurienne, 1348," *Collegium Medievale* 4: 7–45

Getting, Robert McC. 1981. *Balancing on an Alp: Ecological Change and Continuity in a Swiss Mountain Community* (Cambridge: Cambridge University Press)

Glénisson, Jean. 1968. "La Second peste: l'épidémie de 1360–1362 en France et en Europe," *Bulletin de la Société de l'histoire de France, Annuaire*: 27–38

Gottschall, Dagmar. 2003. "Scienza in volgare: Corrado di Megenberg e la peste del 1348," in *Filosofia in volgare nel medioevo*, ed. Nadia Bray and Loris Sturlese, 107–31 (Louvain-la-Neuve: Fédération internationale des instituts d'études médiévales)

Green, Monica H. 2014. "Taking 'Pandemic' Seriously: Making the Black Death Global," *The Medieval Globe* 1: 27–61

Grillo, Paolo. 1994. "Il richiamo della metropolis: immigrazione e crescità demografica a Milano nel XIII secolo," in *Demografia e società nell'Italia medievale: secoli IX–XIV*, ed. R. Comba and I. Naso, 441–45 (Cuneo Società per gli studi storici, archeologici ed artistici della provincia di Cuneo; Società italiana di demografia storica)

Grove, A. T., and Oliver Rackham. 2001. *The Nature of Mediterranean Europe: An Ecological History* (New Haven: Yale University Press)

Guerchberg, Seraphine. 1948. "La controverse sur les prétendus semeurs de la *Peste Noire* d'après les traits de peste de l'époque," *Revue des études juives*,108, no. 1: 3–40

Guy de Chauliac. 1363/1997. *Guy de Chauliac: Inventarium sive chirurgia magna*, ed. Michael McVaugh (Leiden: Brill)

Hinnebusch, B. J. 1997. "Bubonic Plague: A Molecular Genetic Case History of the Emergence of an Infectious Disease," *Journal of Molecular Medicine* 75, no. 9: 645–52

Hinnebusch, B. J. 2005. "The Evolution of Flea-Borne Transmission in *Yersinia pestis*," *Current Issues in Molecular Biology* 7, no. 2: 197–212

Hinnebusch, B. J. 2010. "Plague in the 21st Century: Global Public Health Challenges and Goals," in *National Institutes of Allergy and Infectious Diseases vol. 3: Intramural Research*, ed. Vassil St. Georgiev, 87–94 (New York: Springer)

Hoffmann, Richard C. 2014. *An Environmental History of Medieval Europe* (Cambridge: Cambridge University Press)

Horrox, Rosemary (ed. and trans). 1994. *The Black Death* (Manchester: Manchester University Press)

Hufton, Olwen. 1972. "Begging, Vagrancy, Vagabondage and the Law: An Aspect of the Problem of Poverty in Eighteenth-Century France," *European History Quarterly* 2: 97–123

Kacki, S., and D. Castex. 2012. "Réflexions sur la variété des modalities funéraires en temps d'épidémie: l'exemple de la Peste Noire en contexts urbain et rural," *Archéologie Médiévale* 42, no. 1: 1–21

Katritzky, M. A. 2012. *Healing, Performance and Ceremony in the Writings of Three Early Modern Physicians* (Farnham: Ashgate)

Keeling, M. J., and C. A. Gilligan. 2000. "Bubonic Plague: A Metapopulation Model of a Zoonosis," *Proceedings of the Royal Society of London, B* 267, no. 1458: 2219–30

Keim, P. S., and D. M. Wagner. 2009. "Humans and Evolutionary and Ecological Forces Shaped the Phylogeography of Recently Emerged Diseases," *Nature Reviews Microbiology* 7, no. 11: 813–21

Kirkham, Victoria. 2009. "Introduction: A Life's Work," in *Petrarch: A Critical Guide to the Complete Works*, ed. Victoria Kirkham and Armando Maggi, 1–31 (Chicago: University of Chicago Press)

Kirkham, Victoria, and Armando Maggi, eds. 2009. *Petrarch: A Critical Guide to the Complete Works* (Chicago: University of Chicago Press)

Konkola, K. 1992. "More Than a Coincidence? The Arrival of Arsenic and the Disappearance of Plague in Early Modern Europe," *Journal of the History of Medicine and Allied Sciences* 47, no. 2: 186–209

Latour, Bruno. 1988. *The Pasteurization of France* (Cambridge, MA: Harvard University Press)

Leandri-Morin, Marie-Pierre. 1997. "Représentations provençales et piémontaises de la vie de saint Sébastien : procédés narratifs et sources textuelles," *Mélanges de l'École française de Rome. Moyen-Age, Temps modernes* 109, no. 2: 569–601

Lebègue, Raymond. 1975. "L'ancien théâtre religieux dans les Alpes françaises," *Journal des savants* 3–4: 213–24

Little, Lester K. 2011. "Plague Historians in Lab Coats," *Past and Present* 213: 267–90

Lucenet, Monique. 1986. "La peste inspiratrice," *Bulletins de la Société française d'histoire de la médecine*, [proceedings of the meeting held on 25 January 1986], 49–50

Mallet, Michael, and Christine Shaw. 2012. *The Italian Wars, 1494–1559* (Harlow, UK: Pearson)

Malou, N., et al. 2012. "Immuno-PCR: A New Tool for Paleomicrobiology; The Plague Paradigm," *PLoS One* 7, no. 2: e0031744

McCormick, Michael. 1998. "Bateaux de vie, bateaux de mort," *Settimane di studio-centro italiano di studi alto medioevo* 45: 35–118

McCormick, Michael. 2001. *Origins of the European Economy: Communications and Commerce, AD 300–900* (Cambridge: Cambridge University Press)

McCormick, Michael. 2003. "Rats, Communications and Plague: Towards an Ancient and Medieval Ecology," *Journal of Interdisciplinary History* 34: 1–25

McCormick, Michael, et al. 2012. "Climate Change during and after the Roman Empire: Reconstructing the Past from Scientific and Historical Evidence," *Journal of Interdisciplinary History* 43: 169–220

McMichael, A. J. 2010. "Paleoclimate and Bubonic Plague: A Forewarning of Future Risk?" *BioMed Central Biology* 8, no. 1: 108

Mengel, David. 2011. "A Plague on Bohemia? Mapping the Black Death," *Past and Present* 211: 3–34

Michaud, Francine. 1998. "La peste, la peur et l'espoir: le pélerinage jubilaire de romeux marseillais en 1350," *Le Moyen Âge* 104: 399–434

Michaud, Francine. 1999. "Travail et mouvements migratoires avant et après la Peste Noire à Marseille," *Provence historique* 49: 367–83

Milano, Archivio di Stato , Conservatori alla Sanità, p.a. [parte antiqua], n. 279

Naphy, William G. 2002. *Plagues, Poisons and Potions: Plague-Spreading Conspiracies in the Western Alps, c. 1530–1640* (Manchester: Manchester University Press)

Naphy, W. G. 2002. "An Outline of Europe's Alpine areas," in *Alpine Biodiversity in Europe*, ed. L. Nagu, G. Grabherr, and D. B. A. Thompson, 3–12 (Berlin: Springer)

Nirenberg, David. 1998. *Communities of Violence: Persecution of Minorities in the Middle Ages* (Princeton, NJ: Princeton University Press)

Ostfield, R. S. 2011. *Lyme Disease: The Ecology of a Complex System* (Oxford: Oxford University Press)

Parker, Geoffrey. 2013. *Global Crisis: War, Climate Change, and Catastrophe in the Seventeenth Century* (New Haven, CT: Yale University Press)

Perry, R. D., and J. D. Fetherston. 1997. "*Yersinia pestis:* Etiologic Agent of Plague," *Clinical Microbiology Reviews* 10, no. 1: 35–66

Petrarca, Francesco. 1361–73/1992. *Letters of Old Age, vol. I*, trans. Aldo S. Bernardo, Saul Levin, and Reta A. Bernardo (Baltimore: Johns Hopkins University Press)

Phillips, William D. 1998. "*Peste Negra:* The Fourteenth-Century Plague Epidemics in Iberia," in *On the Social Origins of Medieval Institutions: Essays in Honor of Joseph F. O'Callaghan*, ed. Donald J. Kagay and Theresa M. Vann, 47–62 (Brill: Leiden)

Pollitzer, Robert. 1954. *Plague* (Geneva: World Health Organization)

Pracchi, Roberto. 1971. *Lombardia* (Turino: Unione Tipografico)

Prentice, Michael B., and Lila Rahalison. 2007. "Plague," *Lancet* 369, no. 9568: 1196-207

Preto, Paolo. 1987. *Epidemia, paura e politica nell'Italia moderna* (Bari: Editori Laterza)

Price, P. A., J. Jin, and W. E. Goldman. 2012. "Pulmonary Infection by *Yersinia pestis* Rapidly Establishes a Permissive Environment for Microbial Proliferation," *Proceedings of the National Academy of Sciences* 109, no. 8: 3083–88

Quammen, D. 2012. *Spillover: Animal Infections and the Next Human Pandemic* (New York: Norton)

Rabut, François. 1872. *Le mystère de Monseigneur Saint Sébastien, première journée.* Extract published in Chambéry, *Mémoires et Documents*, 13: 259–452

Racine, Pierre. 2004. "Le col du Saint-Gothard, maillon du grand commerce international (1260–1320)," in *Montagnes médiévales: XXXIVe Congrès de la SHMES, Chambéry, 23–25 May 2003*, 63–82 (Paris: Publications de la Sorbonne)

Rahelinirina, S., J. M. Duplantier, J. Ratovonjato, O. Ramilijaona, et al. 2010. "Study on the Movement of Rattus rattus and Evaluation of the Plague Dispersion in Madagascar," *Vector-Borne and Zoonotic Diseases* 10, no. 1: 77–84

Randall, J. A., et. al. 2005. "Flexible Social Structure of a Desert Rodent, *Rhombomys opimus:* Philapatry, Kinship, and Ecological Constraints," *Behavioral Ecology* 16, no. 6: 961–73

Raverat, Achile. 1872. *Haute Savoie: Genevois, Sémine, Faucigny et Chablais* (Lyons: Meton)

Royer, Katherine. 2014. "The Blind Men and the Elephant: Imperial Medicine, Medieval Historians, and the Role of Rats in the Historiography of Plague," in *Medicine and Colonialism: Historical Perspectives in India and South Africa*, ed. Poonam Bala, 99–110 (London: Pickering & Chatto)

Salkeld, D., M. Salathé, P. Stapp, and J. H. Jones. 2010. "Plague Outbreaks in Prairie Dog Populations Explained by Percolation Thresholds of Alternate Host Abundance," *Proceedings of the National Academy of Sciences* 107, no. 32: 14247–50

Shatzmiller, Joseph. 1974. "Les juifs de Provence pendant la peste noire," *Revue des études juives* 133: 457–80

Shopkow, Leah. 2010. "Three Stories about Life along the Road: The Survival of the Benedictine Monastery of Andres," *Viator* 41: 227–56

Smail, Daniel L. 1996. "Accommodating Plague in Medieval Marseille," *Continuity and Change* 11: 11–41

Soldi Rondinini, Gigliola. 1989. "Milano tra XIV e XVI secolo," in *Florence and Milan: Comparisons and Relations, vol. I*, ed. Nicolai Rubenstein, Sergio Bertelli and Craig Hugh Smyth, 163–85 (Firenze: a Nuova Italia Editrice)

Squatriti, Paolo. 2010. "The Floods of 589 and Climate Change at the Beginning of the Middle Ages: An Italian Microhistory," *Speculum* 85: 799–826

Stenseth, N. Chr., N. I. Samia, H. Viljugrein, K. L. Kausrud, et al. 2006. "Plague Dynamics are Driven by Climate Variation," *Proceedings of the National Academy of Sciences* 103, no. 35: 13110–15

Stenseth, Nils Chr., Bakyt B. Atshabar, Mike Begon, Steven R. Belmain, et al. 2008. "Plague: Past, Present, and Future," *PLoS Medicine* 5: e0009–13

Summers, W. C. 2012. *The Great Manchurian Plague of 1910–1911: The Geopolitics of an Epidemic Disease* (New Haven: Yale University Press)

Sumption, Jonathan. 2001. *The Hundred Years War, Volume 2: Trial by Fire* (Philadelphia: University of Pennsylvania Press)

Suntsov, V. V. 2012. "Origin of the Plague Microbe *Yersinia pestis:* Structure of the Process of Speciation," *Biology Bulletin* 39, no. 1: 1–9

Symes, Carol. 2011. "'The Medieval Archive and the History of Theatre: Assessing the Written and Unwritten Evidence for Premodern Performance," *Theatre Survey* 52: 1–30

Theurillat, J.-P., and A. Guisan. 2001. "Potential Impact of Climate Change on Vegetation in the European Alps: A Review," *Climatic Change* 50: 77–109

Tomé, C., and L. Chaix. 2003. "Marmot's Hunting and Exploitation in the Western Alps and the Southern Jura from Late Pleistocene to Holocene," in *Adaptive Strategies and Diversity in Marmots*, D. Allainé and M. Le Berre (ed.), 77–84 (Lyon: International Network on Marmots)

Tomich, P. Q., and et al. 1984. "Evidence for the Extinction of Plague in Hawaii," *American Journal of Epidemiology* 119: 261–73

Tropeano, D., and L. Turconi. 2004. "Using Historical Documents for Landslide, Debris Flow, and Stream Flood Prevention: Applications in Northern Italy," *Natural Hazards* 31: 663–79

Tschudi, Friedrich von. 1870. *Le monde des Alpes: Description pittoresque des montagnes de la Suisse et particulièrement des animaux qui les peuplent* (Basle: Georg)

Twigg, Graham. 1984. *The Black Death: A Biological Reappraisal* (London: Schocken)

Ugolini, Piero. 1985. "La formazione del sistema territoriale e urbano della Valle Padana," in *Storia d'Italia, Annali, 8: Insediamento e territorial*, ed. Cesare De Seta, 159–240 (Turino: Einaudi)

United States. 1907. *Public Health Reports*, 22: 50

Varlık, Nükhet. 2012. "Conquest, Urbanization and Plague Networks in the Ottoman Empire, 1453–1600," in *The Ottoman World*, ed. Christine Woodhead, 251–63 (New York: Routledge)

Varlık, Nükhet. 2014. "New Science and Old Sources: Why the Ottoman Experience of Plague Matters," *The Medieval Globe* 1: 193–227

Vester, Matthew. 2013. "Introduction," in *Sabaudian Studies: Political Culture, Dynasty and Territory (1400–1700)*, ed. Matthew Vester, 1–36 (Kirksville, MO: Truman State University Press)

Vogler, A. J., et al. 2013. "A Decade of Plague in Mahajanga, Madagascar: Insights into the Global Maritime Spread of Pandemic Plague," *mBio* 4: e00623-12

Walsh, K., et al. 2013. "A Historical Ecology of the Ecrins (Southern French Alps): Archaeology and Palaeoecology of the Mesolithic to the Medieval Period," *Quaternary International*, 30: 1–22

Wilschut, L. I., et al. 2013. "Potential Corridors and Barriers for Plague Spread in Central Asia," *International Journal of Health Geographics* 12: 15pp

Wimsatt, J., and D. E. Biggins. 2009. "A Review of Plague Persistence with Special Emphasis on Fleas," *Journal of Vector Borne Diseases* 46: 85–99

Zanetti, Dante. 1977. "A Milano nel 1524: i sospetti del Gentilino," in *Fatti e idee di storia economica nei secoli XII-XX: studi dedicati a Franco Borlandi* 105–15 (Bologna: il Mulino)

Ziegler, Michelle. 2014. "The Black Death and the Future of the Plague," *The Medieval Globe* 1: 259–283

Zimina, R.P., and I. P. Gerasimov. 1973. "The Periglacial Expansion of Marmots (*Marmota*) in Middle Europe during the Late Pleistocene," *Journal of Mammalogy* 54: 327–40

Ann G. Carmichael (carmicha@indiana.edu) is an historical epidemiologist originally trained in medicine and now emerita at Indiana University. She specializes in the history of plague and other infectious diseases, particularly in late medieval and Renaissance Italy. She is currently completing a study of mortality and public health in Sforza-era Milan (1450–1535).

Abstract Historical sources documenting recurrent plagues of the "Second Pandemic" usually focus on urban epidemic mortality. Instead, plague persists in remote, rural hinterlands: areas less visible in the written sources of late medieval Europe. Plague spreads as fleas move from relatively resistant rodents, which serve as "maintenance hosts," to an array of more susceptible rural mammals, now called "amplifying hosts." Using sources relevant to plague in thinly populated Central and Western Alpine regions, this paper postulates that Alpine Europe could have been a region of plague persistence via its population of wild rodents, particularly the Alpine marmot.

Keywords Plague, vector-borne disease, Alpine Europe, *Marmota marmota*, Milan, Savoy, Petrarch.

NEW SCIENCE AND OLD SOURCES: WHY THE OTTOMAN EXPERIENCE OF PLAGUE MATTERS

NÜKHET VARLIK

THIS IS A historic moment for plague historians and scientists. At present, a growing consensus in the international scholarly community identifies the Black Death as a pandemic of plague caused by *Yersinia pestis*.[1] This consensus marks the end of a long controversy over the pathogenic agent of the pandemic—a controversy that occupied the front stage of scholarship for decades.[2] Having left this behind, plague historians can now afford to explore new issues as well as revisit old questions with a fresh eye. They can draw from a wealth of research supplied by the "new science" of plague—by which I refer to the flurry of studies in the last decade or two in fields such as bioarcheology, microbiology, genetics, and epidemiology—and seek novel ways of integrating it into historical inquiry. In effect, this moment heralds the beginning of a new chapter in plague scholarship as it invites new avenues of inquiry (see Green 2014, in this issue). One such pathway worth pursuing is the task of calibrating the relationships between the new science of plague and the "old sources"—by which I mean the written sources historians are trained to use.

The new science and the old sources do not always concur, unless the historian makes an effort to make them speak to each other. With this in view, this essay will draw from the Ottoman experience during the so-

I owe a tremendous debt of gratitude to Monica Green, who has provided inspiration and encouragement throughout the process of writing this essay. I would also like to acknowledge Ann Carmichael, George Sussman, Carol Symes, Michelle Ziegler, and the anonymous reviewers of *The Medieval Globe*, with thanks for their invaluable comments and suggestions.

1 The consensus is firmly in place in the geneticist community. Multiple groups of researchers have confirmed *Y. pestis* as the causative agent of the Black Death (e.g., Haensch et al. 2010; Tran et al. 2011). Sequences of *Y. pestis* genomes have been reconstructed from the ancient DNA recovered from the Black Death cemeteries in London (Bos et al. 2011). Informed by recent scientific studies, a growing number of historians have acknowledged this consensus (e.g. Little 2011; Bolton 2013). For its significance in bioarcheology see DeWitte (2014, in this issue).

2 A concise presentation of the controversy can be found in Little 2011. Most recently, historian Samuel K. Cohn (2013) remains unconvinced that any currently existing strain of *Y. pestis* caused the Black Death.

called Second Plague Pandemic (i.e., the Black Death and its recurrent waves) and seek to highlight the critical importance of the historian's craft in working with sources that can shed light beyond the spotlight of scientific research. In order to demonstrate why the Ottoman plague experience matters for an understanding of the Second Pandemic, the essay will tackle two sets of intertwined problems. On the one hand, it will engage with a historical and historiographical discussion of why the Ottoman epidemiological experience has been imagined as the European alterity and how this legacy has obstructed this experience from being studied as part of the larger Afro-Eurasian disease zone of the Second Pandemic. My goal here is to underscore the Eurocentric nature of plague studies by demonstrating how spatio-temporal epidemiological boundaries were constructed in the scholarship. On the other hand, this essay will examine the Ottoman plague experience during the Second Pandemic with a view to offering observations and insights about the Ottoman disease ecologies that sustained plague. More specifically, three aspects of this experience are explored in detail: *persistence*, *foci/focalization*, and *patterns of transmission of plague.* My goal here is to illustrate how the new science of plague can be put in dialogue with historical sources.

Part I. New Science and Old Sources: Challenges and Opportunities

From where we stand today, some may believe that the new science of plague puts an end to historical inquiry.[3] Because the new science can explain the pathogen and its genetic history, one may wonder why we still need to study the old sources. The reasons for this are to be sought in the very etiology of plague that involves a complex system of entanglements in which every organism (as host, vector, or pathogen) constantly interacts with other organisms, as well as the surrounding environment. Thus historians must now account for variations between the specific ways the disease manifests itself at local and regional levels. Such ecological and environmental variations make it all the more compelling to pay attention to the "local knowledge" of plague, in the form it appears in the historical sources.[4]

---

3 The recent engagement of the geneticist community in the debate seems to have been taken by some historians as a threat to the territory of their discipline and led them to react. A recent article written with that conviction has suggested: "Historians are uniquely qualified to assess the value and analyse the content of medieval primary sources and should not allow the glamour of science to make us forget our own expertise" (Pobst 2013: 814).

4 The emphasis on the "local knowledge" of plague and "plague experience" in

It is now clear that plague studies will have to transcend the boundaries of individual disciplines; adopting an interdisciplinary approach is practically inevitable. The student of plague therefore needs to face up to the stipulations of interdisciplinary work. For example, there is a pressing need to keep up with the all-too-quickly-changing findings of the scientific literature, especially in the fields of genomics and evolutionary biology. It is necessary to understand, interpret, and utilize the research findings supplied by allied disciplines and fields, ranging from climate history to bioarcheology. It also means reckoning with what appears to be a growing imbalance between the new science of plague and the old sources. Even if one leaves aside differences in content, the disparity between publication cultures in the sciences and in the humanities cannot be overlooked. The former prefers short, rapidly-produced, multi-authored technical notices that may seem impenetrable to the nonspecialist; the characteristics of humanist publications are almost the opposite (except, in some cases, for their degree of impenetrability). Motivated by different questions, concerns, and agendas, the historical and scientific scholarship of plague do not produce research that can be easily reconciled. How, then, can this new science be used in conjunction with historical accounts? How can the historian put them into dialogue? This imbalance becomes all the more challenging in those fields where the historical scholarship of plague is still relatively undeveloped. There is a wealth of primary sources pertaining to plague in non-Western languages, but it is still in manuscript form. Until these sources are edited, published, and translated in a manner accessible to researchers, our knowledge of past plagues will continue to suffer from this imbalance.

As a result, there remain a number of important gaps in the scholarship of historical plague epidemics that need to be filled. One is the Ottoman experience of plague during the Black Death and its recurrent waves. Judging from modern Ottomanist scholarship, the vast area that came under Ottoman control—stretching at its height from southeast Europe to the Persian Gulf and from the Black Sea basin to the Yemen—did not figure as a breeding ground for plague until the last centuries of the empire's history: the only extensive study covers the period between 1700 and 1850 (Panzac 1985).[5] For the plague outbreaks before this era (i.e., from

---

this essay has benefited from the concept of "local biologies" developed by medical anthropologist Margaret Lock and the recent discussions of this concept in the context of global health. See, for example, Lock 1993 and 1995; Brotherton and Nguyen 2013.

5 Panzac's study has been largely ignored by mainstream historical scholarship. While it was unanimously recognized as a great accomplishment with respect to its

1347 to 1700), no systematic study has hitherto surveyed their temporal and spatial scope or effects, or even considered how the Ottoman epidemiological experience may be integrated into the broader history of the Second Pandemic in the Afro-Eurasian zone.[6]

This is curious because the spatial and temporal correspondence between the empire and the plague can hardly be ignored. Ottoman history almost squarely coincides with the time frame of the Second Plague Pandemic, and evidence suggests that Ottoman power and the plague coexisted for half a millennium, from the Black Death of the mid-fourteenth century to the mid-nineteenth century or so. Yet the ubiquitous presence of plague in the Ottoman world over that half millennium has remained mostly invisible in both historical and scientific scholarship. In what follows, we shall seek to disentangle the web of historical and historiographical problems that have obstructed the Ottoman plague experience from becoming visible. A critical reading of scientific and historical studies of plague sheds light on how European epidemiological imaginaries fashioned the Ottoman experience as the "other" by constructing spatial and temporal epidemiological boundaries; so it is to the construction of these boundaries that we turn now.

The Historical Fiction of Epidemiological Boundaries

The historical scholarship on the Black Death is largely Eurocentric. In this body of scholarship, Europe has occupied a privileged position, compared to other parts of the world that may have been at least as badly affected by plague, if not more so. Our current knowledge about the plague in East Asia, South Asia, Central Asia, the Middle East, and North Africa before the Third Pandemic is at best fragmentary and disconnected.[7] As such, extant

---

documentation of the occurrences of plague outbreaks, their frequency, and methods of spread, its representation of the demographic and economic effects of plague was debated. Historians of the Ottoman empire and the Middle East have been especially critical of the absence of Ottoman sources (e.g., Owen 1986; Dols 1987; Issawi 1988; Fisher 1992). For its absence from European scholarship, see also below.

6 See, e.g., Ünver 1935; Panzac 1973, 1986, 1987, and 2009; Jennings 1993; Lowry 2003; Schamiloglu 2004; Kılıç 2004; Mikhail 2008; 2012; Shefer-Mossensohn 2009 and 2012; White 2010; Varlık 2011; Bulmuş 2012. For a study of the outbreaks between 1347 and 1600, see Varlık (forthcoming). For a call to study the Second Pandemic in this larger Afro-Eurasian disease zone, see Green (2014, in this issue).

7 Even though there are fine historical studies devoted to the epidemiological experience of these areas during the Second Pandemic, they are difficult to bring together in view of their temporal and spatial breadth of coverage. See, e.g.,

scholarship has cultivated a lasting impression that the Black Death was a European phenomenon and that the European epidemiological experience was to be studied *sui generis*. In this epidemiological imagination, non-European epidemiological experiences would only be worthy of scholarly attention if commensurate with that of Europe. In other words, the lacunae in historical plague scholarship are not haphazard; what was studied and what was not can be best understood in the light of European notions of public health and efforts for disease control that came in the form of quarantines, plague commissions, sanitary missions, and international conferences at the dawn of the modern era. Those areas whose plague experience was believed, in the twentieth century, to have been of direct relevance to that of Europe (and perceived as having an impact on European public health concerns) came under the spotlight of scholarship while others remained rather obscure.

The European epidemiological experience thus came to be understood within certain temporal and spatial boundaries, and both are reflected in the periodization of plague, a system that purports to be global but which actually situates Europe at the center and only captures European experiences. By now, it has become commonplace to study three discrete pandemics: the First Pandemic, known as the Justinianic Plague and its recurrent waves (541–*c.*750); the Second Pandemic, known as the Black Death (1346–53) and its recurrent waves that continued for several centuries; and the Third Pandemic that spread globally in a few years after its appearance in Hong Kong in 1894.[8] Although the idea that the Plague of Justinian and the Black Death were two separate waves of epidemic

Hrabak 1957; Krekic 1963; Langer 1975; Dols 1977; Norris 1977; Alexander 1980; Schamiloglu 1993; Ansari 1994; Kōstēs 1995; Manolova-Nikolova 2004; Anandavalli 2007; Stearns 2009 and 2011; Frandsen 2010; Buell 2012. Also see works cited in notes 5 and 6 above. For a study that ambitiously tries to offer a wider (but still Eurocentric) scope, see Benedictow 2004. For studies that have adopted larger or comparative perspectives, see Biraben 1975; Borsch 2005; Sussman 2011. There is also a substantial body of literature devoted to the First Pandemic, including but not limited to Biraben and Le Goff 1969; Dols 1974; Conrad 1981, 1982, and 2000; Christensen 1993; Stathakopoulos 2000 and 2004; van Ess 2001; Little 2007.

8 For this conventionally accepted periodization, see Little 2011. The term "pandemic" appears to have been used infrequently before 1894: Creighton (1891) references it only three times in over seven hundred pages: for example, "there are instances of what are called pandemics, or universal epidemics, of sickness. The Black Death was one such" (p. 397). Interestingly enough, it was the cholera and influenza pandemics that helped spread its use, and by 1918 the term had become common parlance (Morens, Folkers, and Fauci 2009).

activity was becoming common in the nineteenth century, it was not until the outbreak of plague in (British) Hong Kong and the discovery of the plague bacillus that these epidemics were retrospectively placed in a historical timeline. Twentieth-century epidemiologists and epidemiological historians alike seem to have subsequently adopted this schema.[9] Nevertheless, this vision of past plagues can hardly be taken to represent the rhythm of plagues as experienced across the Afro-Eurasian zone. It offers little insight for the ebb and flow of epidemic waves in other areas, especially with regard to the "in-between" outbreaks.

The Ottoman case in particular seems to complicate this periodization, as it blurs the assumed boundaries between the end of the Second Pandemic and the beginning of the Third—just as it blurs a supposed distinction between West and East. After plague receded from Western Europe early in the eighteenth century, sporadic outbreaks continued to occur in Southern and Eastern Europe (e.g., 1743 in Messina, 1815 in Bari), in Russia (e.g., 1770–72 in Moscow), and more persistently in the Middle East until the nineteenth century. Those occurrences were noted in many late nineteenth- and early twentieth-century works (e.g., Simpson 1905: 36–39; Sticker 1908). Modern scholarship has also convincingly shown that plague persisted in the Ottoman empire and Russia (Alexander 1980; Panzac 1985; Robarts 2010). Nevertheless, the Great Plague of London (1665) and that of Marseille (1720–22) continued to be seen as marking the end of the Second Pandemic. Plague outbreaks in the eighteenth and nineteenth centuries, outside of Europe, were only recently recognized as being part of the Second Pandemic (Walløe 2008; Cohn 2008; Bolton 2013: 15).[10]

---

9 It appears for the first time around the turn of the twentieth century. For example, Simpson (1905) identified three pandemics: "The first [. . .] recorded to have originated in Pelusium in Egypt" (p. 5); "The second [. . .] later called the Back Death" (p. 21); and "The pandemic of the present day" (p. 6). Other early twentieth-century works used the term "pandemic" without a system of enumeration (e.g., Eager 1908; Sticker 1908), but by the mid-twentieth century this system of periodization seems to be in place (see e.g., Hirst 1953). However, it probably did not become conventional until the 1970s (Ziegler 1969: 25; Dols 1977: 14).

10 A similar pattern of persistence of plague can be observed between the First and the Second Pandemic, roughly in areas where the Ottomans would come to rule. These recurrent outbreaks also complicate the parameters of these earlier pandemics. See Dols 1974 and 1977: 13–35; McNeill 1976: 70; Conrad 1981. For a list of outbreaks in Anatolia under Seljuk rule (though the diagnosis of these outbreaks is not always clear), see Arık 1991. For a brief description of an outbreak in Tunisia in 1004–05, see Talbi 1981: 223. For a critique of the year 750 as the definite end of the First Pandemic, see Morony 2007.

The question of when the last outbreak of the Second Pandemic took place therefore seems difficult to answer based on extant sources and prevailing habits of thought. Plague continued in Ottoman areas until the mid-nineteenth century, if not longer, since recorded cases in Mesopotamia and the Arabian peninsula appear until the turn of the twentieth century (Simpson 1905: 38–39).[11] Especially in view of the fact that the Third Pandemic also made its appearance around the same time, the question of when the Second Pandemic ended may need to be re-evaluated with the help of scientific studies. In effect, it is possible that the strains of *Y. pestis* involved in the Second Pandemic are still with us today, as demonstrated in the example of a recent outbreak in Libya.[12]

Shifting our focus from temporal to spatial boundaries may also involve questioning what we think we know about plague's past. Once again, the Ottoman case is telling, and it underscores the degree to which the new plague science has maintained or reproduced these spatial boundaries. As noted above, the scarcity of historical studies on Ottoman plagues has rendered it invisible to practitioners of the new science. In the absence of historical studies to guide bioarcheological research, there is no evidence from former Ottoman areas comparable to what has been found for Western Europe.[13] Obviously, this has implications for studying the genetic history of the pathogen. In the absence of aDNA specimens, the plague history of this particular area/era cannot be integrated into the narrative of the new science because the aDNA specimens of *Y. pestis* mostly come from excavations in Europe (France, Germany, Italy, England, and the Netherlands)—places close to centers of molecular biology, centers of information and calculation (Latour 1987).[14] Reconstructing the phy-

11 Twentieth-century scholarship seems to have grown more confident about announcing the "end of plague." For example, Pollitzer (1951: 478) hailed "the gradual disappearance of the disease first from Western and then from Eastern Europe until in 1841 Turkey, the last stronghold of the pest, became free." Drawing from this scholarship, Panzac (1985: 446–517) also held that the last plague was in the 1840s. But at the turn of the twentieth century, news of plague in Istanbul was noteworthy enough to receive international coverage (*British Medical Journal* 1900, 1902a, and 1902b).

12 Recent genetics research on the 2009 Libyan outbreak has demonstrated that a branch of the *medievalis* strain (2.MED) was involved. This strain, independent of the Third Pandemic, could be one that was active during the Second Pandemic (Cabanel et al. 2013; Green 2014, in this issue).

13 Bioarcheology and aDNA research have only recently started being used in the field of Near Eastern studies. For a discussion of the state-of-the-field, including reasons for its belated development, see, e.g., Sołtysiak 2007; Baca and Molak 2008.

14 For a list of the areas of excavation, see "Toward a Molecular History of *Yersinia*

logenetic history of the pathogen depends on identifying modern *Y. pestis* isolates. Some of these specimens have been preserved since the late nineteenth century, others have been isolated more recently. The majority of these modern specimens come from places where plague is (or has until recently been) enzootic. Among these, a large number come from the United States, Russia, Mongolia, and China; fewer from India, Madagascar, Eastern and Central Africa, and elsewhere.[15] For our immediate area of interest, only a small number of isolates from former Ottoman areas (including Turkey, northern Iraq, and western Iran) have been included in recent phylogenetic analyses and studied in relation to where they stand within the evolutionary subdivision of *Y. pestis.*[16] Owing to this imbalance in data collection and analysis, the new science of plague—along with the historical scholarship that informs it—privileges some areas over others.[17]

This ongoing Eurocentricity of plague scholarship has been largely determined by research produced in the nineteenth and twentieth centuries—research with a strong colonial pedigree. On the eve of the Third

pestis," available online at <http://contagions.wordpress.com/2013/01/05/toward-a-molecular-history-of-yersinia-pestis-aha/> [accessed September 19, 2014]. See also Haensch et al. 2010: fig. 1. Especially in view of regulations restricting the shipping of pathogenic specimens across national borders, specimens are currently extracted and processed in places close to the centers of molecular biology. For the most recent regulations issued by the World Health Organization (WHO) regarding the transport of infectious substances, see WHO 2012. According WHO's protocol, *Y. pestis* is listed as a "Category A" infectious substance whose transport is strictly regulated.

15 For information on these isolates and their provenances, see the phylogenetic tree in Cui et al. 2013, reproduced in Green 2014, in this issue; also see Morelli et al. 2010.

16 2.MED1, isolated from this region, evolved sometime before 1775, i.e., before the Third Pandemic. 1.ORI3 is thought to have come from Madagascar during the Third Pandemic, most probably via the pilgrimage route (Morelli et al. 2010: fig. 1). Of the four *Y. pestis* isolates that were preserved in Turkey, three were defined as biotype *orientalis* (Golem and Özsan 1952). One of the four was known to have been isolated from a human case of plague in the Akçakale (Urfa) outbreak of 1947: a small plague outbreak in two Turkish villages on the Syrian border. In the months of February and March, a total of thirteen deaths took place out of a total of eighteen persons affected. This appears to be the last recorded outbreak of plague in Turkey.

17 Either resulting from current concerns about the disease's reemergence and the assessment of its risks or due to privileging areas that can produce aDNA specimens, the "molecular politics" of *Y. pestis* reflect past and current global inequalities of health rather than representing the breadth and intensity of past plagues as experienced across different areas. For an insightful exposition of the "molecular politics" of HIV demonstrating how the global inequalities of the AIDS epidemic can be observed at the molecular level, see Crane, 2011.

Pandemic, European scientists were concerned with "unusual" plague activity in East and South Asia (Creighton 1891: 166–70, 172–73; Sussman 2011: 324). What they considered a new pandemic then signaled new opportunities for research: as soon as plague broke out in (British) Hong Kong in 1894, as noted above, scientists from different countries rushed there to study the epidemic on site; the discovery of the pathogen followed shortly. In 1896, plague was reported in British India (Bombay, then in Pune, Karachi, and Calcutta, soon to be followed by many major port cities across continents).[18] This situation alarmed European colonial governments, which sent plague researchers and public health officials to the colonies. For example, a special committee was formed to investigate plague in India: observing the plague, producing laboratory experiments, and publishing their findings. The result was an immense body of scholarship that continued to develop over the course of the last century. Both historians and scientists are still dealing with the effects of this problematic legacy in one way or another.

From the Ottoman "Laboratory" of Plague to the Colonial Science of Plague

The body of knowledge drawn from the Third Pandemic, as much as it has informed current research, has also hindered it (Royer 2014). This plague science was the product of a certain configuration of power, which is still reflected in some critical assumptions about plague's origins and spread. The legacy of colonial plague science also has important implications for the study of Ottoman plagues, because it retrospectively shaped the perception of Ottoman experience in historical scholarship. To understand how this occurred, we need to recognize that early modern observations of Ottoman plague had come to constitute a working knowledge of the disease in Europe. When the Third Pandemic broke out, this body of knowledge lost its primacy at the expense of colonial plague science, backed by the germ theory of disease. And yet, certain epidemiological assumptions drawn from European analysis of Ottoman plague continued to be used in modern scholarship.

Before the Third Pandemic, both scholarly and lay opinion in Europe maintained that the "seat of the plague" was the Near East, the "Orient" which, at that time, largely coincided with dominions of the Ottoman

18 For the origins and spread of the epidemic in China, see Benedict (1996: 1–130). For its global spread, see Echenberg 2007. For plague in India, see Arnold (1993: chap. 5).

empire (Sussman 2011: 324). From the late seventeenth and early eighteenth centuries onwards, Europeans observed that devastating plague epidemics were becoming less frequent on the continent. When Marseille witnessed what is regarded as the last major outbreak of plague in Western Europe, in 1720, this experience only confirmed the already widespread belief that the disease was being imported from the eastern Mediterranean port cities of the Ottoman empire, such as Constantinople (Istanbul), Smyrna (İzmir), and Alexandria (Takeda 2011: 115–17). The writings of early modern European travelers, merchants, diplomats, and naturalists had no small share in shaping this belief. But above all, we can point to the influence of a substantial number of Western European physicians who, after major plague outbreaks receded from Western Europe, went to Ottoman cities to observe plague, gather firsthand information, and write about their experiences.

Among the most prominent of these physicians were the Russell brothers from Edinburgh, who spent several years in Aleppo and published their observations on plague in the latter half of the eighteenth century.[19] Similarly, Mordach Mackenzie, who worked as the physician of the Levant Company in mid-eighteenth-century Istanbul, regularly reported his observations about plague in the Ottoman capital (Mackenzie 1752 and 1764). Such accounts continued to be published in the nineteenth century.[20] For example, William Wittman, a Royal Artillery surgeon sent to the Ottoman empire following Napoleon's invasion of Egypt, published his observations on the plague in 1804. A more detailed testimony comes from A. Brayer, a French physician residing in Istanbul between 1815 and 1824, who composed a comprehensive two-volume work, which includes his observations on the causes, types, and treatment of plague (Brayer 1836).

The knowledge acquired in the Ottoman "laboratory" of plague appears to have been well received in Europe, since most of these physicians pub-

19 Alexander Russell worked as physician of the Levant Company in Aleppo from about 1740 to 1753. In 1756, soon after his return to London, the first edition of his *Natural History of Aleppo*—including a special section on plague—appeared in print, going through several editions afterwards. His younger brother Patrick followed in his footsteps, practicing medicine in Aleppo where he lived between 1750 and 1772. In 1791, he published his *Treatise of the Plague*, in which he included his observations during the outbreak of 1760–62 and 120 individual case studies in Aleppo. On the life and works of the Russell brothers, see van den Boogert (2010).

20 Two Italian physicians, Eusebio Valli and Antonio Pezzoni, who served in the Greek hospitals of Istanbul during an outbreak of plague in 1803-4, published their individual observations (Valli 1805; Pezzoni 1842 and 1847). See Sarı and Etker (2000) and Yıldırım (2010: 59); see also below.

lished their work promptly and some of those publications went into several editions and translations. Their impact on European scholarly circles is also discernible in the way that these authors used their knowledge to acquire recognition and advance their careers. For example, Alexander Russell's experience in Aleppo, advertised in his writings, helped him to be elected to the Royal Society of London. Later on, his brother Patrick also became a member. Mackenzie's account of the plague in Istanbul was not only published by the Royal Society, it also opened the doors of membership to him (van den Boogert 2010: 146). A more remarkable case in point is that of Charles Maclean, an English physician whose career stagnated until he traveled to the Ottoman capital in 1815 to observe the plague. His observations were swiftly published in London (Maclean 1817). Since plague had receded from Western Europe, this body of firsthand knowledge was especially valuable in promoting the empirical approach to medicine that was flourishing in early nineteenth-century England; hence the direct observations of physicians with overseas experience came to acquire more weight than theoretical knowledge (Kelly 2008: 569). It was in this context that cases from the Ottoman laboratory, that "last vestige of plague," continued to be observed, studied, and discussed—until the Third Pandemic broke out.[21]

When this occurred, the attention of European scholarship largely shifted from Ottoman areas to European colonies in South and East Asia. (The fact that plague had largely disappeared in the Ottoman empire by this time may have also contributed to this shift.) Nevertheless, certain assumptions about the origins, movement, and directionality of epidemic diseases which had been drawn from the Ottoman laboratory were now being transplanted into a colonial context. One such assumption was that the geographic origin of epidemics could be traced to remote areas, far away from centers of knowledge. The nineteenth-century English physician and medical historian Charles Creighton aptly observed:

> According to the dominant school of epidemiologists it is always enough to have traced a virus to a remote source, to the "roof of the world" or to the back of the east wind, and there to leave it, in the full assurance that there must have been circumstances to account for its engendering there, perhaps in an equally remote past, if only we knew them. (Creighton 1891, 1:149; also quoted in Norris 1977: 10)[22]

21 There were a series of international "sanitary" conferences from the mid-nineteenth century to the mid-twentieth, although their main focus was cholera rather than plague. The third was held in Constantinople in 1866 (Howard-Jones 1975).

22 In this era, discussion of plague's "origin" usually meant the geographic origin,

From this it followed that disease would spread in a particular direction and, not surprisingly, this spread was conceptualized as being unidirectional: plague flowed from "less civilized" places to the "centers of civilization." Colonial anxieties thus found a scientific justification in this emphasis on the disease's place of origin, which confirmed that there was something inherently wrong with such lands or peoples and that their contagion could affect civilized peoples and places. [23]

While this framework could conveniently be adopted to explain plague epidemics outside of Europe, it was still difficult to explain past cases of plague in Europe itself. It was not easy to elucidate whether plagues had occurred there spontaneously due to local, regional, or underlying universal circumstances, or whether they had been transmitted from certain "endemic" areas outside Europe.[24] It may help to remember that throughout the early modern era, the European imagination of plague's origin was being constantly replenished by news of plague from the port cities of the eastern Mediterranean, which led to durable associations between plague and the Ottomans. The implications were twofold. On the one hand, the European imagination dissociated itself from plague by projecting the locus of the disease somewhere outside; on the other, it fashioned the Ottoman empire as a plague-exporter, against which Europe had to protect itself. By the Enlightenment, this paradigm was ingrained in scholarly writings and popular opinion alike (Gordon 1999; Lammel 2010; Varlık, forthcoming)—even as the Ottomans ceased to be seen as a military threat in Europe, a turn typically associated with their defeat at the second siege of Vienna in 1683. As the empire's landholdings in Europe shrank through the course of the eighteenth and nineteenth centuries, it came to be seen as a dead or dying body in the European geopolitics: "the sick man of Europe." In the contemporary European imagination, the empire's healthscape not only represented a sickened land and peoples but also an inability to deal with ill-health in a rational and orderly manner.

---

the "endemic focus," not the biological origin of the "virus" later named *Y. pestis*.

23 For a discussion of how the site of the plague shifted from the landscape to the human body (the colonized body) in India, see Arnold (1993: 200–39).

24 For example, J. F. C. Hecker (1859: 17–19) attributed plague-causation to atmospheric changes that would have made "spontaneous plagues" possible everywhere, even in Europe. Towards the end of the century, physician Adrien Proust (1897: 113)—father of the celebrated French novelist—did not deny the possibility of spontaneous plagues in Europe altogether, but did not dwell on it much either (see also Panzac 2003).

Some of these nineteenth-century conceptions continue to be reproduced in historical scholarship of the twentieth century. For example, the absence of a known plague reservoir in modern Europe seems to have retrospectively erased that possibility from Europe's medieval past. Modern scholarship has treated plague as a temporary "invasion" or "alien" presence and has focused heavily on the effects of this "foreign" visitor, instead of examining plague's interaction with the natural and built environment. The enduring vision of the European epidemiological past is one of *difference* that singled it out from the rest of the larger disease zone (Carmichael 2014, in this issue; see also Bolton 2013: 34). Historical scholarship accordingly had to develop ways of explaining this difference. Most visibly, since the 1970s, plague scholarship has approached the Mediterranean world with epidemiological divisions in mind, such as "Christian *vs.* Muslim" or "Oriental *vs.* Occidental." For example, in his authoritative work on the history of plague, Jean-Noël Biraben posited a divide between regions he calls "north-occidental" and "south-oriental" and legitimized this bipartite view by citing differences in climate, fauna, and attitudes toward disease (Biraben 1975: 106).

Subsequent scholarship seems to have maintained epidemiological zones corresponding to those of the early modern period: that of the Ottomans (read: Muslims) and that of the Europeans (read: Christians), with religion as the single most dividing factor (see, e.g., McNeill 1976; Dols 1977; Panzac 1985).[25] These imagined divisions of epidemiological experience have resulted in separate histories of plague in Europe and the Middle East/Islamic world. Even in studies that encompass the Mediterranean, these divisions play an important role in explaining the very differences in the spread of plague and the responses it engendered. This bipartite epidemiological imaginary not only sustains essentialist binaries, it regards the Ottoman epidemiological experience as timeless, uniform, and thus unworthy of historical inquiry.

Part II: The Problem of Plague Persistence in Ottoman Lands

As noted above, plague persisted in Ottoman areas for at least half a millennium: a phenomenon that requires a closer look. By persistence, I refer to recurrences of plague in a given area, resulting from local, regional, or long-distance spread of the infection, either imported from outside or transmitted from local enzootic reservoirs. In studying the persistence

25 Recent studies have shown that religion cannot be accepted as the sole determinant in responses to epidemic diseases (Stearns 2009 and 2011).

of plague, we are at the mercy of our sources. There was no systematic recording of plagues in the Ottoman empire before the eighteenth century, when Western diplomats started regular reporting to quarantine authorities in Europe.[26] For earlier centuries, the nature of the sources rarely affords observations on plague's persistence at the local level. First, there is the problem of plague's visibility. In its enzootic form (when the infection is transmitted between partially resistant rodent hosts and their fleas), there is no substantial rodent "die off," which makes it difficult to detect.[27] Only when the disease assumes epizootic and epidemic form, causing rodent and human mortality, can historical sources make plague visible to us. Second, only rarely do premodern accounts mention where plague came from, so as to enable us to trace the known (or suspected) origin. Even then, this reflects local rumors and reports, which may result from imprecise knowledge. Third, the importation of the infection to port cities as a result of maritime contacts with other infected cities makes it even more difficult to trace the origins of a particular outbreak. This is further complicated by the likelihood of the infection being introduced from multiple areas and/or through multiple channels. For any given outbreak, it is possible that we are looking at more than one strain of the pathogen circulating through different channels.

Indeed, what can be more confidently ascertained from the sources is that plague spread across the empire along complex sets of trajectories that developed and consolidated over the course of the fifteenth and sixteenth centuries (Varlık 2011). This resulted in the repeated exposure of Ottoman cities to the infection throughout the Second Pandemic, turning them into established centers of plague. For example, Istanbul witnessed at least 230 outbreaks during the Second Pandemic, recurring about 2.2 years on average over half a millennium. Similarly, Salonica witnessed outbreaks about 142 times over the course of the same period, about every 3.5 years on average. Other major urban centers of the empire, such as Alexandria, Cairo, Aleppo, Damascus, and Trabzon all experienced frequently recurring outbreaks (Varlık, forthcoming). It is possible that some of those cities sustained the plague on their own, independent from

---

26 It was mainly this body of documentation that Panzac (1985) used to reconstruct the Ottoman plagues of the eighteenth and nineteenth centuries.

27 Scientific studies inform us about the critical importance of rodent hosts and vectors for the maintenance of plague. As long as there is a sufficient number of rodents and fleas, plague seems to be maintained indefinitely in enzootic form (Gage and Kosoy 2005). Other ecological factors such as climate also matter significantly (Nakazawa et al. 2007; Stenseth et al. 2006; Ben Ari et al. 2011)

incoming infection—that is, they functioned as urban reservoirs of plague. Some Ottoman cities (or their immediate hinterlands) may have kept the disease alive from one epidemic season to the next, sustained by commensal rodents and/or ectoparasites.[28]

At this point, it may be helpful to consider whether commensal rodents (specifically colonies of *Rattus rattus*) are capable of sustaining plague over time and can therefore function as temporary reservoirs. The ecological scholarship has placed greater emphasis on the role of ground-burrowing wild rodents in sustaining infection over the long term, and commensal rodents' ability to function in the same manner has not been sufficiently explored (e.g., Keim and Wagner 2009). Nevertheless, there are promising studies which suggest that plague can be maintained over long time periods in small commensal rat subpopulations, without any contact with wild rodents. For example, plague is calculated to persist for a hundred years in a commensal rat population of 60,000, without the need of importing new infection (Gage and Kosoy 2005; Keeling and Gilligan 2000a and 2000b). In other words, even if plague killed a certain population of rats, the infection could be kept alive for a long time. This research also suggests that plague would persist even if quarantine measures were in place, and thus has tremendous implications for explaining the historical persistence of plague in large urban centers such as Istanbul. This means that urban areas with significant commensal rodent populations may have become their own self-perpetuating engines of epidemic activity and as such served as temporary reservoirs of plague.

Plague Foci and the Process of Focalization

But even if urban reservoirs could independently sustain the disease, they were never isolated. On the contrary, early modern Ottoman towns were connected both to their immediate hinterland and to more distant areas through a complex network of maritime and overland routes. It was this set of connections that facilitated the circulation of plague within the empire and beyond it, since at least some of those connections linked the urban areas to rural plague reservoirs (foci). As mentioned above, areas where a sufficient number of wild rodents and ectoparasites live can maintain the disease indefinitely in its enzootic form. Hence, it is important to identify where such foci were located in the empire's vast reach.

28 For example, Panzac (1973) showed that İzmir received the infection from its hinterland in the eighteenth century.

At present, we know of several plague foci in or around former Ottoman areas such as Libya, Yemen, Iran, the Transcaucasian and the northwest Caspian regions (WHO 1999: 16; Anisimov, Lindler, and Pier 2004). These were active plague reservoirs during the Third Pandemic, and perhaps even before. According to Panzac, the highlands between western Iran, northern Iraq, and southeastern Turkey, as well as the mountainous areas of Hijaz and Yemen were *permanent* plague foci that caused outbreaks in the eighteenth and nineteenth centuries. Panzac equally identified what he thought were *temporary* plague foci, including the western Balkans, Moldavia and Wallachia, Istanbul, the Anatolian peninsula, and Egypt (Panzac 1985: 105–33). However, he did not offer an explanation as to when each of these foci came to existence.[29]

Identifying pre-eighteenth-century Ottoman plague foci is challenging. The fragmentary nature of modern *Y. pestis* specimens isolated from these regions does not allow us to determine how old the foci were and how long they remained active.[30] Plague science informs us that enzootic foci are not to be taken as timeless; rather they are dynamic entities that emerge, expand, shrink, or disappear over time. Myriad changes ranging from rodent migration to changes in their predator population, and from fluctuations in climate to modifications in landscape, can affect plague foci (Gratz 1999; Li et al. 2009; Karimova et al. 2010; Eisen and Gage 2012).[31] All these factors make it necessary to pay attention to the circumstances that favor their formation, that is, the process of focalization—the process by which plague forms reservoirs in the natural environment to perpetuate itself, independent of imported infection.

29 Panzac (1985: 128–33) singles out the focus of Egypt ("le foyer égyptien") as a nineteenth-century phenomenon. He postulates that plague had been an "importation" to Egypt until the 1820s when it went through a process of focalization. He noted that both permanent and temporary foci in or near Ottoman areas were concentrated in the highlands (Panzac 1985: 105–33). See further discussion below.

30 However, it is interesting to note that most of modern *Y. pestis* isolates of the biovar *medievalis* (2.MED) come from former Ottoman territories or its neighboring areas, such as Turkey, Iraq, Iran, and Libya. These scattered isolates seem to represent a genetically related cluster of strains even though they were isolated from different areas at different times. The links between these strains should be sought in the region's history during the Second Pandemic, i.e., in the Ottoman plague experience. See for example Cabanel et al. 2013: fig. 4; Achtman et al. 2004: supplementary fig. 7. See nn. 12 and 16 above.

31 For a discussion of problems and biases involved in determining historical foci, see Ben Ari et al. (2012: 8200).

Since the beginning of the twentieth century, there was a certain understanding that at least some plague foci were situated in highlands. Writing in 1905, for instance, English epidemiologist W. J. Simpson suggested that plague originated in some highland areas such as in Assyr in the western Arabian peninsula and in the highlands of what is today southeast Turkey and northern Iraq: "[t]he endemic areas [. . .] are chiefly distinguished for their high altitudes." But the reason he offered was more a cultural construct of highlanders' customs than a real observation about the disease ecology of those areas that differentiated them from that of the lowlands. Simpson reasoned that plague occurred in those areas "for the poverty and filth of the inhabitants, and for the promiscuous manner in which the cattle, fowls, and domestic animals are permitted to live in close association with human beings, the former often occupying the same room as the latter" (Simpson 1905: 38, 117–18). About two decades later, the renowned Chinese epidemiologist Wu Lien-Teh regarded highland locations as "endemic" foci. In reference to the Kumaon and Garwhal areas of northern India, in the foothills of the Himalayas, for example, he wrote, "[t]his locality is highly situated and sparsely populated, most of the inhabitants [. . .] are poor and dwell promiscuously with their cattle" (Lien-Teh 1924: 292).

Looking exclusively for human cases of plague, these epidemiologists failed to see enzootic plague in these highland foci and the disease ecologies that governed them. Hence, no clear explanation (free of cultural bias) could be offered as to why focalization took place in highlands. Recent research from Madagascar has since shed light on the mechanisms that support this process. In this island's ecology, plague is sustained in the highlands (above 800 meters) where flea vectors *(Xenopsylla cheopis* and *Synopsyllus fonquerniei*) are more abundant (Vogler et al. 2011; Andrianaivoarimanana et al. 2013). This research offers new insights for understanding the focalization of plague and the transmission of enzootic plague from the highlands to the lowlands (see also Green 2014 and Carmichael 2014, both in this issue). Certain types of landscapes across all continents favor a high number of rodent reservoirs and their fleas. Most plague reservoirs, including those located on higher altitudes, are found in places with "low annual precipitation, or where dry seasons inhibit the growth of thick woody vegetation and lead to the formation of deserts, semi-deserts and steppes (savannas, prairies, pampas and so on)" (WHO 1999: 13-14). Drawing from this, it is possible to discern the basic outlines of plague foci among diverse eco-regions across the reach of Ottoman domains. The mountain ranges of the Anatolian and Balkan peninsulas, as well as the neighboring highlands of the Caucasus and the Persian plateau, may be identified as areas with ecological factors suitable for the focalization of plague, once introduced. As we shall see below, several rodent species—currently known to be plague hosts—inhabited these highlands, making them likely ecological zones for plague maintenance.

What remains to be identified is how the plague ecologies of the sparsely populated Ottoman highlands were connected to the densely populated lowlands. One possible link bridging these disease ecologies was the seasonal movement of pastoralist nomads of Anatolia and the Balkans between highland summer pastures and lowland winter encampments. The customs and economic activities of pastoralist nomads could have brought them in close contact with plague-hosting animals and their ectoparasites. An Ottoman document from 1571, reporting high plague mortality among the nomads, may be taken as evidence that plague's focalization had already taken a strong hold in the empire's highlands.[32] Despite the general belief expressed in current scholarship, that nomads of Anatolia and the Balkans remained mostly free from plague (e.g., Schamiloglu 2004; McNeill 2012), recent research on North Africa highlights not only their risk of contracting the disease but also of propagating it across considerable distances (Bitam et al. 2010; Ben Néfissa and Moulin 2010). A similar suggestion was made by the nineteenth-century French physician J. D. Tholozan (1874) with regard to the movement of nomads and the spread of plague in eastern Anatolia, western Persia, and Mesopotamia.

There were myriad ways in which nomads interacted with settled societies in the Ottoman domain, directly or indirectly. For example, nomads were not only indispensable for supplying raw materials for the textile and leather industries (e.g., wool, dyes, and hides), they were also involved in the process of producing carpets, rugs, and various other textile products. Similarly, they were the suppliers of transportation animals, such as donkeys, horses, mules, oxen and buffaloes, and camels—a known plague carrier (Faroqhi 1984: 49–50; de Planhol 1969). They would participate in harvests in western Anatolia, as migrant workers, or could serve in various military undertakings of the Ottoman state (Kasaba 2009: 31–35). Nomads came into contact with town-dwellers most repeatedly in the outskirts of Ottoman towns, where businesses such as tanneries, soap factories, and slaughterhouses were located, and low-income families and day laborers resided (Ayalon, forthcoming). These businesses attracted a great number of commensal rodents, exposed laborers to potentially infected materials, and thus functioned as possible gateways of infection leading to urban outbreaks.[33]

---

32 Document from Mühimme Defteri, dated 14 March 1571, published in Yılmaz and Yılmaz (2006, 2: 60).

33 It is generally held that some professionals in premodern cities were at higher

Patterns of Plague Transmission

Recent research has demonstrated that a number of media and forms of mediation might be concurrently involved in plague transmission—especially during pandemics—along with the basic rodent host-vector-human transmission. For example, it has been shown that *Y. pestis* survives in flea feces, in post-mortem hosts, in soil, and in plants (Gage and Kosoy 2005; Drancourt, Houhamdi, and Ranoult 2006; Eisen et al. 2008; Ayyadurai et al. 2008; Easterday et al. 2012; Pawlowski et al. 2011). Also, it has been recognized that humans may become infected by plague as a result of consumption of infected food, wounds (such as those caused by animal bites or scratches), or exposure to airborne bacteria. With this in mind, there is a growing awareness of the need to complicate the patterns of plague transmission, with a recent plea being that "the epidemiology of plague must be seen in a much less diagrammatic manner than in the past" (Raoult et al. 2013: 19).

Similarly, historical scholarship on plague has very recently moved beyond an exclusive reliance on models of rodent-host-vector-to-human transmission. In particular, the recent turn in the humanities toward recognizing the role of animals and other nonhuman agents has stimulated novel avenues of inquiry in plague historiography (e.g., Catanach 2001; Stathakopoulos 2011; Campbell 2010 and 2011; Kelly 2013). A comparable change can be observed in Ottomanist historiography, which has informed recent studies of Ottoman environmental history (White 2011; Mikhail 2011, 2013a, 2013b). In particular, a recent case study of the 1791 plague outbreak in Egypt illustrates this trend well, by exploring plague's connections to flooding, rodent behavior, and other climatic conditions, so as to situate it in its environmental context (Mikhail 2008, 2012). While it is imperative to recognize the role of human agency in the spread of plague, it is equally important to broaden our vision to the larger environment.

This is another problem for the historian: the ground-burrowing rodents of the early modern Ottoman landscape are barely visible in the sources.[34] An interesting piece of anecdotal evidence comes from the six-

risk of infection. Among these were butchers, bakers, millers, artisans of cloth and paper, by virtue of their handling meat, grains, and textiles, all instrumental media in the dissemination of plague. See Audoin-Rouzeau 2003: 233-8.

34 Further research is needed to clarify the taxonomy of rodents in the Ottoman landscape. A nineteenth-century Ottoman Turkish lexicon (Redhouse 1880) includes the following species: short-tailed field mouse (*arvicola arvalis*); jerboa (*dipus aegyptius*); water vole (*arvicola amphibius*); marmot (*arclomys marmotta*); lemming (*myodes lemmus*); and bank vole (*myodes glareolus*).

teenth-century German traveler Hans Dernschwam, who left a detailed description of an animal he saw in northwest Anatolia:

> It is slightly larger than a mouse, smaller than a vole, with delicate and well-proportioned limbs. It looked like a hare. Its head, mouth, and ears were well-balanced; its back was rather long and elegant. It had a very long tail. The tail was like a lion's tail with a little ball on its end. It held up its tail in the air. This way it looked like an African monkey. (Dernschwam [1553–55]/1987: 307–08)

This depiction brings to mind the jerboa, which is known to be a plague carrier. Yet, it is difficult to identify what type of jerboa it may have been. Jerboas do not occur in this part of Anatolia today; only the *Euphrates jerboa* (*Allactaga euphratica*) can be found marginally in southeastern Turkey (Arslan et al. 2012). If this species were indeed a type of jerboa that inhabited Anatolia in the sixteenth century but is now extinct, it would be interesting to reflect on the relationship between the extinction of this animal and the disappearance of plague.

The seventeenth-century Ottoman traveler Evliya Çelebi (*c.* 1630–83/1996) documented the types of rodents he encountered, such as the bank vole, the ground squirrel, the water vole, and probably the Persian jird (*Meriones persicus*)—known to be a plague carrier.[35] Writing in the eighteenth century, Alexander Russell (1794, 2: 180–82) listed different species of rodents occurring in Aleppo at the time, along with their names in Arabic and Latin. Not seeing any reason to discuss commensal rodents, Russell simply noted: "There is nothing remarkable in the Rat, and the Mouse. Most of the houses are infested with them." As for wild rodents, he mentioned the short-tailed field mouse, the dormouse, the hamster, the water rat, and the jerboa (which supports the above-mentioned observations of Dernschwam). Furthermore, an English traveler in Anatolia testified to seeing marmot-like rodents in Ilgın (modern day Konya, in Turkey) during a plague epidemic in 1836:

> The plain swarmed with a species of burrowing animal about the size of a squirrel, which I had also seen in other parts of Asia Minor; but whether a species of marmotte, jerboa, lemming, or hamster, I could not ascertain. . . . Their colour is a light yellowish brown, and they abound in the southern provinces of Russia, where the variety or species is known by the name of "Rat des steppes." (Hamilton 1842, 2: 189; cf. Panzac 1985: 123)

35 The Persian jird (*meriones*) has been identified as a "real reservoir of plague" by Baltazar et al. (1952), who believed that they were able to keep plague "permanently enzootic." See also Green 2014 and Carmichael 2014, both in this issue.

This rodent species may be identified as the white-throated woodrat (*Neotoma albigula*), which no longer occurs in this part of the world (Wrobel 2006: 339). What is important to note here is that several rodent species documented by early modern sources are currently known to be plague carriers. The fact that most of those species have now become extinct in Anatolia and the Balkans, where plague no longer occurs, invites further questions. Whether those rodent species became extinct due to plague or by other causes, it may be valuable to consider this connection.

Along with rodents, a number of animals (e.g., cats, dogs, rabbits, camels, and goats) can become infected by plague and transmit it to humans (Fedorov 1960; Ell 1979 and 1980; Christie, Chen, and Elberg 1980; Salkeld and Stapp 2006; Raoult et al. 2013). Some premodern observers of plague may have noticed this phenomenon. One such testimony comes from the English physician Charles MacLean, albeit to mock and discredit such beliefs. In 1815, in Istanbul, he claims to have heard that "Of all quadrupeds, the shaggy horse, or horse with long hair, is alone exempt from contracting the infection of plague. Other animals, and birds of every kind, can receive, and communicate the infection" (Maclean 1817: 202). This point deserves some attention, because Maclean's informants believed that a wide variety of animals were known to contract the infection and recognized their role as intermediaries in its transmission. At least one other nineteenth-century testimony identified a dog as a putative transmitter of plague. This keen observation comes from the memoirs of H. G. O. Dwight, an American missionary in Istanbul who lost his wife and son to plague during an outbreak in 1837. In one of his letters, Dwight noted that the dog of their neighbor—a family that had recently lost a child to plague—often came to their house yard to play with his youngest son, John, who later contracted the disease and died (Dwight 1840: 23). Such testimonies are rare, yet deserve further attention considering the notoriously large street dog population in Ottoman cities, above all in Istanbul. European travelers often commented on the street dogs of the Ottoman capital as a typical feature of the city until the modern era. Perhaps the best known of these accounts is that of the Italian writer Edmondo de Amicis (1896: 108–13), who noted that "the dogs constitute a second population of the city."[36] This does not necessarily mean that dogs were the principal hosts to plague, but their presence may be taken

36 Their presence, however, came to be seen (at the turn of the twentieth century) as a sign of the Ottoman incapacity to regulate a sanitary urban space. For a discussion of street dogs of Istanbul and the efforts to eliminate them as a "measure of progress," see Brummett 1995.

into consideration when thinking about the patterns of plague transmission in early modern Ottoman towns.

In addition, the role of mammalian carnivores (feeding on rodents, such as marmots, ground squirrels, and voles) may require further consideration. It has been noted that carnivores can act as transitory hosts, transporting infected arthropods between different rodent populations. Recent research also suggests that mammalian carnivores exhibit some characteristics as plague hosts that can sustain the infection in enzootic form (Salkeld and Stapp 2006). In the Ottoman landscape, these carnivores would include wolves, foxes, jackals, and hyenas. Although these species mostly avoided crowded human settlements, there are references to foxes and jackals sighted in the outskirts of Ottoman towns by early modern observers (Russell 1794, 2: 183–85). Perhaps more to the point is the infamous tendency of hyenas to dig up and desecrate graves. Hyenas were surprisingly common in parts of Eurasia (Meserve 2012), including areas governed by the Ottoman empire, and may deserve closer attention in the context of plague studies. One sixteenth-century testimony comes from the account of the Habsburg ambassador Ogier Ghiselin de Busbecq, who mentioned hyenas that dug up human bodies from graves in Anatolia. Busbecq (1554–62/2005: 48–49) notes that locals of that area placed heavy stones on top of graves to protect them from hyenas. Hyenas were also observed by the Russell brothers in Aleppo and its surroundings in the eighteenth century, where they were commonly known by the locals who sometimes caught them alive "in the hills at no great distance from town" (Russell 1794, 2: 186–88). It appears that the threat of hyenas was still known to the late nineteenth-century town-dwellers on the northern coast of Anatolia, as suggested by an official document.[37] Another example of a mammalian carnivore that fed on small rodents is the weasel. The fifteenth-century Spanish traveler Pero Tafur commented on the abundance of weasels—presumably the Egyptian weasel (*Mustela subpalmata*)—in Damietta both in the streets and inside the house (1926: 68). Even though the historical evidence is fragmentary, both intra- and inter-species interactions of carnivores are important for the local transmission of plague, especially in linking the plague ecologies of urban areas to their hinterlands.

37 According to this document, dated 1872, the population of the town Çatalzeytin, west of Sinop, claimed that "a hyena monster was stealing children from houses." See "The Hyena Monster of Sinop and the Vagaries of Ottoman Population Accounts," available online at <http://www.docblog.ottomanhistorypodcast.com/2012/08/the-art-of-not-being-seen-hyena-monster.html> [accessed September 19, 2014].

Even more significant is the case of animals that can potentially transport infected fleas over long distances and cause metastatic leaps of plague. These are predator birds that feed on rodents, including large birds of prey (such as hawks, falcons, and owls) and migratory birds (Benedictow 2004: 47). Sixteenth-century Ottoman plague treatises loosely observed a connection between the behavior of migratory birds and epidemics. For example, the plague treatise composed by İlyas bin İbrahim, an Iberian Jewish physician who came to Istanbul in the early sixteenth century, reports that outbreaks of disease were preceded by environmental events (e.g., earthquakes, astrological and meteorological events) and the flight of certain animals and birds (1894: 28). Increased visibility of certain species of burrowing animals and insects was also regarded as a sign of a coming plague.

The plague treatise of the sixteenth-century Ottoman theologian and biographer Ahmed Taşköprizade mentioned the arrival of migratory birds, especially that of the white stork, as a precursor to plague (Taşköprizade 1875; Ünver 1935: 70–71). This association between the arrival of migratory birds and that of the plague was a keen observation in the absence of the linking knowledge about the transfer of fleas. White storks (*Ciconia ciconia*) are predatory birds that feed on small rodents (such as voles, and possibly rats) in addition to various sorts of insects. They also feed at garbage dumps and nest on roofs, poles, and straw stacks, making them a prime candidate for carrying diseases (van den Bossche et al. 2002; Hubálek 2004; Malkinson et al. 2001 and 2002). Recent research also suggests that migratory birds can be a factor in disseminating plague-infected fleas (Heier et al. 2011). Furthermore, in the Ottoman case, the trajectories of their migration seem to have coincided with those of plague. The migratory route followed by the white stork from Europe to Southeast Africa crisscrossed the Ottoman lands from northwest to southeast, and largely corresponded to the main pilgrimage and caravan route in the eastern Mediterranean, before crossing over the Sinai peninsula to Egypt, Sudan, and further south into Africa (van den Bossche et al. 2002). Incidentally, this migratory route passed right over Istanbul and across the Bosphorus. Historical sources sometimes mention flocks of storks. For example, Hans Dernschwam ([1553–55]/1987: 44) notes seeing flocks of thousands of storks near Edirne in the mid-sixteenth century. This correspondence between the trajectories of migratory birds and that of pilgrimage and caravan routes seems to further complicate the pathways of plague's diffusion. Given both scientific and anecdotal evidence, it should be possible to surmise that migratory birds can be associated with metastatic leaps of the infection between remote and isolated enzootic foci and urban areas.

This does not suggest that they were the sole agents for transmitting the infection; rather this was one among many routes that helped circulate plague over land, sea, and air. This reminds us of the importance of expanding our vision to develop a "bird's-eye view" of plague's diffusion, in addition to envisioning its spread along trade routes or by other means that place human agency at the center.

Conclusion

Studying the Ottoman plague experience during the Second Pandemic offers three important insights. First, it underscores the critical importance of focalization. Such processes may be helpful in studying the plague experience of even those areas that are historically imagined to have received the infection from outside: for example, Europe. Second, it draws attention to the necessity of adopting more complex models of plague transmission, with a special emphasis on interspecies dynamics and the local species that serve as hosts, vectors, and as intermediaries. In order to better understand local plague ecologies, it may be invaluable to expand our vision to include a wider spectrum of rodent species and consider the role of domestic and commensal mammals, mammalian carnivores, predator and migratory birds in plague transmission. Third, it urges the elimination of old models of assumed/imagined epidemiological boundaries and trajectories that have been built on flawed historical constructs, such as those that have been inherited from nineteenth-century Eurocentric notions and colonial plague science. Instead, it highlights the importance of adopting more unified epidemiological perspectives for studying larger disease zones, such as the Afro-Eurasian zone during the Second Pandemic. The Ottoman epidemiological experience is not only eminently comparable to those other contemporaneous experiences, but also indispensable for a full understanding of plague in this larger disease ecology. Finally, the new plague science, as valuable as it is, should be considered as a set of guidelines in studying the plague. Historical sources suggest that the disease could manifest itself in different forms and have different effects, depending on local circumstances. As lesser-known epidemiological experiences are recovered from the past, this evidence will supply increased opportunities not only for the plague historian but for the plague scientist as well.

Bibliography

Achtman, Mark, Giovanna Morelli, Peixuan Zhu, Thierry Wirth, et al. 2004. "Microevolution and History of the Plague Bacillus, *Yersinia pestis*," *Proceedings of the National Academy of Sciences* 101, no. 51: 17837–42

Ágoston, Gábor, and Bruce Alan Masters. 2009. *Encyclopedia of the Ottoman Empire* (New York: Facts on File)

Alexander, John T. 1980. *Bubonic Plague in Early Modern Russia: Public Health & Urban Disaster* (Baltimore: Johns Hopkins University Press)

Amicis, Edmondo de. 1896. *Constantinople*, trans. by Maria Hornor Lansdale (Philadelphia: Coates)

Anandavalli, Lakshmikanthan. 2007. "The Black Death in Medieval India: A Historical Mystery," *Tangents: The Journal of the Master of Liberal Arts Program at Stanford University* 6: 20–25

Andrianaivoarimanana, V., K. Kreppel, N. Elissa, J.-M. Duplantier, et al. 2013. "Understanding the Persistence of Plague Foci in Madagascar," *PLoS Neglected Tropical Diseases* 7, no. 11: e2382

Anisimov, A. P., L. E. Lindler and G. B. Pier. 2004. "Intraspecific Diversity of *Yersinia pestis*," *Clinical Microbiology Reviews* 17, no. 2: 434–64

Ansari, B. M. 1994. "An Account of Bubonic Plague in Seventeenth Century India in an Autobiography of a Mughal Emperor," *Journal of Infection* 29: 351–52

Arık, Feda Şamil. 1991. "Selçuklular Zamanında Anadolu'da Veba Salgınları," *Tarih Araştırmaları Dergisi* 15, no. 26: 27–57

Arnold, David. 1993. *Colonizing the Body: State Medicine and Epidemic Disease in Nineteenth-Century India* (Berkeley: University of California Press)

Arslan, A., T. Yorulmaz, K. Toyran, İ. Albayrak, et al. 2012. "C-Banding and Ag-NOR Distribution Patterns in Euphrates Jerboa, *Allactaga euphratica* (Mammalia: Rodentia), from Turkey," *Mammalia* 76: 427–34

Audoin-Rouzeau, Frédérique. 2003. *Les Chemins de la peste: le rat, la puce et l'homme* (Rennes: Presses universitaires de Rennes)

Ayalon, Yaron. Forthcoming. "When Nomads Meet Urbanites: The Outskirts of Ottoman Cities as a Venue for the Spread of Epidemic Diseases," in *Plagues in Nomadic Contexts: Historical Impact, Medical Responses, and Cultural Adaptations in Ancient to Mediaeval Eurasia*, ed. Kurt Franz et al. (Leiden: Brill)

Ayyadurai, S., L. Houhamdi, H. Leipidi, C. Nappez, et al. 2008. "Long-Term Persistence of Virulent *Yersinia pestis* in Soil," *Microbiology* 154: 2865–71

Baca, M., and M. Molak. 2008. "Research on Ancient DNA in the Near East," *Bioarchaeology of the Near East* 2: 39–61

Baltazard, M., M. Bahmanyar, Ch. Mofidi, and B. Seydian. 1952. "Le foyer de peste du Kurdistan," *Bulletin of the World Health Organization* 5: 441–72

Ben Ari, T., S. Neerinckx, K. L. Gage, K. Kreppel, et al. 2011. "Plague and Climate: Scales Matter," *PLoS Pathogens*, 7, no. 9: e1002160

Ben Ari, T., S. Neerinckx, L. Agier, B. Cazelles, et al. 2012. "Identification of Chinese Plague Foci from Long-Term Epidemiological Data," *Proceedings of the National Academy of Sciences* 109: 8196–8201

Ben Néfissa, K., and A. M. Moulin. 2010. "The North African Plague and Charles Nicolle's Theory of Infectious Diseases," *Gesnerus-Swiss Journal of the History of Medicine and Sciences* 67: 30–56

Benedict, Carol Ann. 1996. *Bubonic Plague in Nineteenth-Century China* (Stanford: Stanford University Press)

Benedictow, Ole J. 2004. *The Black Death, 1346–1353: The Complete History* (Woodbridge: Boydell)

Biraben, Jean-Nöel. 1975. *Les hommes et la peste en France et dans les pays européens et méditerranéens* (Paris: Mouton)

Biraben, Jean-Nöel, and Jacques Le Goff. 1969. "La peste dans le haut Moyen-Âge," *Annales. Économies, Sociétés, Civilisations* 24: 1484–1510

Bitam, I., S. Ayyadurai, T. Kernif, M. Chetta, et al. 2010. "New Rural Focus of Plague, Algeria," *Emerging Infectious Diseases* 16: 1639–40

Bolton, J. L. 2013. "Looking for *Yersinia pestis:* Scientists, Historians and the Black Death," in *The Fifteenth Century, XII: Society in an Age of Plague*, ed. Linda Clark and Carole Rawcliffe, 15–38 (Woodbridge: Boydell)

Boogert, Maurits van den (ed.). 2010. *Aleppo Observed: Ottoman Syria through the Eyes of Two Scottish Doctors, Alexander and Patrick Russell* (Oxford: Oxford University Press)

Borsch, Stuart J. 2005. *The Black Death in Egypt and England: A Comparative Study* (Austin: University of Texas Press)

Bos, K. I., V. J. Schuenemann, G. Brian Golding, H. A. Burbano, et al. 2011. "A Draft Genome of *Yersinia pestis* from Victims of the Black Death," *Nature* 478, no. 7370: 506–10

Bossche, Willem van den, et al. 2002. *Eastern European White Stork Populations: Migration Studies and Elaboration of Conservation Measures* (Bonn: Bundesamt für Naturschutz [BfN]/German Federal Agency for Nature Conservation)

Brayer, A. 1836. *Neuf années à Constantinople: observations sur la topographie de cette capital, l'hygiène et les mœurs de ses habitants, l'Islamisme et son influence: la peste, ses causes, ses variétés, sa marche et son traitement: la non-contagion de cette maladie: les quarantaines et les lazarets* (Paris: Ballizard, Barthès, Dufour et Lowell)

British Medical Journal. 1900. "The Plague: Plague and Plague Measures in the Turkish Empire," *British Medical Journal* 2, no. 2086 (December 22): 1810–11

British Medical Journal. 1902a. "Literary Notes," *British Medical Journal* 2, no. 2167 (July 12): 142

British Medical Journal. 1902b. "The Destruction of Rats on Ship-Board," *British Medical Journal* 1, no. 2144 (February 1): 294–95

Brotherton, P. Sean, and Vinh-Kim Nguyen. 2013. "Revisiting Local Biology in the Era of Global Health," *Medical Anthropology* 32: 287–90

Brummett, Palmira. 1995. "Dogs, Women, Cholera, and Other Menaces in the Streets: Cartoon Satire in the Ottoman Revolutionary Press, 1908–11," *International Journal of Middle East Studies*, 2: 433–60

Buell, Paul D. 2012. "Qubilai and the Rats," *Sudhoffs Archiv* 96, no. 2: 127–44

Bulmuş, Birsen. 2012. *Plague, Quarantines, and Geopolitics in the Ottoman Empire* (Edinburgh: Edinburgh University Press)

Busbecq, Ogier Ghiselin de. 1554–62/2005. *The Turkish Letters of Ogier Ghiselin de Busbecq, Imperial Ambassador at Constantinople, 1554–1562: Translated from the Latin of the Elzevir Edition of 1663*, trans. Edward Seymour Forster (Baton Rouge: Louisiana State University Press)

Cabanel, N., A. Leclercq, V. Chenal-Francisque, B. Annajar, et al. 2013. "Plague Outbreak in Libya, 2009, Unrelated to Plague in Algeria," *Emerging Infectious Diseases*, 19, no. 2: 230–36

Campbell, Bruce M. S. 2010. "Physical Shocks, Biological Hazards, and Human Impacts: The Crisis of the Fourteenth Century Revisited," in *Economic and Biological Interactions in Pre-Industrial Europe, from the Thirteenth to Eighteenth Centuries*, ed. Simonetta Cavaciocchi, 13–32 (Florence: Firenze University Press)

Campbell, Bruce M. S. 2011. "Panzootics, Pandemics and Climate Anomalies in the Fourteenth Century," in *Beiträge zum Göttinger Umwelthistorischen Kolloquium, 2010–2011*, ed. B. Hermann, 177–216 (Göttingen: Universitätsverlag)

Carmichael, Ann G. 2014. "Plague Persistence in Western Europe: A Hypothesis," *The Medieval Globe* 1: 157–191

Catanach, I. J. 2001. "The 'Globalization' of Disease? India and the Plague," *Journal of World History*, 12: 131–53

Çelebi, Evliya. *c.* 1630–83/1996. *Seyahatname*, ed. Robert Dankoff, Seyit Ali Kahraman, Yücel Dağlı, Zekeriya Kurşun, et al., 10 vols. (Istanbul: Yapı Kredi Yayınları)

Christensen, Peter. 1993. *The Decline of Iranshahr: Irrigation and Environments in the History of the Middle East, 500 B.C. to A.D. 1500* ([Copenhagen]: University of Copenhagen)

Christie, A. B., T. H. Chen, and Sanford S. Elberg. 1980. "Plague in Camels and Goats: Their Role in Human Epidemics," *Journal of Infectious Diseases* 141, no. 6: 724–26

Cohn, Samuel Kline, Jr. 2008. "Epidemiology of the Black Death and Successive Waves of Plague," in *Pestilential Complexities: Understanding Medieval Plague*, ed. Vivian Nutton, 74–100 (London: Wellcome Trust Centre for the History of Medicine at University College London)

Cohn, Samuel Kline, Jr. 2013. "The Historian and the Laboratory: The Black Death Disease," in *Society in an Age of Plague (The Fifteenth Century, XII)*, ed. Linda Clark and Carole Rawcliffe, 195–212 (Woodbridge: Boydell)

Clark, Linda, and Carole Rawcliffe (eds.). 2013. *Society in an Age of Plague (The Fifteenth Century, XII)* (Woodbridge: Boydell)

Conrad, Lawrence. 1981. "The Plague in the Early Medieval Near East" (PhD dissertation, Princeton University)

Conrad, Lawrence. 1982. "*Tāʿūn* and *Wabāʾ*: Conceptions of Plague and Pestilence in Early Islam," *Journal of the Economic and Social History of the Orient* 25: 268–307

Conrad, Lawrence, and Dominik Wujastyk. 2000. *Contagion: Perspectives from Pre-Modern Societies* (Aldershot: Ashgate)

Crane, J. T. 2011. "Viral Cartographies: Mapping the Molecular Politics of Global HIV," *BioSocieties* 6: 142–66

Creighton, Charles. 1891. *A History of Epidemics in Britain* (Cambridge: Cambridge University Press)

Cui, Y., C. Yu, Y. Yan, D. Li, et al. 2013. "Historical Variations in Mutation Rate in an Epidemic Pathogen, *Yersinia pestis*," *Proceedings of the National Academy of Science* 110, no. 2: 577–82

Dernschwam, Hans. [1553–55]/1987. *İstanbul ve Anadolu'ya seyahat günlüğü*, trans. Yaşar Önen (Ankara: Kültür ve Turizm Bakanlığı)

DeWitte, Sharon N. 2014. "The Anthropology of Plague: Insights from Bioarcheological Analyses of Epidemic Cemeteries," *The Medieval Globe* 1: 97–123

Dols, Michael. 1974. "Plague in Early Islamic History," *Journal of the American Oriental Society* 94: 371–83

Dols, Michael. 1977. *The Black Death in the Middle East* (Princeton, NJ: Princeton University Press)

Dols, Michael. 1987. "Review of Daniel Panzac, *La peste dans l'empire Ottoman, 1700–1850*," in *Medical History* 31: 109–10

Drancourt, M., L. Houhamdi, and D. Raoult. 2006. "*Yersinia pestis* as a Telluric, Human Ectoparasite-Borne Organism," *Lancet Infectious Diseases* 6: 234–41

Dwight, H. G. O. 1840. *Memoir of Mrs. Elizabeth B. Dwight, Including an Account of the Plague of 1837* (New York: Dodd)

Eager, John Macauley. 1908. *The Present Pandemic of Plague* (Washington: Government Printing Office)

Easterday, W. R., K. L. Kausrud, B. Starr, L. Heier, et al. 2012. "An Additional Step in the Transmission of *Yersinia pestis*?," *ISME Journal* 6: 231–36

Echenberg, Myron J. 2007. *Plague Ports: The Global Urban Impact of Bubonic Plague, 1894–1901* (New York: New York University Press)

Eisen, R. J., and K. L. Gage. 2012. "Transmission of Flea-Borne Zoonotic Agents," *Annual Review of Entomology* 57: 61–82

Eisen, R. J., J. M. Petersen, C. L. Higgins, D. Wong, et al. 2008. "Persistence of *Yersinia pestis* in Soil Under Natural Conditions," *Emerging Infectious Diseases* 14: 941–43

Ell, S. R. 1979. "Some Evidence for Interhuman Transmission of Medieval Plague," *Review of Infectious Diseases* 1: 563–66

Ell, S. R. 1980. "Interhuman Transmission of Medieval Plague," *Bulletin of the History of Medicine* 54: 497–510

Ess, Josef van. 2001. *Der Fehltritt des Gelehrten: Die "Pest von Emmaus" und ihre theologischen Nachspiele* (Heidelberg: Winter)

Faroqhi, Suraiya. 1984. *Towns and Townsmen of Ottoman Anatolia: Trade, Crafts, and Food Production in an Urban Setting, 1520–1650* (Cambridge: Cambridge University Press)

Fedorov, V. N. 1960. "Plague in Camels and its Prevention in the USSR," *Bulletin of the World Health Organization* 23: 275–81

Fisher, Alan. 1992. "Review of *La peste dans l'Empire ottoman, 1700–1850* (Collection Turcica, 5) by Daniel Panzac," *Middle East Studies Association Bulletin* 26: 72–74

Frandsen, Karl-Erik. 2010. *The Last Plague in the Baltic Region, 1709–1713* (Copenhagen: Museum Tusculanum Press)

Gage, K. L., and M. Y. Kosoy. 2005. "Natural History of Plague: Perspectives from More than a Century of Research," *Annual Review of Entomology* 50: 505–28

Golem, Bilal, and Kemal Özsan. 1952. "Türk Veba Suşlarında Biyoşimik Karakter Farkları," *Türk İjiyen ve Tecrübi Biyoloji Dergisi* 12: 29–51

Gordon, Daniel. 1999. "Confrontations with the Plague in Eighteenth-Century France," in *Dreadful Visitations: Confronting Natural Catastrophe in the Age of Enlightenment*, ed. Alessa Johns, 3–29 (New York: Routledge)

Gratz, N. 1999. "Rodent Reservoirs and Flea Vectors of Natural Foci of Plague," in *Plague Manual: Epidemiology, Distribution, Surveillance and Control*, 63–96 (Geneva: World Health Organization)

Green, Monica H. 2014. "Taking 'Pandemic' Seriously: Making the Black Death Global," *The Medieval Globe* 1: 27–61

Haensch, S., R. Bianucci, M. Signoli, M. Rajerison, et al. 2010. "Distinct Clones of *Yersinia pestis* Caused the Black Death," *PLoS Pathogens* 6, no. 10: e1001134

Hamilton, William John. 1842. *Researches in Asia Minor, Pontus and Armenia* (London: John Murray)

Hecker, J. F. C. 1859. *The Epidemics of the Middle Ages*, trans. B. G. Babington (London: Trübner)

Heier, L., G. O. Storvik, S. A. Davis, H. Vilhugrein, et al. 2011. "Emergence, Spread, Persistence and Fade-out of Sylvatic Plague in Kazakhstan," *Proceedings of the Royal Society B: Biological Sciences* 278, no. 1720: 2915–23

Hirst, L. 1953. *The Conquest of Plague: A Study of the Evolution of Epidemiology* (Oxford: Clarendon Press)

Howard-Jones, Norman. 1975. *The Scientific Background of the International Sanitary Conferences, 1851–1938* (Geneva: World Health Organization)

Hrabak, Bogumil. 1957. "Kuga u balkanskim zemljama pod Turcima od 1450 do 1600 godine," *Istoriski glasnik* 1–2: 19–37

Hubálek, Z. 2004. "An Annotated Checklist of Pathogenic Microorganisms Associated with Migratory Birds," *Journal of Wildlife Diseases* 40: 639–59

İlyas bin İbrahim. 1894. *Tevfîkâtü'l-hamidiyye fî def'i'l-emrâzi'l-vebâ'iyye*, trans. Ahmedü'ş-Şami Ömeri (Istanbul University, Cerrahpaşa History of Medicine Library, MS 105)

Issawi, Charles. 1988. "Review of *La peste dans l'Empire ottoman* by Daniel Panzac," *International Journal of Middle East Studies* 20: 115–16

Jennings, Ronald C. 1993. "Plague in Trabzon and Reactions to It according to Local Juridical Registers," in *Humanist & Scholar: Essays in Honor of Andreas Tietze*, ed. Heath W. Lowry and Donald Quataert, 37–46 (Istanbul: Isis Press)

Karimova, T. Yu, V. M. Neronov, and V. P. Popov. 2010. "Development of Views on Natural Focality of Plague," *Biology Bulletin*, 37: 725–32

Kasaba, Reşat. 2009. *A Moveable Empire: Ottoman Nomads, Migrants, and Refugees* (Seattle: University of Washington Press)

Keeling, M. J., and C. A. Gilligan. 2000a. "Metapopulation Dynamics of Bubonic Plague," *Nature* 407, no. 6806: 903–06

Keeling, M. J., and C. A. Gilligan. 2000b. "Bubonic Plague: A Metapopulation Model of a Zoonosis," *Proceedings of the Royal Society of London. Series B: Biological Sciences* 267, no. 1458: 2219–30

Keim, P. S., and D. M. Wagner. 2009. "Humans and Evolutionary and Ecological Forces Shaped the Phylogeography of Recently Emerged Diseases," *Nature Reviews Microbiology* 7: 813–21

Kelly, Catherine. 2008. "'Not From the College, But through the Public and the Legislature": Charles Maclean and the Relocation of Medical Debate in the Early Nineteenth Century," *Bulletin of the History of Medicine* 82: 545–69

Kelly, Kathleen Coyne. 2013. "Flea and ANT: Mapping the Mobility of the Plague, 1330s–1350s," *Postmedieval: A Journal of Medieval Cultural Studies* 4: 219–32

Kılıç, Orhan. 2004. *Eskiçağdan Yakınçağa Genel Hatlarıyla Dünyada ve Osmanlı Devletinde Salgın Hastalıklar* (Elazığ: Fırat Üniversitesi Rektörlüğü)

Kōstēs, Kōstas. 1995. *Ston kairo tēs panōlēs: eikones apo tis koinōnies tēs Hellēnikēs chersonēsou, 14os–19os aiōnas* (Hērakleio: Panepistēmiakes Ekdoseis Krētēs)

Krekic, B. 1963. "Europe centrale et balkanique," *Annales: Économies, Sociétés, Civilisations* 8: 594–95

Lammel, Hans-Uwe. 2010. "Western European Perception and Representation of Plagues in Eastern Europe, the Ottoman Empire and the Near East, 1650–1800," in *Economic and Biological Interactions in Pre-Industrial Europe from the Thirteenth to Eighteenth Centuries*, ed. Simonetta Cavaciocchi, 399–421 (Florence: Firenze University Press)

Langer, Lawrence N. 1975. "The Black Death in Russia: Its Effects upon Urban Labor," *Russian History* 2: 53–67

Latour, Bruno. 1987. *Science in Action: How to Follow Scientists and Engineers through Society* (Cambridge, MA: Harvard University Press)

Li, Y., Y. Cui, Y. Hauck, N. E. Platonov, et al. 2009. "Genotyping and Phylogenetic Analysis of *Yersinia pestis* by MLVA: Insights into the Worldwide Expansion of Central Asia Plague Foci," *PLoS ONE* 4, no.6: e6000

Lien-Teh, W. 1924. "The Original Home of Plague," in *Far Eastern Association of Tropical Medicine, Transactions of the Fifth Biennial Congress Held at Singapore, 1923*, ed. A. L. Hoops and J. W. Scharff, 286–304 (London: Bale & Danielsson)

Little, Lester K. 2011. "Plague Historians in Lab Coats," *Past and Present* 213: 267–90

Little, Lester K. (ed.). 2007. *Plague and the End of Antiquity: The Pandemic of 541–750* (Cambridge: Cambridge University Press)

Lock, Margaret. 1993. "Cultivating the Body: Anthropology and Epistemologies of Bodily Practice and Knowledge," *Annual Review of Anthropology* 22: 133–55

Lock, Margaret. 1995. *Encounters with Aging: Mythologies of Menopause in Japan and North America* (Berkeley: University of California Press)

Low, Michael Christopher. 2008. "Empire and the Hajj: Pilgrims, Plagues, and Pan-Islam under British Surveillance, 1865–1908," *International Journal of Middle East Studies* 40: 269–90

Lowry, W. Heath. 2003. "'Pushing the Stone Uphill: The Impact of Bubonic Plague on Ottoman Urban Society in the Fifteenth and Sixteenth Centuries," *Osmanlı Araştırmaları* 23: 93–132

Mackenzie, Mordach. 1752. "Extracts of Several Letters of Mordach Mackenzie, M. D. Concerning the Plague at Constantinople," *Philosophical Transactions (1683–1775)* 47: 384–95

Mackenzie, Mordach. 1764. "An Account of the Plague at Constantinople in a Letter from Mordach Mackenzie, M. D. to Sir James Porter, His Majesty's Envoy Plenipotentiary at Brussels, and F. R. S.," *Philosophical Transactions (1683–1775)* 54: 69–82

Maclean, Charles. 1817. *Results of an Investigation, Respecting Epidemic and Pestilential Diseases; Including Researches in the Levant, Concerning the Plague* (London: Underwood)

Malkinson, M., C. Banet, Y. Weisman, S. Pokamunski, et al. 2002. "Introduction of West Nile Virus in the Middle East by Migrating White Storks," *Emerging Infectious Diseases* 8: 392–97

Malkinson, M., Y. Weisman, S. Pokamunski, R. King, et al. 2001. "Intercontinental Transmission of West Nile Virus by Migrating White Storks," *Emerging Infectious Diseases* 7, no. 3 (supp.): 540

Manolova-Nikolova, Nadja I. 2004. *Čumavite vremena (1700–1850)* (Sofia: IF-94)

McNeill, J. R. 2012. "The Eccentricity of the Middle East and North Africa's Environmental History," in *Water on Sand: Environmental Histories of the Middle East and North Africa*, ed. Alan Mikhail, 27–50 (Oxford: Oxford University Press)

McNeill, William H. 1976. *Plagues and Peoples* (New York: Anchor)

Meserve, Ruth I. 2012. "Striped Hyenas and 'Were-Hyenas' in Central Eurasia," in *Archivum Eurasiae Medii Aevi*, ed. Th. T. Allsen, P. B. Golden, R. K. Kovalev, and A. P. Martinez, 199–220 (Wiesbaden: Harrassowitz)

Mikhail, Alan. 2008. "The Nature of Plague in Late Eighteenth-Century Egypt," *Bulletin of the History of Medicine* 82: 249–75

Mikhail, Alan. 2011. *Nature and Empire in Ottoman Egypt: An Environmental History* (Cambridge: Cambridge University Press)

Mikhail, Alan. 2012. "Plague and Environment in Late Ottoman Egypt," in *Water on Sand: Environmental Histories of the Middle East and North Africa*, ed. Alan Mikhail, 111–32 (Oxford: Oxford University Press)

Mikhail, Alan. 2013a. *The Animal in Ottoman Egypt* (Oxford: Oxford University Press)

Mikhail, Alan. 2013b. "Unleashing the Beast: Animals, Energy, and the Economy of Labor in Ottoman Egypt," *American Historical Review* 118: 317–48

Morelli, G., Y. Song, C. J. Mazzoni, M. Eppinger, et al. 2010. "*Yersinia pestis* Genome Sequencing Identifies Patterns of Global Phylogenetic Diversity," *Nature Genetics* 42, no. 12: 1140–43

Morens, D. M., G. K. Folkers, and A. S. Fauci. 2009. "What Is a Pandemic?," *Journal of Infectious Diseases* 200, no. 7: 1018–21

Morony, Michael G. 2007. "'For Whom Does the Writer Write?' The First Bubonic Plague Pandemic According to Syriac Sources," in *Plague and the End of Antiquity: The Pandemic of 541–750*, ed. Lester K. Little, 59–86 (Cambridge: Cambridge University Press)

Nakazawa, Y., R. Williams, A. Townsend Peterson, P. Mead, et al. 2007. "Climate Change Effects on Plague and Tularemia in the United States," *Vector-Borne and Zoonotic Diseases* 7: 529–40

Norris, J. 1977. "East or West? The Geographic Origin of the Black Death," *Bulletin of the History of Medicine* 51: 1–24

Nutton, Vivian (ed.). 2008. *Pestilential Complexities: Understanding Medieval Plague* (London: Wellcome Trust Centre for the History of Medicine at University College London)

Owen, Roger. 1986. "Review of *La peste dans l'Empire ottoman, 1700–1850* by Daniel Panzac," *Bulletin (British Society for Middle Eastern Studies)* 13: 210–12

Panzac, Daniel. 1973. "La peste à Smyrne au XVIIIe siècle," *Annales. Histoire, Sciences Sociales* 28: 1071–93

Panzac, Daniel. 1985. *La peste dans l'empire ottoman, 1700–1850* (Leuven: Peeters)

Panzac, Daniel. 1986. *Quarantaines et lazarets: l'Europe et la peste d'Orient, XVIIe–XXe siècles* (Aix-en-Provence: Édisud)

Panzac, Daniel. 1987. "Alexandrie: peste et croissance urbaine (XVIIe–XIXe siècles)," *Revue de l'Occident musulman et de la Méditerranée* 46: 81–90

Panzac, Daniel. 2003. *Le docteur Adrien Proust: père méconnu, précurseur oublié* (Paris: L'Harmattan)

Panzac, Daniel. 2009. "Plague," in *Encyclopedia of the Ottoman Empire*, ed. Gábor Ágoston and Bruce Alan Masters, 462–63 (New York: Facts on File)

Pawlowski, D. R., D. J. Metzger, A. Raslawsky, A. Howlett, et al. 2011. "Entry of *Yersinia pestis* into the Viable but Nonculturable State in a Low-Temperature Tap Water Microcosm," *PLoS ONE* 6, no.3: e17585

Pezzoni, A. 1842. "Notice of Cases of Plague Contracted in the Lazeretto of Constantinople, in a Letter Addressed to Dr. Davy," *Medico-Chirurgical Transactions* 25: 167–91

Pezzoni, A. 1847. *De la contagionabilité de la peste, fondée principalement sur les résultats obtenus par les quarantaines en turquie* (Constantinople: Impr. du Journal de Constantinople)

Planhol, Xavier de. 1969. "Le boeuf porteur dans le proche-Orient et l'Afrique du nord," *Journal of the Economic and Social History of the Orient* 12: 298–321

Pobst, Phyllis. 2013. "Should We Teach That the Cause of the Black Death Was Bubonic Plague?," *History Compass* 11: 808–20

Pollitzer, R. 1951. "Plague Studies. 1. A Summary of the History and Survey of the Present Distribution of the Disease," *Bulletin of the World Health Organization* 4: 475–533

Proust, Adrien. 1897. *La défense de l'Europe contre la peste: et la Conférence de Venise de 1897* (Paris: Masson)

Raoult, D., N. Mouffok, I. Bitam, R. Piarroux, et al. 2013. "Plague: History and Contemporary Analysis," *Journal of Infection* 66: 18–26

Robarts, Andrew. 2010. "A Plague on Both Houses? Population Movements and the Spread of Disease across the Ottoman-Russian Black Sea Frontier, 1768–1830s" (PhD dissertation, Georgetown University)

Royer, Katherine. 2014. "The Blind Men and the Elephant: Imperial Medicine, Medieval Historians, and the Role of Rats in the Historiography of Plague," in *Medicine and Colonialism: Historical Perspectives in India and South Africa*, ed. Poonam Bala, 99–110 (London: Pickering & Chatto)

Redhouse, Sir James W. 1880. *A Turkish and English Lexicon* (Beirut: Librarie du Liban)

Russell, Alexander. 1794. *The Natural History of Aleppo. Containing a Description of the City, and the Principal Natural Productions in Its Neighbourhood; Together with an Account of the Climate, Inhabitants, and Diseases; Particularly of the Plague*, 2nd ed., 2 vols. (London: Millar)

Russell, Patrick. 1791. *A Treatise of the Plague: Containing an Historical Journal, and Medical Account, of the Plague, at Aleppo, in the Years 1760, 1761, and 1762; Also, Remarks on Quarantines, Lazarettos, and the Administration of Police in Times of Pestilence. To Which Is Added, an Appendix, Containing Cases of the Plague; and an Account of the Weather, during the Pestilential Season* (London: Robinson)

Sarı, Nil, and Şeref Etker. 2000. "19.yy. Başında İki İtalyan Hekimin Türkiye'de İlaç Araştırmaları," V. Türk Eczacılık Tarihi Kongresi (İzmir, May 25–26, 2000)

Salkeld, D. J., and P. Stapp. 2006. "Seroprevalence Rates and Transmission of Plague (*Yersinia pestis*) in Mammalian Carnivores," *Vector Borne and Zoonotic Diseases (Larchmont, N.Y.)* 6: 231–39

Schamiloglu, Uli. 1993. "Preliminary Remarks on the Role of Disease in the History of the Golden Horde," *Central Asian Survey* 12: 447–57

Schamiloglu, Uli. 2004. "The Rise of the Ottoman Empire: The Black Death in Medieval Anatolia and its Impact on Turkish Civilization," in *Views from the Edge: Essays in Honor of Richard W. Bulliet*, ed. Neguin Yavari, Lawrence G.Potter, and Jean-Marc Ran Oppenheim, 255–79 (New York: Columbia University Press)

Shefer-Mossensohn, Miri. 2009. *Ottoman Medicine: Healing and Medical Institutions, 1500–1700* (Albany: SUNY Press)

Shefer-Mossensohn, Miri. 2012. "Communicable Disease in Ottoman Palestine: Local Thoughts and Actions," *Korot* 21: 19–49

Simpson, William John Ritchie. 1905. *A Treatise on Plague, Dealing with the Historical, Epidemiological, Clinical, Therapeutic and Preventive Aspects of the Disease* (Cambridge: Cambridge University Press)

Slack, Paul. 2012. *Plague: A Very Short Introduction* (Oxford: Oxford University Press)

Sołtysiak, Arkadiusz. 2007. "Editorial," *Bioarchaeology of the Near East* 1: 1–3

Stathakopoulos, Dionysios. 2000. "The Justinianic Plague Revisited," *Byzantine and Modern Greek Studies* 24: 255–76

Stathakopoulos, Dionysios. 2004. *Famine and Pestilence in the Late Roman and Early Byzantine Empire: A Systematic Survey of Subsistence Crises and Epidemics* (Aldershot: Ashgate)

Stathakopoulos, Dionysios. 2011. "Invisible Protagonists: The Justinianic Plague from a Zoocentric Point of View," in *Animals and Environment in Byzantium (7th–12th c.)*, ed. Ēlías Anagnōstákēs, Taxiarchēs G. Kollas, and Eutychia Papadopoulou, 87–95 (Athens: Centre for Byzantine Research, National Hellenic Research Foundation)

Stearns, Justin K. 2009. "New Directions in the Study of Religious Responses to the Black Death," *History Compass* 7: 1363–75

Stearns, Justin K. 2011. *Infectious Ideas: Contagion in Premodern Islamic and Christian Thought in the Western Mediterranean* (Baltimore: Johns Hopkins University Press)

Stenseth, N. Chr., N. I. Samia, H. Viljugrein, K. Linné Kausrud, et al. 2006. "Plague Dynamics are Driven by Climate Variation," *Proceedings of the National Academy of Sciences* 103, no. 35: 13110–15

Sticker, Georg. 1908. *Abhandlungen aus der Seuchengeschichte und Seuchenlehre* (Gießen: Töpelmann)

Sussman, George D. 2011. "Was the Black Death in India and China?," *Bulletin of the History of Medicine* 85: 319–55

Tafur, Pero. 1926. *Travels and Adventures, 1435–1439*, ed. Malcolm Letts (New York: Harper)

Takeda, Junko Thérèse. 2011. *Between Crown and Commerce: Marseille and the Early Modern Mediterranean* (Baltimore: Johns Hopkins University Press)

Talbi, Mohamed. 1981. "Laws and Economy in Ifrīqiya (Tunisia) in the Third Islamic Century: Agriculture and the Role of Slaves in the Country's Economy," in *The Islamic Middle East, 700–1900: Studies in Economic and Social History*, ed. Abraham Udovitch, 209–49 (Princeton: Darwin)

Taşköprizade, Ahmed. 1875. *Risalah al-Shifa li-Adwa al-Waba'* ([Cairo]: al-Matba'ah al-Wahbiyah)

Tholozan, Joseph Désiré. 1874. *Histoire de la peste bubonique en Perse; ou, Détermination de son origine, de sa marche, du cycle de ses apparitions et de la cause de sa prompte extinction* (Paris: Masson)

Tran, T.-N.-N., M. Signoli, L. Fozzati, G. Aboudharam, et al. 2011. "High Throughput, Multiplexed Pathogen Detection Authenticates Plague Waves in Medieval Venice, Italy," *PLoS ONE* 6, no. 3: e16735

Ünver, Süheyl. 1935. "'Türkiyede Veba (Taun) Tarihçesi Üzerine," *Tedavi Kliniği ve Laboratuvarı Mecmuası* 5: 70–88

Valli, Eusebio. 1805. *Sulla peste di Costantinopoli del MDCCCIII; giornale* ([Mantova?]: Società tip. all'Apollo)

Varlık, Nükhet. 2011. "Conquest, Urbanization, and Plague Networks in the Ottoman Empire, 1453–1600," in *The Ottoman World*, ed. Christine Woodhead, 251–63 (New York: Routledge)

Varlık, Nükhet. Forthcoming. *Plague and Empire in the Early Modern Mediterranean World: The Ottoman Experience, 1347–1600* (Cambridge: Cambridge University Press)

Vogler, A. J., F. Chan, D. W. Wagner, P. Roumagnac, et al. 2011. "Phylogeography and Molecular Epidemiology of *Yersinia pestis* in Madagascar," *PLoS Neglected Tropical Diseases* 5. no. 9: e1319

Walløe, Lars. 2008. "Medieval and Modern Bubonic Plague: Some Clinical Continuities," in *Pestilential Complexities: Understanding Medieval Plague*, ed. Vivian Nutton, 59–73 (London: Wellcome Trust Centre for the History of Medicine at University College London)

White, Sam. 2010. "Rethinking Disease in Ottoman History," *International Journal of Middle East Studies* 42: 549–67

White, Sam. 2011. *The Climate of Rebellion in the Early Modern Ottoman Empire* (Cambridge: Cambridge University Press)

WHO [World Health Organization]. 1999. "Plague Manual: Epidemiology, Distribution, Surveillance and Control" WHO/CDS/CSR/EDC/99.2

WHO [World Health Organization]. 2012. "Guidance on Regulations for the Transport of Infectious Substances 2013–2014 (Applicable as from 1 January 2013)" WHO/HSE/GCR/2012.12

Wittman, William. 1804. *Travels in Turkey, Asia Minor, Syria, and across the Desert into Egypt during the Years 1799, 1800, and 1801, in Company with the Turkish Army, and the British Military Mission. To Which Are Annexed, Observations on the Plague, and on the Diseases Prevalent in Turkey, and a Meteorological Journal* (Philadelphia: Humphreys)

Wrobel, Murray (ed.). 2006. *Elsevier's Dictionary of Mammals* (Amsterdam: Elsevier)

Yıldırım, Nuran. 2010. *A History of Healthcare in Istanbul: Health Organizations, Epidemics, Infections and Disease Control, Preventive Health Institutions, Hospitals, Medical Education* (Istanbul: Istanbul University)

Yılmaz, Coşkun, and Necdet Yılmaz, (eds). 2006. *Osmanlılarda Sağlık*, 2 vols. (Istanbul: Biofarma)

Ziegler, Philip. 1969. *The Black Death* (New York: Harper & Row)

Nükhet Varlık (varlik@andromeda.rutgers.edu) is Assistant Professor of History at Rutgers University-Newark in New Jersey. She studies the early modern history of medicine, epidemic diseases, and the rise of public health in the Mediterranean world. She is the author of several articles and her first book, entitled *Plague and Empire in the Early Modern Mediterranean World: The Ottoman Experience, 1347–1600*, is forthcoming from Cambridge University Press. She is also editing a collection of articles entitled *Plague and Contagion in the Islamic Mediterranean* (contracted by Ashgate Press). In conjunction with this research, she teaches courses on epidemic diseases in world history, with a particular focus on plague. In her teaching, she incorporates research findings from bioarcheology, genetics, and climate history. She is the recipient of an NEH Fellowship for study at the American Research Institute in Turkey, a Senior Fellowship from Koç University's Research Center for Anatolian Civilizations, and a Turkish Cultural Foundation Post-Doctoral Fellowship. She holds a PhD from the University of Chicago.

Abstract Reconstructing the Ottoman plague experience is vital to understanding the larger Afro-Eurasian disease zone during the Second Pandemic. This essay deals with two different aspects of this experience. On the one hand, it discusses the historical and historiographical problems that rendered this epidemiological experience mostly invisible to previous scholars of plague. On the other, it reconstructs the empire's plague ecologies, with particular attention to plague's persistence, focalization, and transmission. Further, it uses this epidemiological experience to offer new insights and complicate some commonly held assumptions about plague history and its relationship to plague science.

Keywords Anatolia, Black Death, Mediterranean, pandemic, periodization, hyena, *Ciconia ciconia*.

HETEROGENEOUS IMMUNOLOGICAL LANDSCAPES AND MEDIEVAL PLAGUE: AN INVITATION TO A NEW DIALOGUE BETWEEN HISTORIANS AND IMMUNOLOGISTS

FABIAN CRESPO and MATTHEW B. LAWRENZ

> I have been asked by some of my friends to write something about the cause of this general pestilence, showing its natural cause, and why it affected so many countries, and why it affected some countries more than others, and why in some countries it affected some cities and towns more than others, and why in one town it affected one street, and even one house, more than another, and why it affected nobles and gentry less than other people.

WHEN THE FRENCH astrologer and physician Geoffrey de Meaux (fl. 1310–49) wrote these words around 1349, he was trying to assess, from a scientific perspective, the great challenge of applying the universal principles of the science of the stars to the very particular task of explaining why some people survived while others around them died in the wake of the Black Death (Horrox 1994: 165). His close contemporary, the Florentine author Giovanni Boccaccio (1313–75) similarly wrote that "not all those who adopted these diverse opinions died, nor did they all escape" (Boccaccio [1353]/1982: 9): suggesting, as Geoffrey did, that a complex selective process was at work during a plague outbreak.

In his treatise on surgery, Guy de Chauliac (d. *c.* 1368), a leading medical authority and physician to three successive popes, described the causes of mortality as twofold in his discussion of the bubonic plague: one active and universal, one passive and particular. Regarding the latter, Guy wrote: "The particular, passive case was the disposition of each body, such as cachocymia, debility, or obstruction, whence it was that the working men and those living poorly died" (1363/1974: 774). In other words, we can argue that Guy explained that cases of heterogeneous mortality were

The authors would like to thank three anonymous reviewers whose comments helped to improve this article significantly. We would also like to thank Monica Green for all her help and constant feedback; her support made this project possible. Finally, we would like to thank Ann Carmichael, Gregory Demas, Sharon DeWitte, Michelle Ziegler, and Carol Symes for their suggestions and valuable comments on earlier versions of this paper.

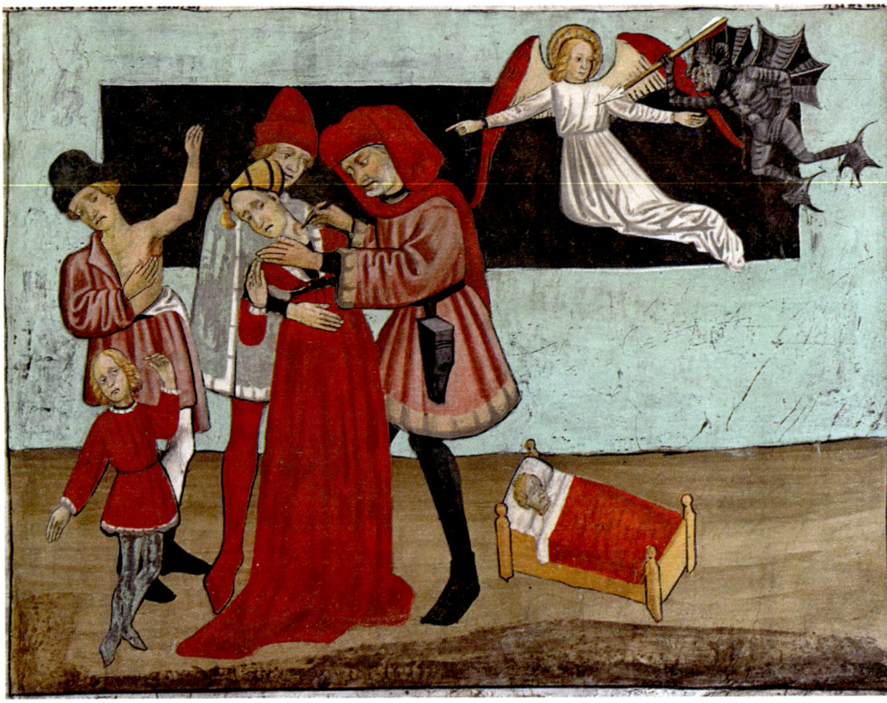

Plate 2. Lancing a Bubo (Chapel of Saint-Sébastien, Lanslevillard)

The image above shows a physician (with a case for medical implements hanging at his belt) lancing a bubo on the neck of a woman afflicted with plague. A young man (probably his assistant) steadies the patient; meanwhile, her husband strips off his tunic to reveal a bubo under his arm, readying himself for the same lancet. A small boy also holds up his arm, perhaps indicating that he, too, feels a bubo developing. A smaller child lies in bed, ill or asleep. Above the scene, a devil brandishes a lancet of his own—one that will inflict plague, rather than treat it—but an angel deflects his aim.

This is one of a series of extraordinary murals that decorate a chapel dedicated to St. Sebastian and located in the remote Alpine village of Lanslevillard, in the Haute-Maurienne region (modern département of Savoie, France), where plague became endemic in the later Middle Ages (see Carmichael 2014, in this issue). The murals were painted between the years 1446 and 1518. St. Sebastian (like St. Roch) was venerated by those seeking to be cured or spared from plague. According to legend, Sebastian had suffered martyrdom at the hands of the Roman emperor Diocletian. Because he had died from the wounds of numerous arrows, his intercession was sought by those who wanted to ward off the sting of deadly pestilence. *Caption: Carol Symes. Photo: Paul Smit.*

due to the previous biological conditions of infected individuals. Moreover, Guy's description of his own infection offers clear evidence that not all exposed individuals died: "I was ill for six weeks, in such a great danger that all my friends believed I would die; but the aposteme ripened, and was treated as I have described, and by God's will I survived." A contemporary physician and poet from Almeria (Spain), Abū Ja'far Ahmad Ibn Khātima, also described several cases where the individual "was rid of his pains and fully healed" after different treatments (cited in Aberth 2005: 60). All of these witnesses were well aware that different individuals responded differently to the plague.

During the Black Death, not every person within a family, town, or region was exposed to the plague pathogen. Moreover, if we accept that the major causative organism was *Yersinia pestis*, we must assume that exposure to the bacillus depended upon a complex interplay of factors: the presence of pathogen-bearing fleas (or possibly lice) and rodents, exposure to another human being who had expelled *Y. pestis*-ridden aerosolites from their lungs, or exposure to the lancet of a surgeon who had just lanced the buboes of another patient (a common practice) (see **Plate 2**). These factors suggest that those exposed to the fourteenth-century plague probably did not experience the same symptoms and/or disease progress.

In this essay, we accordingly focus our attention on those individuals who were exposed to the pathogen but had differing fates: survival or death. Paleo-epidemiologist Sharon DeWitte, with other colleagues, has carefully explored Black Death mortality using bone markers that indicate degrees of physiological stress and health, finding that the Black Death was not an indiscriminate killer. This research showed that people varied in risk mortality during the epidemic, and that the medieval plague especially targeted individuals in poor health (DeWitte and Wood 2008; DeWitte 2010; DeWitte and Hughes-Morey 2012; DeWitte 2014, in this issue). Some individuals survived and others not. But why were some people more at risk than others? We could argue, in keeping with common epidemiological assumptions, that babies, elders, or weak adults would normally not survive, once infected. Usually, we suggest that "weak" individuals (or even populations) would have had a higher mortality rate during plague epidemics because of poor nutrition, stress, and prior disease assaults or ongoing co-morbidities. How can we link (biologically speaking) all these factors together with poor health and higher risk of death when infected by plague? Clearly, we must explore with more nuance the specific factors that differentiated historical epidemics from one another, and that differentiated human responses to them.

But is today's science any better at answering such questions than the science of the medieval practitioners? We need to probe more deeply into the human immune system in order to discover how different biological, environmental, and social factors could have affected its function and impacted human health. For part of the answer to the conundrum of differential mortality could depend on which individuals (once infected) were able to mount an appropriate immune response. This is especially important because it is not a problem isolated in the past. When talking about plague, we are talking about a pathogen and its interaction with several hosts (not only humans), and about a pathogen-host interaction that has a common universal pattern which determines how the pathogen tries to survive and spread,[1] and how the host will contain or stop that process. However, each exposed human host is immersed in a specific environment and social context that could have a significant impact on her/his capacity to counter the plague pathogen. We must therefore attempt to reconstruct medieval environments and demographics with the understanding that they changed constantly in time and space, as did host-pathogen interactions.

In the last century, many historians and scientists have studied the problem of immunological responses to plague by focusing on "immunity" as an acquired and long-lasting response.[2] The historical and scientific evidence is strong enough to show that exposure to plague does not generate a long-lasting immunological memory that will protect the exposed individuals from future plague infections. It is time for a more comprehensive approach to the role of the immune system. In order to explain the differential mortality detected during medieval plague, we must consider the immunological status of individuals when exposed to the plague pathogen.

To answer (or try to answer) the question of who died when exposed to the plague pathogen, we propose that studying the individual immune system's responsiveness, or *immune competence* (IC), can help to explain differential mortality during medieval plague. In this essay, IC represents the capacity of an individual to generate an appropriate immune response involving innate and/or acquired mechanisms (we will explain these differences below). However, IC is not only a biological concept. As noted above, humans are immersed in specific environments and social contexts

1 That is, all interactions taking place between a pathogen and its host (i.e., human, animal, plant). Host-pathogen interactions can be described at the population, individual, or molecular levels. See Casadevall and Pirofski (2000) for a more comprehensive analysis of this concept.

2 Contributions to the discussion of human immunity and plague include: Hirst 1953; Pollitzer 1954; Ziegler 1969; McNeill 1976; Appleby 1980; Ell 1984; Scott and Duncan 2001; Cohn 2002; Sallares 2007; Benedictow 2010. The acquired immune response involves two different processes: *clonal selection* of B lymphocytes (heightened production of those that have the "right recipe" to combat the pathogen antigens); and the development of *immunological memory* (meaning that specific lymphocytes will retain and remember the "recipe" in case of a future encounter with the same infection).

that can be heterogeneous within the same populations, towns, and even within the same families. During the fourteenth century, some individuals infected with plague survived without modern antibiotics and modern medical treatments: how and why?

We must reconcile historical and scientific information to answer these questions. Some historians study nutrition, stress, and health in medieval daily life; and scientists should take account of these historical findings when attempting to understand who had higher risk of dying during plague epidemics due to a lower IC. Simply put, immunologists should be aware of the heterogeneous environments and social contexts of human populations across time and space, and how these factors can influence the IC of individuals. Historians, for their part, should be aware of the complexity of the immune system, and the fact that it does not only consist of acquired immunity but also changes constantly. Neither populations nor individuals are fixed entities, either biologically or culturally. Demographic variables such as age, sex, socio-economic status, and living conditions can play a significant role in shaping the IC of individuals and populations, and we must also consider environmental and ecological factors. Assuming that all populations had (and have) the same IC before an epidemic is as misleading as assuming that all populations will develop the same type of immunity or immunological memory after exposure to a pathogenic insult. We can't hypothesize a uniform IC for all individuals and human populations.

Therefore, the goals of this essay are: to reformulate the immunological questions regarding differential mortality in those individuals and populations exposed to plague in order to consider the role of immunological competence in determining their fate; and to define a new theoretical framework in which historians and scientists can meet and collaborate on a more comprehensive approach to immunity and plague.

The Later Middle Ages as a "Great Transition"

In the introduction to his recent lectures, "The Great Transition: Climate, Disease and Society in the Thirteenth and Fourteenth Centuries,"[3] Bruce Campbell (a specialist in medieval economic history) observes: "Across the Old World, the late thirteenth and fourteenth centuries witnessed profound and sometimes abrupt changes in the trajectory of established

3 The Ellen McArthur Lectures in Economic and Social History at the University of Cambridge, 2013: <http://www.econsoc.hist.cam.ac.uk/podcast-campbell.html> [accessed September 19, 2014].

historical trends." Specifically, Campbell points out that environmental changes induced "ecological dislocation" across Eurasia. They also affected human biology, probably imposing a significant stress on the individual capacity to develop normal physiological functions. When Campbell calls attention to the "burden of structural poverty," "climatically induced ecological dislocation and political collapse," and the fact that there was "no return to the ecological *status quo ante*," immunologists should be compelled to explore how these catastrophic developments affected the IC of medieval populations, and how changes in IC could have conditioned individual immune responses to plague.

For example, famines could have played a crucial role in the evolution of IC in human populations. As the historian William Chester Jordan (1996: 186) suggests in his book on the Great Famine of the early fourteenth century:

> The horrendous mortality of the Black Death in northern Europe in part should reflect the fact that poor people who were in their thirties and forties during the plague had been young children in the period 1315–1322 and were differentially more susceptible to the disease than those who had been adults during the famine or were born after the famine abated.[4]

Jordan clearly invites scientists to join him in substantiating his hypothesis. Why and how did some individuals present higher susceptibility? Did climate influence IC? What kinds of social and biological differences can we find between populations of high and low susceptibility?

Emerging scientific disciplines such as developmental biology and ecological immunology are helping us to connect the dots and explain how health, nutrition, stress, and climate can affect immunological fitness. These findings should inform our understanding of plague during the Middle Ages, as should consideration of the complex transition that medieval populations faced and its subsequent impact on their IC.

The Human Immune Response and *Yersinia pestis*: Cytokines as Crucial Players and Markers for Immune Competence

As we explained above, IC represents the capacity of an individual to generate an appropriate immune response involving all immunological barriers and mechanisms, innate and/or acquired. While the first line of defense against pathogens are simple physical barriers (skin and mucous membranes), a complex network of immunological responses deflects

4 Jordan arrived at these conclusions based on studies of nutritional biology during famines (e.g., Rivers 1988).

pathogens if the physical barriers fail (Sompayrac 2008). In general, the immune system reacts to infection via two mechanisms: *the cellular response*, which is commonly associated with the *innate immune response* and involves white blood cells (called phagocytes) that recognize, engulf, and destroy pathogens; and *the humoral response*, which is commonly associated with the *acquired immune response*, and involves the secretion of protective molecules (called antibodies). These two responses work in concert and effectively protect us from infection through a complex multilayered network of cooperation that blurs the distinction between innate and acquired responses (Danilova 2008). The power of the immune system lies in the comprehensive capacity of the system to recognize and respond quickly to different pathogens. To achieve this, the immune system depends on fine tuning and a high degree of "immunological plasticity": the capacity to change and adjust responses depending on intra- and extracellular conditions and/or environmental circumstances. Extensive genetic and experimental data (of which we will present only a fraction in this essay) demonstrate that, when facing a pandemic event and its successive manifestations, all individuals who are exposed to the pathogen will not have a similar immune system responsiveness or IC.

Plague is a zoonotic infectious disease, caused by the bacterium *Yersinia pestis*.[5] If we consider the classic ecological model of plague outbreaks, *Y. pestis* is maintained in the wild, mostly in rodent populations, and transmitted by flea vectors; humans are incidental victims of the disease (Perry and Fetherston 1997; Gage and Kosoy 2005). To survive inside the mammalian host, *Y. pestis* utilizes a variety of mechanisms to evade or overcome the immune system (Li and Yang 2008). At the site of infection (e.g., a flea bite), the cells of the innate immune response (neutrophils and macrophages) try to control the infection. Although many invading bacteria are killed by neutrophils, *Y. pestis* is able to survive when ingested by macrophages and can be transported to other tissues, especially the lymph nodes. Eventually, *Y. pestis* escapes from these macrophages and begins to proliferate, ultimately entering into the blood stream to cause a systemic infection and death of the host (Amadei et al. 2011).

Normally, when invading bacteria are recognized by cells of the innate immune system, these cells produce proteins called cytokines.[6] Cytokines

5 *Yersinia pestis* is a gram-negative facultative intracellular bacterium, mostly living intracellularly (usually within macrophages), but after proliferation can be released into the extracellular environment.

6 The term "cytokine" usually refers to hormone-like messengers which facilitate communication between cells of the immune system (Sompayrac 2008).

signal to other cells that an infection is in progress and recruit additional immune cells to the site of infection to help fight the invading bacteria. However, *Y. pestis* has developed mechanisms to inhibit or alter the production of these cytokines, essentially allowing the bacterium to hide or evade recognition by the innate immune system. For example, proteins produced by the plague pathogen have been shown to inhibit the expression of an important cytokine: tumor necrosis factor-alpha (TNFα),[7] produced by host macrophages where TNFα is a crucial pro-inflammatory cytokine involved in the innate response (Boland and Cornelis 1998). A virulence factor named LcrV also enhances the release of interleukin-10 (IL-10) by host immune cells,[8] where IL-10 is being exploited to down-regulate or decrease the production of pro-inflammatory cytokines such as TNFα and interferon-gamma (IFNγ)[9] (Brubaker 2003). Interestingly, treatment with exogenous IFNγ and TNFα have inhibited the multiplication of *Y. pestis* in a mouse model, showing that both cytokines were crucial for the absolute or longer survival of infected hosts (Lukaszewski et al. 2005; Nakajima and Brubaker 1993).

In recent years, additional research has further suggested that the individual capacity of the host to produce the cytokines TNFα and IFNγ in response to plague infection is an important co-determinant in the ability of the individual to mount an effective immune response (Lin et al. 2011).[10] Most human populations differ in the type and intensity of their immunological responses, which can be observed by differences in the expression of different immune proteins, such as cytokines.[11] Cytokines profoundly

---

7 TNFα was originally identified and named after a molecule that caused the necrosis of tumors *in vivo* within specific experimental conditions. Today, TNFα is considered the principal mediator involved in most acute inflammatory responses to gram-negative bacteria such as *Y. pestis* (Abbas and Lichtman 2005).

8 The term "interleukin" refers to the chemical way that different leukocytes communicate with each other. It is now recognized that many interleukins can also communicate with other non-immune cells. Different interleukins have been classified using numbers. IL-10 is one of the main inhibitors (within the immune system) of activated immune cells, controlling most innate immune reactions and cell-mediated immunity (Abbas and Lichtman 2005).

9 IFNγ is a crucial cytokine that mediates cell immunity against intracellular microbes. The term *interferon* derives from the ability of these molecules to *interfere* with the infection.

10 Therefore, we can consider that having an appropriate production of TNFα and IFNγ is a significant immunological component of the host IC when fighting *Y. pestis*.

11 We will expand on this below in the section entitled "Lessons from Immunogenetics Studies."

influence growth, differentiation, and activation functions that determine and regulate the immune response, and ultimately affect the states of health and disease (Borish and Steinke 2003). The types of cytokines that are produced during an immune response determine the effector mechanisms that will predominate. The development of appropriate cytokine networks to combat infections depends on the nature of the pathogen, the genetic background of the individual (Wilson, Seymour, and Henderson 1998), as well as developmental factors during growth and environmental factors (Nelson et al. 2002).

At the end of the last century, the study of cytokine genetic variants or single nucleotide polymorphisms (hereafter SNPs)[12] captured the attention of many researchers trying to explain differences in the success of human tissue transplants (Hutchinson et al. 1998a; Hutchinson et al. 1998b; Sankaran et al. 1999). Preliminary results showed that ethnicity influences cytokine genetic variation at the level of single nucleotide polymorphisms (SNPs) (Hoffman et al. 2002; Meenagh et al. 2002; Delaney et al. 2004; Raj, Govindaraju, and Chakraborty 2007). In some regions, significant cytokine SNP variation was observed in tribes and/or ethnic groups within the same region, suggesting that moderate differentiation among disease-causing factors could occur even among evolutionarily and geographically related ethnic populations (Gadelha et al. 2005; Raj, Govindaraju, and Chakraborty 2007). The cytokine genetic make-up thus has a significant impact on the immune response that is mounted,[13] and this must be understood as a crucial factor for IC. For example, a study conducted by Linda Larcombe and colleagues found that some Canadian aboriginal populations present a high frequency of cytokine SNPs commonly associated with the low expression of cytokines that promote inflammation (Larcombe et al. 2005). The authors postulated that the evolution of that unique cytokine genetic profile may be linked to aboriginal adaptation to an environment in which helminthic, parasitic, and fungal infections predominated. Therefore, depending on the regional interaction of host and pathogens, we find different immunological profiles among human populations. We can assume that, during the Middle Ages, not all populations were exposed to the same pathogenic experience, and the consequence of that is the emergence of different immunological backgrounds in different regions and populations.

12 Most genetic variants are associated with "point" or single mutations that affect the genetic code ("recipe") for the corresponding cytokine.

13 The cytokine genetic make-up is the observed differential cytokine SNPs distribution in human populations.

Yet we must recognize that because plague has such an inherently complex ecology, it is exceedingly difficult to reconstruct all of the factors that would have gone into determining whether a given individual was even exposed to the disease. Despite all that we know today about the transmission of *Y. pestis* between arthropod vectors and mammalian hosts, we cannot necessarily explain, as Geoffrey de Meaux put it, "why in one town it affected one street, and even one house, more than another." Beyond those basic epidemiological variables of exposure to the pathogen, however, there are also questions arising from the differing immune responses among those who did have the bad luck to be bitten by an infected flea. Not all populations, or even individuals, are able to generate the same immune responses when encountering an infection (Nelson et al. 2002; McDade 2005; French, Moore, and Demas 2009; Martin, Hawley, and Ardia 2011). Therefore, it is possible that, assuming equal risk of infection, different individual capacities to generate an appropriate immune response against pathogens can help us to understand the differential mortality within and between populations during plague outbreaks.

Historical Perspectives on Human Immunity and Medieval Plague: The First Dialogue between Historians and Immunologists

Many historians and scientists of the plague have recognized that the study of the immune system and its corresponding mechanisms could be an important factor in understanding the differential mortality exhibited by medieval plague outbreaks. However, such studies have not focused on IC. As noted above, these early studies were focused on *acquired immunity* due to previous exposure to the plague pathogen (Hirst 1953; Pollitzer 1954; Ziegler 1969; McNeill 1976). Indeed, we must make a clear statement here: most historians use the term "immunity" to mean *acquired immune response* (explained above) without considering the *innate or cellular response* (also explained above) that is a crucial immunological barrier, especially when mounting an effective and fast response to the plague pathogen. To take an example: Andrew Appleby, a historian specializing in agrarian history and demography, suggested a hypothetical scenario in which "those people with little natural resistance died when they caught plague, while those with greater resistance lived, and passed on their natural resistance to their children" (Appleby 1980). But for those populations that were not previously exposed to plague, what does it mean to have a "natural" or "greater" resistance? It is important to highlight again that, from an immunological perspective, the term "resistance" does not solely imply the physiological capacity to recognize a pathogenic antigen (a non-self molecule) and to mount an appropriate immune response that usually leads to a short- or long-term memory (i.e., acquired immune response). The innate or cellular response is also an important component of the individual IC and must also be taken into consideration when conducting historical research on past plagues.

Until very recently, this type of scholarship was stymied because arguments over human immunity and medieval plague also revolved around a different kind of debate: what disease was plague? This question has since been resolved, yet it is worth revisiting how historians' understanding of "acquired immunity" has impacted that debate to date. In fact, one powerful argument against *Y. pestis* as the pathogen that caused the Black Death has been based on the human lack of a capacity to develop immunological memory once exposed to the plague pathogen (again, "immunity" in this case has been understood solely as *acquired* immunity). Most notably, Samuel Cohn has insisted that medieval plague cannot be compared with modern bubonic plague, citing early bacteriological studies (e.g., Burgess 1930) which pointed out that humans (unlike rats) cannot develop immunity to plague (Cohn 2002: 33). Moreover, he has been skeptical about the possibility of differential immunity when comparing the medieval "Second Pandemic" with the "Third Pandemic" that began in the late nineteenth century:

> Why would human populations that once possessed natural immunity to a bacillus with the ability to adapt to it with remarkable speed in the fourteenth to eighteenth centuries have then lost all traces of that ability by the end of the nineteenth century? (Cohn 2002: 249)

But if our approach to IC is correct, we must expect that not all individuals within and between populations will be able to develop the same type of immunological memory, thus enabling the same disease to flourish even in the same population at a later time.

When the medieval historian and demographer Ole Benedictow tried to answer and critique Cohn's arguments in an extensive monograph, he referred to acquired immunity and pointed out that

> epidemic diseases which do not produce good persistent immunity in survivors will have much larger powers of spread, recurrence and mortality than diseases conferring persistent immunity. Consequently, other factors being equal, they will also tend to produce much higher mortality rates over time, since the whole population will be at risk every time they recur. (Benedictow 2010: 207)

Stephen Ell, a medievalist and specialist on plagues, may have been one of the first historians to employ a more nuanced concept of immunity as a factor in the epidemiology of medieval plague (Ell 1984).[14] He suggested that "Human immunity to plague probably helps to account for much of the age and sex distribution and geographical variation of plague." While Ell focused his attention on the human host's capacity to develop immunological memory (acquired immunity) after exposure to the plague pathogen, he argued against the idea of "uniform immunity or resistance," meaning that not all populations were able to develop the same type of immunity. Scientist Robert Sallares followed this line of thought when he wrote that "the fact that different plague epidemics were caused by essentially the same organism at the DNA level does not necessarily mean that the epidemiology of plague must always be the same" (Sallares 2007: 256). And it is worth remembering that, in the mid-twentieth century, microbiologist G. B. Mackaness clearly pointed out that the process involved in the development of acquired immunity also depends on the "state of immunological reactivity" of the host (Mackaness 1964), or what we now refer to as IC.

As we have now established, instead of focusing on one aspect of the immune response—either as a genetic legacy or as an acquired long-lasting response—historians and scientists can adopt a more comprehensive and collaborative approach, analyzing and estimating the IC of medieval populations and their susceptibility to plague. These findings, in turn, can be used to help us understand and respond to future outbreaks. The challenge that remains is how to study variation in IC within and between historical populations, and to determine how we can apply modern immunological models while carefully considering that populations do not represent fixed entities.

Lessons from Immunogenetic Studies: Can We See the Whole Picture without Looking at Historical Contexts?

We have already established that the most common immunological reasoning employed by historians and scientists to explain the differences in mortality during plague epidemics is a diverse history of exposure to plague (resulting or not in acquired immunity) between populations in different regions. In response, we have argued that differences in IC could help to explain differential plague mortality. This means that we must search for evidence that human populations present different immunological profiles, and the first evidence will come from genetic analyses of genes that code for cytokines and other immune proteins. As we explained

14 Stephen Ell received a Master's degree and PhD in medieval history from the University of Chicago, and later he received a medical degree from Loyola University.

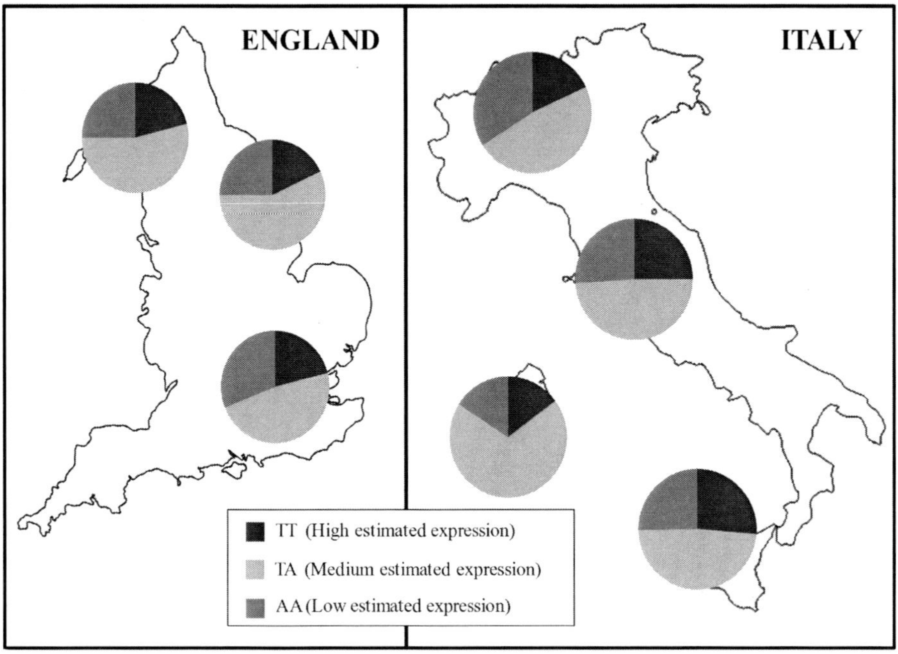

Map 5. Distribution of Genetic Variants for IFN γ (+874). Based on Contemporaneous Populations (www.allelefrequencies.net).

above, heritable cytokine SNPs are common in human populations, and some SNPs can alter how much of that cytokine will be produced (either at a basal level or in response to infection). Since the levels of cytokines, such as IFNγ, are targeted and reduced by *Y. pestis* during infection (Brubaker 2003), differences in the basal level of cytokine production by individuals could be an important contributing factor in mounting an effective innate immune response against the plague pathogen (again, without necessarily implying acquired immune responses).[15] To demonstrate cytokine genetic variation in human populations we used a worldwide database of modern populations to calculate the genetic variants in IFNγ distribution for England and Italy.[16] The goal here is not to attempt an historical

15 While these studies were conducted on animal models (mouse and rat) we could potentially extrapolate these findings to generate novel hypotheses on humans.

16 *Allelefrequencies.net* is an internet database maintained by a consortium composed of the Royal Liverpool and Broadgreen University Hospitals and the University of Liverpool in the United Kingdom. Most samples come from regional hospital and clinical studies all around the globe. While these samples do not represent past demographic scenarios and can show high admixture levels, they can be used to show regional trends for immunological profiles. One of these variants has a specific

reconstruction using modern populations but to highlight the heterogeneity of any population (**Map 5**).

For example, combined modern populations in northern Italy show a higher frequency of individuals with low IFNγ systemic expression (possibly associated with a weaker innate inflammatory response). Meanwhile, modern populations in England show regional differences in IFNγ, indicating that we should not underestimate regional immunological variation. Another cytokine, such as IL-10, presents genetic variability that can impact the amount of cytokine an individual can express (Turner et al. 1997).[17] IL-10 is also exploited by the plague pathogen to inhibit the immune response (Brubaker 2003). Interestingly, the genetic variation for IL-10 also shows high variability within the same region and among the neighboring cities of Milan, Torino, and Pavia (**Map 6**).

This analysis demonstrates that not all modern populations have the same baseline production of IFNγ, and IL-10, two cytokines crucial to generating an appropriate immune response to *Y. pestis*. Since this data highlights regional differences, we must consider historical and demographic contexts to make sense of this regional diversity. Moreover, we cannot extrapolate from this data to make assumptions about past populations in the same regions. Therefore, this is a perfect example of one of our key points: historians must step in and help scientists put all these biological differences into context.

But let us now pose a new question: how do we translate these immunogenetic maps into epidemiological scenarios for a historical plague epidemic? The most simplistic approach is to consider that a population combining a high frequency of individuals who are high producers of IL-10 (an anti-inflammatory cytokine that usually tries to counterbalance an excessive inflammatory response) with a high frequency of individuals who are low producers of IFNγ and/or TNFα (both pro-inflammatory cytokines) could face a weak innate (cellular) response at the site of the infection (e.g., the site of a flea bite), thus facilitating the replication and spread of the pathogen in their bodies and the community at large.

"address" in the IFNγ gene: +874. In that specific position (+874), human populations can differ in one chemical component: nitrogen base T (thymine) or nitrogen base A (adenine). Because each human has two copies for each nitrogen base (what in biology is called "diploidy") an individual can be coded AA, TT, or TA. If a human possesses AA, the baseline production of IFNγ is low; if a human has TT, then baseline production of IFNγ is high; finally, TA represents an intermediate production of IFNγ (Pravica et al. 2000).

17 In this case, the specific genetic "address" for the SNP in this cytokine is -1082.

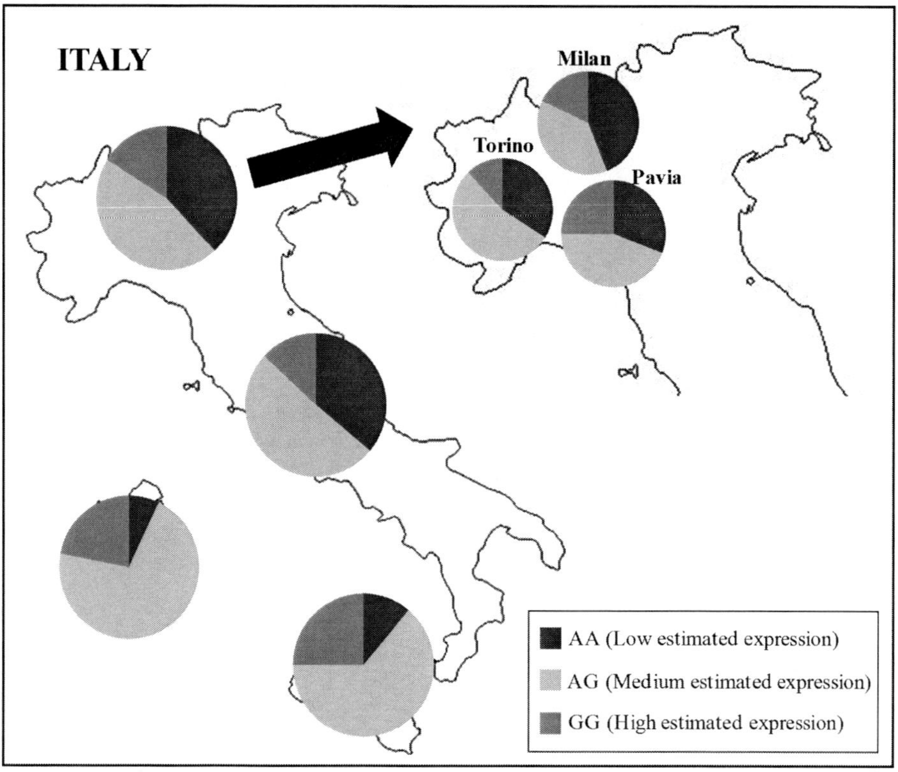

Map 6. Distribution of Genetic Variants for IL-10 (-1082) Based on Contemporaneous Populations (www.allelefrequencies.net).

As we've made clear, these maps represent modern genetic data, and we cannot argue that a similar genetic distribution pertained during the Middle Ages. The challenge that remains is to study the cytokine SNPs in medieval populations in conjunction with the distribution and impact of plague in those populations. But the challenge could be met if techniques of ancient DNA (aDNA) analysis are applied. Similar molecules, such as CCR5,[18] have been analyzed in this way, using data from medieval populations. CCR5 belongs to a group of immune proteins similar to cytokines. Called "chemokines," most act to induce "chemotaxis" or chemical-induced cell movement. (Basically, immune cells that release chemokines will call for "help" to other immune cells, which will migrate to the site of infection). The research conducted on CCR5Δ32 and plague resistance over the past ten years is both interesting and controversial, but it does establish the technological foundation for studying and expanding the genetic analysis of other immune genes, such as those producing cytokines.

---

18 CC stands for "Chemo-Kine," and R stands for "Receptor."

CCR5 has a SNP named Δ32 that is commonly associated with human immunodeficiency virus (HIV) resistance. Initially, some researchers suggested that the high frequency of CCR5Δ32 detected in modern European populations can't be explained by HIV's recent arrival and selective process. It was further suggested that past epidemics of plague (especially the Black Death) generated the selective process that can explain the high frequency of CCR5Δ32 (Stephens et al. 1998). But this argument was contested, due to ambiguous results and the uncertainty as to whether CCR5Δ32 really offers some type of resistance to plague (Mecsas et al. 2004; Elvin et al. 2004). It did not take too long for researchers to apply aDNA technologies to the problem and to estimate the frequency of CCR5Δ32 in the past (Hummel et al. 2005; Kremeyer, Hummel, and Herrmann 2005). Preliminary results have (so far) rejected the idea that the increased frequency of CCR5Δ32 in European populations was due to plague, but ongoing studies have revived the debate (Biloglav et al. 2009). As historian Samuel Cohn and scientist L. T. Weaver have put it: "The exciting correlations discovered by geneticists and epidemiologists between present-day genotypes in human populations, and varying levels of resistance to diseases, now demand a new cooperation between scientists and historians" (Cohn and Weaver 2006).

Recently, a more complex immunogenetic reconstruction was published using modern populations but inferring a selective process generated by medieval plague (Laayouni et al. 2014). In this study, the authors exploited what they called "a special historic demographic situation in Europe" represented by two populations with different genetic ancestry: European Romanians and the Rroma people (commonly known as "Gypsies"). The authors argue that these two populations, who have ostensibly shared the same geographic region for the past thousand years, have therefore experienced similar environmental conditions, including infectious diseases. The Rroma people migrated into Europe before the last millennium from northern India, but they intermarried little with European Romanians. Even after one thousand years, there is still a clearly detectable genetic similarity between the Rroma people and people from northern India. However, not all genes of these two groups showed that correspondence. Toll-like receptor (TLR) genes are among those genes which differed significantly between the Rroma and present-day north Indians.[19] These immune genes play a crucial role in recognizing and launching an

19 TLRs are proteins localized on the cell membrane of immune cells which recognize (directly or indirectly) molecules that are characteristic of broad classes of invaders (Sompayrac 2008).

immune response, especially in fighting back a broad spectrum of pathogens, such as *Y. pestis*. Conversely, and surprisingly, the authors found strong genetic similarity in TLRs between the Rroma people and European Romanians, despite their distinctiveness. Laayouni and colleagues identified plague as the selective factor that shaped the genetic similarities between the Rroma and the European Romanians, on the grounds that both populations were exposed to the Second Plague Pandemic.[20]

Crucial to this analysis is the assumption that the Second Plague Pandemic did not impact northern India. That assumption may now be open to question (see Green 2014, in this issue). But even though some of this study's findings are controversial, we must welcome this kind of research, in which there is cross-fertilization of biological data and historical evidence. This kind of study can help us to identify specific selective agents (such as plague) when understanding the reshaping of immunological profiles in human populations. Precisely because today's demographic and environmental data does not reflect past population structures and/or dynamics, or past environments, all immunogenetic reconstructions will only make sense within the environmental and historical contexts reconstructed by historians, paleodemographers, and bioarcheologists. Accordingly, to test the hypothesis proposed in this essay, we must understand the complex dynamics of medieval populations and how environmental and social factors affected the IC in those populations. While we can argue that different factors at different times can have different impacts on the regional variation of IC, we must consider that climatic fluctuations and famines could have played a significant role in constantly reshaping the IC in human populations.[21]

Differential Immune Competence: The Potential Role of Climate and Famines

The role of seasonality has been the most frequently cited factor when correlating climate with the incidence of plague (Hirst 1953; Pollitzer 1954; Ziegler 1969; McNeill 1976; Slack 1990; Scott and Duncan 2001; Cohn 2002 and 2008; Benedictow 2004; Campbell 2013). However, it is not

20 The authors of this study acknowledge that other infectious diseases (such as tuberculosis and leprosy) were common in the region at that time; but they argue that these infections were as common in India as in Europe.

21 We must understand that climatic fluctuations (for example, environmental temperature) could represent seasonal variation within the same year, as well as long-lasting climatic shifts with longer and probably more significant stress on the IC.

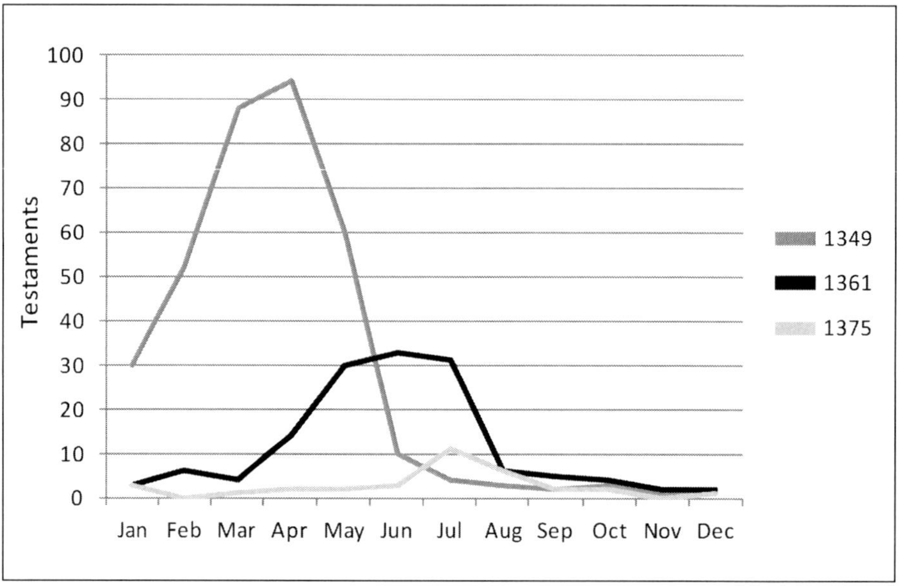

Graph 5. The Plague in London (1349–1361–1375): Data Based on Wills and Testaments. *Modified from Cohn 2002: 184–85.*

fully clear that all plague outbreaks followed a seasonal pattern. Basing his assessments on the study of medieval testaments, Cohn asserted that plague in Mediterranean Europe was a "summer event" peaking either in June or July (Cohn 2002: 28). But when we inspected the data used by Cohn, we found a different seasonal pattern throughout the northern hemisphere, exemplified by data from three successive waves of plague in London (**Graph 5**).

Seasonal variation in infection and disease prevalence may represent fluctuations in either the host, the pathogen, or the vector. But in the last decade, growing evidence based on animal models suggests that seasonal variation is most often due to changes primarily in the host, not the pathogen (Nelson et al. 2002). This is very significant for the historical study of IC. For example, the circulating immune cells helper T-lymphocytes and B-lymphocytes (important for antibody-mediated immunity) are usually elevated in winter, but cell-mediated immunity (which involves key players in immune response to plague, such as phagocytes) is higher in the summer (Nelson et al. 2002). A recent study conducted in Poland, using healthy male subjects, found that a significant seasonal variation was detected in neutrophils (phagocytes that play a key role in killing plague pathogen at the site of infection), with the highest bactericidal activity of these immune cells observable in summer (Klink et al. 2012).[22] Such discrepancies of immune cell function among modern human populations reflect differences in environmental and physiological factors, such as energy balance (Nelson et al. 2002). In this context, "energy" implies the energy that an organism is able to expend for conducting all physiological activities at a specific time, including mounting all necessary immune responses.

Nutrition deficiency is among the most important factors that affect the energetic balance of an organism. Famines or catastrophic subsistence have clearly impacted the energy balance of individuals and populations throughout history, and have consequently impacted the energetic supply of the immune system. Most medieval chroniclers and other witnesses, as well as modern historians, have suggested that human fragility due to famines preceding or coincident with plague outbreaks have accounted for the peak in mortality (Herlihy 1997: 32). However, in some populations, plague followed good harvests, likely because the increase in grain production boosted the rat populations (Cohn 2002: 31). While we cannot rule out the link between famines and plague outbreaks in some European regions, we also need to consider the long-term impact of famines and malnutrition on the immune system, and their contribution to mortality rates.

The age at which individuals experience famines may also contribute to IC: this is demonstrable even before birth. The fetus is not a passive organism, and environmental factors during pregnancy will have a strong influence on the biological profile of the individual. Threatening scenarios encountered by the growing fetus generate immediate adaptive responses that may promote survival but may also leave the individual with a potentially disadvantageous phenotype that s/he must "cope with" for life. Simply put, the fetus will receive environmental signals (through the mother) that can "reprogram" different biological components (such as the immune system) during development (Gluckman, Beedle, and Hanson 2009).[23] As noted above, historian William Chester Jordan cited scientific evidence (Rivers 1988) when he pointed out that "there are long-

22 This study included 155 healthy male subjects who had been donors of neutrophils. It has been conducted by the Institute of Medical Biology at the Polish Academy of Science (Lodowa, Poland) since the year 2000.

23 The discipline of developmental biology is also calling for our attention when we attempt to understand how (and when) environmental factors can impact our biological development. As an example, a fetus whose mother faces famine (as well as other biological stressors, such as infections) will receive different environmental signals compared to a fetus that receives an appropriate food supply and/or is not exposed to infections during pregnancy. (Interestingly, if a fetus will receive more food than necessary, that can also affect the future of the individual.)

term effects in children who survive famines, long term effects that are considerably more severe than those on adults who survive starvation rations" (Jordan 1996: 186). The short-term impact of malnutrition during development of the immune system can have long-term effects on how the immune system will respond to maintain the body's homeostasis and especially how it will fight infections (Suskind, Lachney, and Udall 1994; Chandra 1996; Roseboom et al. 2001).

Jordan's insights have been further supported by more recent work. Paleo-epidemiologist Sharon DeWitte and historian Philip Slavin published an interdisciplinary study on patterns of health in the pre-Black Death population of London by examining the effects of the Great Famine (1315–17) and the Great Bovine Pestilence (1319–20) (DeWitte and Slavin 2013). They focused on health or heterogeneity in health among those who ultimately died during the Black Death, and they included individuals born around the year 1319 because their growth *in utero* might have been negatively impacted by the famine.[24] Preliminary analysis revealed no significant differences in skeletal markers among the pre-famine, famine, and post-famine generations of Black Death victims, 491 of whom were buried in a cemetery at East Smithfield. While DeWitte and Slavin argued that the lack of significant results could be an artifact of the small sample size, they also concluded that

> the Great Famine could have reduced the proportion of the frailest individuals between 1315 and 1317. The Great Bovine Pestilence, which followed soon after and resulted in a catastrophic and long-term dearth of dairy products and fertilizer for crops, did not produce high human mortality, whether selective or indiscriminate, but it could have created a generation of relatively weak people who were less resilient than those who survived the famine. (DeWitte and Slavin 2013: 57)

Here is an important argument that speaks to the central hypothesis of our essay: "weak people who were less resilient" can have a compromised IC, while a weak or compromised immune response could result from infection or disease later in life.

---

24 In this study, adult ages were calculated using a skeletal age-estimation procedure called "transition analysis." This analysis was applied (for adults) on different skeletal-age markers such as the pubic symphysis, iliac auricular surface, and cranial suture closure. For individuals younger than twenty years, the age was estimated using epiphyseal fusion, dental development, and eruption.

Plague Was Not the Only Infectious Disease: Co-Infections and Immune Competence

Most (if not all) mammals are usually co-infected with more than one pathogen, and such a "co-infective state" will condition the IC and immune responses to individual pathogens. We cannot assume that pathogenic loads within and between human populations are always similar over time and space. As Ann Carmichael, a specialist in historical epidemiology, has put it, "All pre-industrial epidemics, including plagues, had multiple infectious diseases exacerbating morbidity and mortality" (Carmichael 2008: 51). Furthermore, a number of ecological factors likely play an important role in determining pathogen distribution and the immunological responses of human populations. A study on human pathogens has suggested that macroscale distribution patterns of human diseases and human populations exposed to a higher diversity of pathogens display higher genetic diversity for some immune proteins (Guegan, Prugnolle, and Thomas 2008). This is the case for the major histocompatibility complex (MHC) or human leukocyte antigen (HLA),[25] where higher genetic diversity is detected in areas with higher pathogen abundance and diversity (Guegan, Prugnolle, and Thomas 2008; Parham 2005).

While not all infectious diseases occur at once in any region, or affect the same populations, we can speculate that co-infections happened frequently during the Middle Ages (as they do today). From an immune-modulatory perspective,[26] perhaps the most significant chronic infection is due to helminths. Helminths are parasitic worms that cause a wide variety of infectious diseases and may be classified into nematodes or roundworms, trematodes or flatworms, and cestodes or tapeworms. Helminth infections cause an overall down-regulation or hypo-responsiveness of the immune system, consequently affecting the immune reaction to concomitant infections that occur with high frequencies in helminth-endemic areas, such as malaria and tuberculosis (Van Riet, Hartgers, and Yazdanbakhsh 2007). Such chronic co-infective scenarios can be very complex and cannot be analyzed apart from their corresponding environmental

25 The MHC proteins (or HLA when specifically applied to humans) are the ones that "present" the non-self antigen (pathogen proteins) to other immune cells, consequently triggering the immune reaction or response. Simply put, more diversity of pathogens implies more antigen diversity that must be recognized by more diverse MHC proteins.

26 That is, considering factors that can "modulate" or alter the systemic immune response, creating a quasi-permanent shift in the immunological response and affecting the IC with respect to other pathogens.

and social contexts. For example, nutritionists have recognized that parasitic infections can have an impact on the nutritional status of the host, but it was also recognized that malnutrition could be a predisposing factor for parasitic infections (Kolski and Scott 2001).

When paleo-parasitologists Evilena Anastasiou and Piers Mitchell analyzed the twelfth-century latrine of a crusader castle on Cyprus, they found eggs of two species of parasitic intestinal helminths. They concluded that "The discovery of these parasites highlights how mediaeval crusaders may have been at risk of malnutrition at times of siege and famine as these worms competed with them for nutrients" (Anastasiou and Mitchell 2013: 218). Shifting the immune response, chronic helminth infections may also affect the IC against *Y. pestis*, exacerbating the production of anti-inflammatory cytokines such as IL-10. This anti-inflammatory scenario could have played a role in the differential mortality detected during medieval plague. It remains to be determined whether populations that had a higher burden of helminthic infection were the ones with higher mortality during plague epidemics. However, not only parasitic (macroparasite) infections should be considered when studying the IC of medieval populations and its potential impact on differential mortality. It has also been suggested that leprosy could, in many instances, generate a "hyper-immune state" (overreactive immune system with increased levels of pro-inflammatory proteins) (Ell 1987) and thus impact the individual IC and the corresponding response to the plague pathogen.

A Historical-Ecological-Immunological Model for Studying Plague

The immune system is characterized by a high degree of plasticity and marked fluctuations can occur as a reaction to environmental factors (French, Moore, and Demas 2009). An emerging discipline such as ecological immunology can therefore help us to understand how ecological and social factors affect and reshape our immune system. While most preliminary studies produced by this young discipline deal with non-human animals, the last decade has seen a growing number dealing with the translation of such findings to human ecology and immunology (McDade 2003, 2005; McDade et al. 2010; Trotter et al. 2013).

However, immunological studies in laboratory settings do not account for social and ecological factors that operate within and between populations. This is problematic, because populations are not static entities fixed in space and time, either biologically and culturally. If malnutrition, climatic fluctuations, and co-infections can have a significant impact on the IC of an individual, how can we apply these findings to past societies?

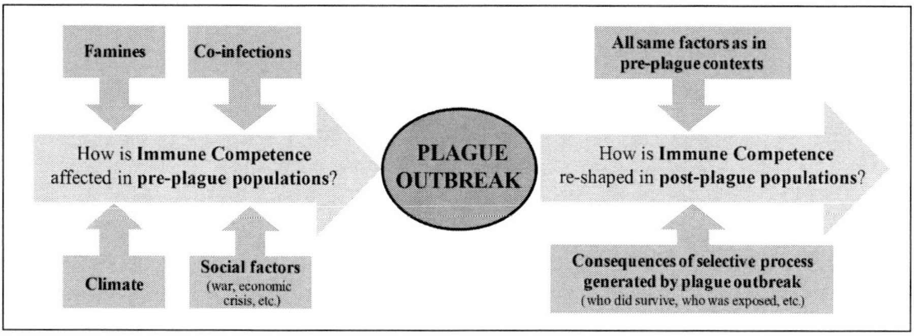

Graph 6. Proposed Multifactorial Model for Understanding the Impact of Biological, Ecological, and Social Factors on Human Immune Competence (IC) before, during, and after Plague Outbreaks

And can we extrapolate from individual data to a population at large, or to an entire region? We have also stressed that the human immunological response is not uniquely conditioned by the acquisition of (or failure to acquire) long-lasting resistance after exposure to a particular pathogen. As we have explained, the innate immune response is crucial to fighting *Y. pestis* at the site of the infection, and the individual's health and IC will play a significant role in determining which individuals will be able to mount a quick and effective primary/innate response, seconds after the infection (for example, by flea bite).

Every plague outbreak occurs within a unique environmental, biological, and social context. Each outbreak then reshapes the environmental, biological, and cultural profile of the affected population and region. A more comprehensive and accurate reconstruction of medieval demography and ecology will be the only way to reconstruct the IC of individuals and populations in this era (**Graph 6**). If this can be achieved, it will enable us to build better models for understanding how and why plague outbreaks occur now, and in the future. The proposed model offers an invitation to medievalists: the opportunity to make a significant contribution to human health by helping us to study the factors that impacted human immunology in the past, thus helping to combine modern immunological knowledge with the disciplines of history, anthropology, bioarcheology, paleoepidemiology, and paleoimmunology.

We are witnesses to an increasing interest in the study of past disease and the search for lessons that we can apply to the future. As this special issue of *The Medieval Globe* insists, scholars and scientists have a unique opportunity to generate a truly interdisciplinary agenda for future research.

Bibliography

Abbas, A. K., and A. H. Lichtman. 2005. *Cellular and Molecular Immunology*, 5th ed. (Philadelphia: Saunders)

Aberth, John. 2005. *The Black Death: The Great Mortality of 1348–1350. A Brief History with Documents* (New York: Palgrave Macmillan)

Amedei, A., E. Niccolai, L. Marino, and M. M. D'Elios. 2011. "Role of Immune Response in *Yersinia pestis* Infection," *Journal of Infection in Developing Countries* 5, no. 9: 628–39

Anastasiou, E., and P. D. Mitchell. 2013. "Human Intestinal Parasites from a Latrine in the 12th Century Frankish Castle of Saranda Kolones in Cyprus," *International Journal of Paleopathology* 3, no. 3: 218–23

Appleby, A. 1980. "The Disappearance of Plague: A Continuous Puzzle," *Economic History Review* 33: 161–73

Benedictow Ole J. 2004. *The Black Death, 1346–1353: The Complete History* (Woodbridge: Boydell)

Benedictow, Ole J. 2010. *What Disease Was Plague? On the Controversy over the Microbiological Identity of Plague Epidemics of the Past* (Leiden: Brill)

Biloglav, Z., L. Zgaga, M. Smoljanovic, C. Hayward, et al. 2009. "Historic, Demographic, and Genetic Evidence for Increased Population Frequencies of CCR5Δ32 Mutation in Croatian Island Isolates after Lethal 15th-Century epidemics," *Croatian Medical Journal* 50, no. 1: 34–42

Bocaccio, Giovanni. [1353]/1982. *The Decameron*, trans. M. Musa and Peter Bondanella (New York: Norton)

Boland, A., and G. Cornelis. 1998. "Role of YopP in Suppression of Tumor Necrosis Factor Alpha Release by Macrophages during *Yersinia* Infection," *Infection and Immunity* 66, no. 5: 1878–84

Borish, L., and J. Steinke. 2003. "Cytokines and Chemokines," *Journal of Allergy and Clinical Immunology* 111, no. 2: S460–S475

Brubaker, R. R. 2003. "Interleukin-10 and Inhibition of Innate Immunity to *Yersinae*: Roles of Yops and LcrV (V Antigen)," *Infection. Immunity* 71, no. 7: 3673–81

Burgress, A. S. 1930. "Virulence, Immunity and Bacteriological Variation in Relation to Plague," *Journal of Hygiene* 30, no.2 : 165–79

Campbell, Bruce M. S. 2013. "The Great Transition: Climate, Disease and Society in the 13th and 14th Centuries," The Ellen McArthur Lectures, University of Cambridge <http://www.econsoc.hist.cam.ac.uk/podcast-campbell.html> [accessed September 19, 2014]

Carmichael, Ann G. 2008. "Universal and Particular: The Language of Plague, 1348-1500," *Medical History Supplement* 27: 17–52

Carmichael, Ann G. 2014. "Plague Persistence in Western Europe: A Hypothesis," *The Medieval Globe* 1: 157–191

Casadevall, A., and L. Pirofski. 2000. "Host-Pathogen Interactions, II: Basic Concepts of Microbial Commensalism, Colonization, Infection, and Disease," *Infection and Immunity* 68, no. 12: 6511–18

Chandra, R. K. 1996. "Nutrition, Immunity and Infection: From Basic Knowledge of Dietary Manipulation of Immune Responses to Practical Application of

Ameliorating Suffering and Improving Survival," *Proceeedings of the National Academy of Sciences* 93, no. 25: 14304–07

Cohn, Samuel K. Jr. 2002. *The Black Death Transformed: Disease and Culture in Early Renaissance Europe* (London: Arnold)

Cohn, Samuel K. Jr. 2008. "Epidemiology of the Black Death and the Successive Waves of Plague," *Medical History Supplement* 27: 74–100

Cohn, Samuel K., and L. T. Weaver. 2006. "The Black Death and AIDS: CCR5-Δ32 in Genetics and History," *Quarterly Journal of Medicine* 99: 497–503

Danilova, N. 2008. "Evolution of the Human Immune System," in *Handbook of Human Molecular Evolution, vol. 1*, ed. D. Cooper and H. Kehrer-Sawatzki, 1068–74 (Chichester: Wiley)

Delaney, N., V. Esquenazi, D. Lucas, A. Zachary et al. 2004. "TNF-α, TGF-β, IL-10, L-6, and IFN-γ Alleles among African Americans and Cuban Americans. Report of the ASHI Minority Workshops: Part IV," *Human Immunology* 65: 1413–19

DeWitte, Sharon N. 2010. "Age Patterns of Mortality during the Black Death in London, A.D. 1349–1350," *Journal of Archaeological Science* 37, no. 12: 3394–3400

DeWitte, Sharon N. 2014. "The Anthropology of Plague: Insights from Bioarcheological Analyses of Epidemic Cemeteries," *The Medieval Globe* 1: 97–123

DeWitte, Sharon N., and J. W. Wood. 2008. "Selectivity of the Black Death with Respect to Preexisting Health," *Proceedings of the National Academy of Sciences* 105, no. 5: 1436–41

DeWitte, Sharon N., and G. Hughes-Morey. 2012. "Stature and Frailty during the Black Death: The Effect of Stature on Risks of Epidemic Mortality in London, A.D. 1348–1350," *Journal of Archaeological Science* 39, no. 5: 1412–19

DeWitte, Sharon N., and Philip Slavin. 2013. "Between Famine and Death: England on the Eve of the Black Death – Evidence from Paleoepidemiology and Manorial Accounts," *Journal of Interdisciplinary History* 44: 37–60

Ell, S. R. 1984. "Immunity as a Factor in the Epidemiology of Medieval Plague," *Review of Infectious Diseases* 6, no. 6: 866–79

Ell, S. R. 1987. "Plague and Leprosy in the Middle Ages: A Paradoxical Cross-Immunity?," *International Journal of Leprosy and Other Mycrobacterial Diseases* 55, no. 2: 345–50

Elvin, S. J., E. D. Williamson, J. C. Scott, J. N. Smith, et al. 2004. "Evolutionary Genetics: Ambiguous Role of CCR5 in *Y. pestis* Infection," *Nature* 430: 417

French, S. S., M. C. Moore, and G. E. Demas. 2009. "Ecological Immunology: The Organism in Context," *Integrative and Comparative Biology* 49, no. 3: 246–53

Gadelha, S. R., L. C. J. Alcantara, G. C. S. Costa, D. L. Rios, et al. 2005. "Ethnic Differences in the Distribution of Interleukin-6 Polymorphisms among Three Brazilian Ethnic Groups," *Human Biology* 77, no. 4: 509–14

Gage, K. L., and M. Y. Kosoy. 2005. "Natural History of Plague: Perspectives from More than a Century of Research," *Annual Review of Entomology* 50: 505–28

Gluckman, P., A. Beedle, and M. Hanson. 2009. *Principles of Evolutionary Medicine* (Oxford: Oxford University Press)

Green, Monica H. 2014. "Taking 'Pandemic' Seriously: Making the Black Death Global," *The Medieval Globe* 1: 27–61

Guegan, J.-F., F. Prugnolle, and F. Thomas. 2008. "Global Spatial Patterns of Infectious Diseases and Human Evolution," in *Evolution in Health and Disease*, ed. S. C. Stearns and J. C. Koella, 19–29 (Oxford: Oxford University Press)

Guy de Chauliac. 1363/1974. "Bubonic Plague," trans. Michael R. McVaugh, in *A Source Book in Medieval Science*, ed. Edward Grant, 773–74 (Cambridge, MA: Harvard University Press)

Herlihy, David. 1997. *The Black Death and the Transformation of the West* (Cambridge, MA: Harvard University Press)

Hirst, L. 1953. *The Conquest of Plague: A Study of the Evolution of Epidemiology* (Oxford: Clarendon Press)

Hoffman, S. C., E. M. Stanley, E. D. Cox, B. S. DiMercurio, et al. 2002. "Ethnicity Greatly Influences Cytokine Gene Polymorphisms Distribution," *American Journal of Transplantation* 2, no. 6: 560–67

Horrox, Rosemary (ed. and trans.). 1994. *The Black Death* (Manchester: Manchester University Press)

Hummel, S., D. Schmidt, B. Kremeyer, B. Herrmann, et al. 2005. "Detection of the CCR5-Δ32 HIV Resistance Gene in Bronze Age Skeletons," *Genes and Immunity* 6: 371–74

Hutchinson I. V., D. M. Turner, D. Sankaran, M. R. Awad, et al. 1998a. "Influence of Cytokine Genotypes on Allograft Rejection," *Transplant Proceedings* 30, no. 3: 862–63

Hutchinson I. V., D. M. Turner, D. Sankaran, M. R. Awad, et al. 1998b. "Cytokine Genotypes in Allograft Rejection: Guidelines for Immunosuppression," *Transplant Proceedings* 30, no. 8: 3991–92

Jordan, William Chester. 1996. *The Great Famine: Northern Europe in the Early Fourteenth Century* (Princeton: Princeton University Press)

Klink, M., K. Bednarska, E. Blus, M. Kielbik, et al. 2012. "Seasonal Changes in Activities of Human Neutrophils *in vitro*," *Inflammation Research* 61: 11–16

Koski, K. G., and M. E. Scott. 2001. "Gastrointestinal Nematodes, Nutrition and Immunity: Breaking the Negative Spiral," *Annual Review of Nutrition* 21: 297–321

Kremeyer, B., S. Hummel, and B. Herrmann. 2005. "Frequency Analysis of the Δ32ccr5 HIV Resistance Allele in a Medieval Plague Mass Grave," *Anthropologischer Anzeiger* 63: 13–22

Laayouni, H., M. Oosting, P. Luisi, M. Ioana, et al. 2014. "Convergent Evolution in European and Rroma Populations Reveals Pressure Exerted by Plague on Toll-Like Receptors," *Proceedings of the National Academy of Sciences* 111, no. 7: 2668–73

Larcombe, L., J. Rempel, I. Dembinski, K. Tinckam, et al. 2005. "Differential Cytokine Genotype Frequencies among Canadian Aboriginal and Caucasian Populations," *Genes and Immunity* 6: 140–44

Li, B., and R. Yang. 2008. "Interaction between *Yersinia pestis* and the Host Immune System," *Infection and Immunity* 76, no. 5: 1804–11

Lin, J. S., S. Park, J. J. Adamovicz, J. Hill, et al. 2011. "TNFα and IFNγ Contribute to F1/LcrV-Targeted Immune Defense in Mouse Models of Fully Virulent Pneumonic Plague," *Vaccine* 29, no. 2: 357–62

Lukaszewski, R., A. Dermot, J. Kenny, R. Taylor, et al. 2005. "Pathogenesis of *Yersinia pestis* Infection in BALB/c Mice: Effects on Host Macrophages and Neutrophils," *Infection and Immunity* 73, no. 11: 7141–50

Mackaness, G. B. 1964. "The Immunological Basis of Acquired Cellular Resistance," *Journal of Exploratory Medicine* 120, no. 1: 105–20

Martin, L. B., D. M. Hawley, and D. R. Ardia. 2011. "An Introduction to Ecological Immunology," *Funcional Ecology* 25, no. 1: 1–4

McDade, T. W. 2003. "Life History Theory and the Immune System: Steps toward a Human Ecological Immunology," *American Journal of Physical Anthropology* supp. 37: 100–25

McDade, T.W. 2005. "The Ecologies of Human Immune Function," *Annual Review of Anthropology* 34: 495–521

McDade, T. W., J. Rutherford, L. Adair, and C. W. Kuzawa. 2010. "Early Origins of Inflammation: Microbial Exposures in Infancy Predict Lower Levels of C-Reactive Protein in Adulthood," *Proceedings of the Royal Society B: Biological Sciences* 277: 1129–37

McNeill, William H. 1976. *Plagues and Peoples* (New York: Anchor)

Mecsas, J., G. Franklin, W. A. Kuziel, R. R. Brubaker, et al. 2004. "Evolutionary Genetics: CCR5 Mutation and Plague Protection," *Nature* 427: 606

Meenagh, A., F. Williams, O. Ross, C. Patterson, et al. 2002. "Frequency of Cytokine Polymorphisms in Populations from Western Europe, Africa, Asia, the Middle East and South Africa," *Human Immunology* 63, no. 11: 1055–61

Nakajima, R., and R. R. Brubaker. 1993. "Association between Virulence of *Yersinia pestis* and Suppression of Gamma Interferon and Tumor Necrosis Factor Alpha," *Infection and Immunity* 61, no. 1: 23–31

Nelson, R. J., G. E. Demas, S. L. Klein, and L. J. Kriegsfeld. 2002. *Seasonal Patterns of Stress, Immune Function, and Disease* (Oxford: Oxford University Press)

Parham, P. 2005. "MHC Class I Molecules and KIRS in Human History, Health and Survival," *Nature Reviews Immunology* 5: 201–14

Perry, R. D., and J. D. Fetherston. 1997. "*Yersinia pestis*-etiologic agent of plague," *Clinical Microbiolology Reviews* 10, no. 1: 35–66

Pollitzer, R. 1954. *Plague* (Geneva: World Health Organization)

Pravica, V., C. Perrey, A. Stevens, J. H. Lee, et al. 2000. "A Single Nucleotide Polymorphism in the First Intron of the Human IFN-g Gene: Absolute Correlation with a Polymorphic CA Microsatellite Marker of High IFN-g Production," *Human Immunology* 61: 863–66

Raj, S., D. Govindaraju, and R. Chakraborty. 2007. "Genetic Variation and Population Structure of Interleukin Genes among Seven Ethnic Populations from Karnataka, India," *Journal of Genetics* 86, no. 3: 189–94

Riet, E. van, F. C. Hartgers, and M. Yazdanbakhsh. 2007. "Chronic Helminth Infections Induce Immunomodulation: Consequences and Mechanisms," *Immunobiology* 212, no. 6: 475–90

Rivers, J. P. W. 1988. "The Nutritional Biology of Famines," in *Famine*, ed. G. A. Harrison, 57–106 (Oxford: Oxford University Press)

Roseboom, T. J., J. H. van der Meulen, C. Osmond, D. J. Barker, et al. 2001. "Adult Survival after Prenatal Exposure to the Dutch Famine, 1944–1945," *Paediatric and Perinatal Epidemiology* 15, no. 3: 220–25

Sallares, Robert. 2007. "Ecology, Evolution, and Epidemiology of Plague," in *Plague and the End of Antiquity: The Pandemic of 541–750*, ed. Lester K. Little, 231–89 (Cambridge: Cambridge University Press)

Sankaran, D., A. Asderakis, S. Ashraf, I. S. Roberts, et al. 1999. "Cytokine Gene Polymorphisms Predict Acute Graft Rejection following Renal Transplantation," *Kidney International* 56, no. 1: 281–88

Scott, Susan, and Christopher Duncan. 2001. *Biology of Plagues: Evidence from Historical Populations* (Cambridge: Cambridge University Press)

Slack, Paul. 1990. *The Impact of Plague in Tudor and Stuart England* (Oxford: Oxford University Press)

Sompayrac, Lauren M. 2008. *How the Immune System Works*, 3rd ed. (Oxford: Blackwell)

Stephens, J. Claiborne, D. E. Reich, D. B. Goldstein, H. Doo Shin, et al. 1998. "Dating the Origin of the CCR5-Δ32 AIDS-Resistance Allele by Coalescence of Haplotypes," *American Journal of Human Genetics* 62, no. 6: 1507–15

Suskind, R. M., C. L. Lachney, and J. N. Udall, Jr. 1994. "Malnutrition and the immune response," in *Dairy Products in Human Health and Nutrition*, ed. M. Serrano Rios et al., 285–97(Rotterdam: Balkema)

Trotter, J. H., A. L. Liebl, E. J. Weeber, and L. B. Martin. 2011. "Linking Ecological Immunology and Evolutionary Medicine: The Case of Apolipoprotein E," *Functional Ecology* 25, no. 1: 40–47

Turner, D. M., D. M. Williams, D. Sankaran, M. Lazarus, et al. 1997. "An Investigation of Polymorphism in the Interleukin-10 Gene Promoter," *European Journal Immunogenetics* 24, no. 1: 1–8

Wilson, M., R. Seymour, and B. Henderson. 1998. "Bacterial Perturbation of Cytokine Networks," *Infection and Immunity* 66, no. 6: 2401–09

Ziegler, Philip. 1969. *The Black Death* (London: Collins)

Fabian Crespo (fabian.crespo@louisville.edu) is a biological anthropologist specializing in human evolutionary immunology. In 2001, he moved from the University of Buenos Aires to the Department of Anthropology at the University of Louisville, Kentucky, where he began to develop the working hypothesis that different pathogenic experiences in the past have shaped the immune systems in different human populations. Since 2010, two experiences have greatly influenced this research: his participation in the Global History of Health Project at the Ohio State University, and the NEH Summer Seminar, "Health and Disease in the Middle Ages," directed by Dr. Monica Green and Dr. Rachel Scott, in 2012. He is currently working on the Black Death's impact on the immune systems of human populations and testing the potential role of cross immunity in the decline of medieval leprosy in Europe.

Matthew B. Lawrenz (matt.lawrenz@louisville.edu) is a microbiologist at the Center for Predictive Medicine for Biodefense and Emerging Infectious Diseases, Department of Microbiology and Immunology, at the University of Louisville's School of Medicine. He is interested in understanding how bacterial pathogens are able to infect and cause disease in humans, and since 2003 he has been studying the interactions between *Yersinia pestis* (the bacterium that causes human plague) and mammalian hosts. Specifically, Dr. Lawrenz's laboratory works to identify the factors that allow *Y. pestis* to cause disease and to understand how the bacillus is able to avoid detection and elimination by the innate immune system (i.e., by macrophages). Dr. Lawrenz's long-term goal is to use the information from these studies to aid in the design of new vaccines and therapeutic treatments to combat bacterial infection. Prior to his work with *Y. pestis*, Dr. Lawrenz studied Lyme Disease, an emerging bacterial infection that is transmitted by ticks, and helped develop the serological test used to diagnosis this infection. In 2012, Dr. Lawrenz began collaborating with Dr. Crespo to understand the potential impact of the Black Death on the evolution of the immune system in human populations.

Abstract Efforts to understand the differential mortality caused by plague must account for many factors, including human immune responses. In this essay we are particularly interested in those people who were exposed to the *Yersinia pestis* pathogen during the Black Death, but who had differing fates—survival or death—that could depend on which individuals (once infected) were able to mount an appropriate immune response as a result of biological, environmental, and social factors. The proposed model suggests that historians of the medieval world could make a significant contribution to the study of human health, and especially the role of human immunology in past environments and societies, by helping to reconstruct these conditions.

Keywords Plague, immunology, differential mortality, medieval Europe, Black Death.

THE BLACK DEATH AND THE FUTURE OF THE PLAGUE

MICHELLE ZIEGLER

THE GRAVITAS OF *Yersinia pestis*, unique among pathogens, is based more on its history than on modern case numbers. When new outbreaks of plague are reported in the media, journalists are quick to link these incidents with the horrors of the medieval Black Death—and then to claim that there is no real threat to society, because we now have modern antibiotics. Walking a thin line between stirring up interest and not causing panic, reporters are only half right on both counts. On the one hand, modern plague cases *are* caused by the same lethal bacterium, *Yersinia pestis*; and yet the phenomenon of the Black Death was far greater than any of the isolated cases or small outbreaks that usually attract such attention today. On the other, antibiotics are not a panacea that can wholly protect us from the next pandemic. Plague is re-emerging in a world of growing antibiotic resistance, economic interdependence, and rapid transit. *Yersinia pestis* is found in enzootic foci on every inhabited continent except Australia, and it was found in the arsenals of some states in the twentieth century. Political instability and weak economies can prevent the growth of adequate public health infrastructures that would enable rapid response to large infectious disease outbreaks, natural or not. Air travel makes pneumonic plague quickly transferable from one site to another. If public health officials and environmental services do their due diligence, an isolated case in the United States (or in most other countries) should not be cause for panic. However, the outbreak of over a hundred pneumonic plague cases, something that occurred in Congo in 2004 and 2005, was almost ignored by the media even though this was a serious risk to regional health. Sensationalizing the plague does not help us to deal with these realities, but neither does the lack of attention given to plague in areas of the world that are often beneath our notice.

This essay addresses three basic questions. First, what does it mean for plague to be classified as a re-emerging infectious disease? Second, what

I would like to express my sincere gratitude to Monica Green and Ann Carmichael, who both took me under their wings and introduced me to the medieval history of medicine. They have had the patience of saints. I am also grateful to Nükhet Varlık, Fabian Crespo, Carol Symes, and the anonymous reviewers for their helpful comments on an earlier draft of this paper.

is the human incidence of plague around the world today? And finally, how do we unite study of the plague in the past and present to create a better understanding of plague dynamics, to better prepare for the future?

A Re-emerging Infectious Disease

Frank Snowden (2008) has argued that the public health successes of the twentieth century led to an era of over-confidence in medical science: many supposed that the conquest and even eradication of pathogens was just a matter of time. Before the AIDs pandemic, it was unthinkable that this progress was illusory or temporary. But the growing awareness of the threat posed by the human immunodeficiency virus (HIV) in the 1980s was the first widely recognized indication that progress was neither inevitable nor irreversible. Then, between 1991 and 1995, the return of two old bacterial foes and the emergence of a terrifying new virus delivered a one-two punch to public confidence. Cholera had been undetected in the western hemisphere for a century when large new epidemics broke out in Central and South America, eventually claiming four thousand lives and raising fears of infrastructure failures. In 1994, a pneumonic plague outbreak in Surat, India, was followed by the discovery, the following year, of antibiotic-resistant strains of plague isolated in Madagascar. In 1995, spread of the Ebola virus in Zaire (now the Democratic Republic of Congo) also gained the attention of the global health community because of its gruesomely high fatality rate in a country without an adequate surveillance network. Within ten years, from the mid-1980s to mid-1990s, modern society's sense of security was shattered; hence, the new focus on "emerging and re-emerging" infectious diseases.

The 1994 plague epidemic in Surat has since become a textbook example of what can happen when a naturally ocurring epidemic is not brought under control. Like many other countries, India had discontinued plague surveillance in the 1980s, believing that it was no longer necessary after the end of the Third Pandemic (Garrett 2000: 5; Barrett 2008; Sivaramakrishnan 2011).[1] As medical anthropologist Ron Barrett (2008) has argued, this outbreak appears to have resulted from a natural spillover, but it was greatly exacerbated by temporary and permanent human settlement patterns, insufficient healthcare and urban infrastructure, and other governmental failures. The outbreak was triggered by an earthquake that reactivated a bubonic plague focus in the rural village of Mamla, in the Breed

1 The Third Pandemic has never been officially declared "over," but there is a general consensus that it ended in the 1950s.

district. Social interactions (probably the movement of migrant workers) then transferred the plague to Surat, a city of over 1.5 million people, where it quickly became a pneumonic epidemic. Plague did not move through the city homogenously: 78% of confirmed cases were first-generation immigrants to the city, living in slum communities (Barrett, 2008).

But India's public health system was not up to the challenge, and officials even struggled to identify the individuals who were infected (Dutt, Akhtar, and McVeigh 2006). Physicians fled clinics in the most affected districts and antibiotic shortages were common (Barrett 2008). Meanwhile, the media—rehashing lore of "the Black Death" and invoking the loss of some ten to twelve million Indians during the plague pandemic of the early twentieth century—helped to spur a mass exodus from the city. Those traveling by train carried the plague to Delhi and Calcutta, 80 and 160 kilometers away from Surat, respectively; eventually, over half a million people fled to all parts of India, potentially bringing plague with them (Dutt, Akhtar, and McVeigh 2006). And yet the extent of the epidemic still cannot be reliably determined: all told, there were 5,150 suspected cases of pneumonic and bubonic plague but only 53 confirmed deaths, which suggests that over-diagnosis inflated the number of cases. During an epidemic, it is not uncommon for only a few cases to be confirmed by laboratory analysis, especially in developing countries, and the absence of adequate laboratory support means that every febrile case is assumed to be pneumonic plague and is treated as such with antibiotics (Barrett 2008: 53). In Surat, pneumonic plague was confirmed in eighteen patients whose cultures tested positive for *Yersinia pestis*, and this finding was confirmed by the World Health Organization in 1994 and then by genetic analysis in 2000 (Dutt, Akhtar, and McVeigh 2006).

That same subsequent analysis in 2000 also confirmed that the Surat outbreak was caused by a strain of *Yersinia pestis* descended from a Third Pandemic strain (1.ORI) now endemic in Indian foci (Kingston et al. 2009). In 1994, however, the U.S. Centers for Disease Control and Prevention (CDC) had reported that the Surat plague was caused by a previously unknown strain of the pathogen—and to Indian officials this unfortunately leant backing to rumors of bioterrorism that had begun to circulate early on. Surat's Muslims were accused of poisoning the city's water system and causing many more deaths than actually occurred (Barrett 2008). Indian officials even blamed a local Islamic group for the epidemic and transferred plague response to the Department of Defense (Price-Smith 2002: 242). Only two years before, Surat had been the scene of Hindu-Muslim clashes that had fueled distrust in the local government, on both sides; the rumor that officials were planning to quarantine the city was therefore another factor that led Surat's citizens to flee. A lack of competent public health measures and pre-existing social tensions, heightened by fear and rumor, therefore exacerbated an outbreak of plague that could have been controlled.

Andrew Price-Smith (2002: 235) has argued that the psychological impact of the Surat plague was so great that it degraded the state capacity of India and impeded or weakened relations with countries around the world.[2] India paid a high price for the panic. Its neighbors (China, Nepal, Bangladesh, and Pakistan) completely closed their borders. Travel restrictions on people, imports, and in some cases mail were also imposed by other countries around the world. India lost an estimated 420 million dollars in trade from the United Arab Emirates alone (Barrett 2008). In the midst of the plague, the Indian stock market plunged, and costs of blocked exports and lost tourism revenues have been estimated at $1.8 billion, a significant blow for a developing country (Price-Smith 2002: 242). Like the plague, an economic collapse in one country becomes rapidly contagious, triggering economic instability and consequently political instability around the world (Price-Smith 2002; Koblentz 2010).

Only one year after the outbreak in Surat, the first antibiotic-resistant strains of *Yersinia pestis* were discovered in Madagascar (Welsh et al. 2007). From 1995 to 1998, more antibiotic-resistant strains were isolated in that same offshore African island, including one that is resistant to all of the known antibiotics used for plague treatment and prophylaxis (Galimand, Carniel, and Courvalin 2006). Like other bacteria, plague gains its resistance from a process called "lateral gene transfer," acquiring genes from other species of bacteria that carry antibiotic resistance plasmids (small circular DNA shuttles). *Yersinia pestis* readily accepts such plasmids from other enteric bacteria like *Escherichia coli* and *Salmonella enterica.* For example, the multi-drug resistant (MDR) plasmid found in *Yersinia pestis* is "nearly identical" to those found in Salmonella (Welsh et al. 2007). Although similar antibiotic resistance has not been found in human cases outside of Madagascar, plague isolates must now be vigilantly screened for naturally occurring antibiotic resistance (Urich et al. 2012; Stenseth et al. 2008). At the media briefing for the CDC's first threat-assessment on antibiotic resistance, in 2013, its director Dr. Tom Frieden warned:

---

2 According to Price-Smith (2002: 339), "State capacity is the capability of the government, and its level determines the state's ability to satisfy the most important needs: survival, protection of its citizens from physical harm as a result of internal or external predation, economic prosperity and stability, power projection, and ideological projection."

"If we are not careful, we will soon be in a post-antibiotic era. . . And for some patients and for some microbes, we are already there" (quoted by McKenna 2013). Although Freiden was not speaking specifically of plague, antibiotics' capacity to play a role in plague containment can no longer be assumed (Oyston and Williamson 2013; Stenseth et al. 2008).

Maintaining State Capacity and the Threat of Plague

Challenges to state capacity (the ability of the state to maintain basic functions) have existed since the beginning of settled civilization. The social and economic costs of these recent plague outbreaks are simply modern manifestations of trends that began with the sixth-century "Plague of Justinian," or First Pandemic. For the premodern world, as for our own, plague was not just a health crisis. All plagues are a threat to civil society; they jeopardize not just individuals but the fabric of communities and the institutions that maintain order. Plagues also decimate workforces, causing transformations in land use and the environment (see, e.g., Borsch 2014, in this issue). In the past, they spread through maritime economic networks: those of the Roman Empire in the sixth century, the mercantile empires of Italian city-states in the fourteenth century (Wheelis 2002; Horrox 1994: 14–26), and the British Empire at the turn of the twentieth (Echenberg 2007). Long-distance transmission of the next pandemic, if there is one, will likely be via airline networks, as was the case for the Severe Acute Respiratory Syndrome (SARS) pandemic in 2003 and which appears to be the case for the unfolding threat of MERS (Middle East Respiratory Syndrome). SARS has also directed our attention to the role played by "super spreaders": individuals who transmit disease to far greater degree than the average infected person (Stein 2011).[3] As Myron Echenberg has observed, "comparisons between the beginnings of the third [plague] pandemic in 1894 and the arrival of severe acute respiratory syndrome, or SARS, in 2003 are remarkable and suggest that we can do better at applying the experience of the past" (Echenberg 2007: 308).

Since the late 1990s, pandemics of all kinds have been considered matters of national and international security on the same level as military and terrorist threats, climate change, and refugee flows (Koblentz 2010). On January 10, 2000, the United Nations (UN) Security Council designated

3 When super-spreading is tied to a particular place, it is designated as a disease hotspot. For example, for plague, sites of grain storage are likely hotspots where infected rats and fleas are found in higher than average numbers, resulting in an increased number of human cases linked to that location. See further discussion below.

the HIV pandemic as a global security issue, moving it beyond the purview of the World Health Organization (WHO) (Price-Smith 2002). This set a precedent for allowing the UN to intervene in the governance of a sovereign state if it does not mount an adequate public health response to disease. Within this international security framework, plague is regarded as both a pandemic threat and a terrorist threat, given its potential to be used as a biological weapon. Indeed, *Yersinia pestis* is one of only three bacteria to have been labeled a "category A" biological weapons agent (the others being anthrax and tularemia). This top-level security designation is also shared by botulinum toxin, along with several hemorrhagic viruses and smallpox. Traits that define a "category A" agent include ease of distribution or transmission, high mortality rate, likelihood of causing social disruption and panic, and the necessity for special public health preparedness (CDC n.d.).

Major American initiatives are currently helping to build up global disease detection and response networks. For example, the United States has upgraded or rebuilt former Soviet anti-plague stations in the now-independent states of Kazakhstan and Uzbekistan, equipping them for improved surveillance and biosecurity (Koblentz 2012: 138; Pasternak 2013). The U.S. government also budgeted $5.54 billion for biodefense and disaster preparedness in 2012–13, of which $574.2 million was specifically dedicated to biodefense (Franco and Sell 2012). Some of this funding has already been used to answer historical questions relating to plague: ancient DNA (aDNA) confirmation of *Yersinia pestis* in specimens from a sixth-century Bavarian cemetery and the reconstruction of the ancient genome were supported in part by the Department of Homeland Security (Harbeck et al. 2013; Wagner et al. 2014). The latest advance in aDNA work, the Microbial Detection Array, which can screen aDNA for multiple pathogens, was developed in conjunction with the Lawrence Livermore National Laboratory (Devault et al. 2014). Of the full-scale federal response drills conducted to date, two of the exercises simulated plague attacks in multi-agent scenario exercises (TOPOFF 1 in May 2000 and TOPOFF 3 in April 2005; Inglesby, Grossman, and O'Toole 2001). These exercises involved thousands of participants, from local "first responders" to cabinet-level officials and governors.[4]

Yet pneumonic plague remains a bioterrorism concern for several reasons. With plague being endemic and enzootic in foci scattered around the world, natural sources cannot be fully identified or effectively controlled.

---

4 For an accessible review of biosecurity drills, see Armstrong (2012).

Furthermore, many enzootic foci in Central Asia, the Middle East, and Africa are located in poor, politically unstable areas where basic national security and public health institutions are already vulnerable or underdeveloped, as well as in several states that have known programs or have used biological or chemical weapons in the past, such as Syria, Iran, and North Korea. Moreover, *Y. pestis* can be processed into a crude weapon without sophisticated technology or expensive equipment. In 2008, forty al-Qaeda operatives in Algeria were discovered to have died of plague, perhaps as the result of a failed experiment in biological weapons development (Lake 2009; "40 al-Qaeda Terrorists" 2009).

But as we have already noted in the case of Surat, plague does not have to be deployed as a weapon to be a threat. War and infectious disease have a reciprocal effect. War weakens a society's ability to respond adequately to infectious disease by disrupting the social order, destroying civic infrastructure, and causing mass movements of people. Conversely, epidemics destabilize society and reduce state capacity, creating the conditions for political and social unrest. A recent instance of the former was the self-limiting outbreak of plague that occurred during the Libyan revolution in 2011, which could not be clinically confirmed or effectively treated because of ongoing hostilities (Cabanel et al. 2013). Plague outbreaks in the Democratic Republic of Congo—over ten thousand cases between 2000 and 2009—were also clearly exacerbated by ongoing political instability (Butler 2013). The violence and social disruption caused by the Vietnam War fostered a plague outbreak from 1966 to 1974, resulting in the loss of thousands of lives and the creation of endemic foci that persist to this day (Price-Smith 2009: 172–73). Outbreaks of plague and smallpox during the Korean War led to accusations that the United States had used biological weapons against North Korean and China. These accusations were later shown to be intentionally false; but here, again, environmental and institutional devastation contributed to the severity and persistence of disease (Hamblin 2013).

Plague Incidence and Causes Today

Plague is considered a re-emerging infectious disease because the number of cases, overall, has been climbing since the 1980s (see, e.g., Neerinckx, Bertherat, and Leirs 2010). Old plague foci are producing new cases after long intervals of quiescence. Moreover, endemic poverty and political unrest in developing countries with plague foci, the appearance of antibiotic-resistant strains of plague, and the potential use of plague as a biological weapon are major concerns.

The incidence, causes, and mortality rate of plague vary widely. Between 2000 and 2009, there were 21,725 cases reported to the WHO, with a case fatality rate of 7.4%. Of all these cases, 97% came from Africa (Butler 2013). Bubonic plague makes up the vast majority of these reported cases, but it can also manifest as primary septicemic plague, primary pneumonic plague, gastrointestinal plague, and plague pharyngitis. The most common of these presentations are perhaps better classified by their primary mode of exposure: insect bite or the entry of infectious bodily fluids through cuts and abrasions (bubonic and septicemic), inhalation (pneumonic), and ingestion (gastrointestinal and pharyngeal), respectively. While the "classic" rat-flea-human pathway is currently dominant, there is well-documented and long-standing evidence that other pathways of human exposure were common in past outbreaks and could become common again under certain conditions (Stenseth et al. 2008; Green 2014, in this issue; Carmichael 2014, in this issue). The human flea, *Pulex irritans*, has been implicated in Tanzanian plague outbreaks between 1986 and 2004 (Laudisoit et al. 2007) and may have been the agent of plague epidemics in medieval northern Europe, as well (Hufthammer and Walløe 2013). The human body louse has also been shown to be capable of transmitting *Yersinia pestis* and is another hypothetical medieval vector (Houhamdi et al. 2006; Drancourt, Houhamdi, and Raoult 2006). Here, it may be significant that combined epidemics of plague and louse-transmitted typhus were reported by contemporary physicians in Seville, in 1582 (Bowers 2013: 50). It may also be significant that aDNA testing of individuals buried in a Venetian mass grave and in graves from Bondy, France, have identified medieval cases of co-infection with *Y. pestis* and louse-transmitted *Bartonella quintana* (trench fever) (Tran et al. 2011a and 2011b).

Like cases of plague transmitted by human ectoparasites (fleas and lice), gastrointestinal plague and pharyngeal plague are relatively rare today. In the past, they may have been more common in areas where camels were the primary beast of burden (Christie, Chen, and Elberg 1980), and even a source of food. An outbreak of pharyngeal plague in 1997 was the first plague occurrence in Jordan since before the foundation of the modern state in 1921 (Arbaji et al. 2005). Three years earlier, a similar outbreak of pharyngeal plague occurred in Saudia Arabia, both caused by the consumption of infected camel meat (Bin Saeed, Al-Hamdan, and Fontaine 2005). An outbreak of gastrointestinal plague in 2007 is the first recorded outbreak in Afghanistan in the modern era and also the largest known outbreak to date. In December of that year, eighty-three individuals developed probable cases, some manifesting pharyngeal lesions, caused by consuming a visibly ill camel. The total case fatality rate was

20.5%, and the attack rate among those who ate the cooked camel meat was approximately 80% (Leslie et al. 2010). Gastrointestinal plague from consumption of camel meat has also been reported in Libya, and from the consumption of guinea pigs in Ecuador and Peru (Leslie et al. 2010; Stenseth et al. 2008). Consumption of diseased meat was not uncommon during the Middle Ages (Newfield 2012), and this should be considered as a possible route of infection for historic plagues, too, especially during food shortages. Moreover, gastrointestinal plague is not necessarily rare among other animals. Carnivores can contract the plague from the blood of their prey as well as from the prey's fleas. Pharyngeal plague is also not uncommon in cats, which can in turn then transmit plague pneumatically to humans (Gage et al. 2000).

Meanwhile, a recent upsurge in cases of bubonic plague heralds the re-emergence of very old plague foci around the Mediterranean and in Central Asia: in Algeria (2003 and 2008), Libya (2009 and 2011), and Kyrgyzstan (2013). The 2009 Libyan outbreak has been shown to be completely distinct from those of Algeria, and also different from those of the entire Third Pandemic (1.ORI strains). Instead, the plague in Libya was caused by the reactivation of an ancient plague focus (Cabanel et al. 2013). Such foci, having gone unmonitored for decades, are now showing signs of life in other places as well: plague has recently been confirmed in a western Iranian focus that had not been surveyed in thirty years (Esamaeili et al. 2013). Currently, the most active plague focus in the world is in the Ituri region of the Democratic Republic of Congo, which produces approximately one thousand bubonic cases per year (Butler 2013; Neerinckx et al. 2010). Large outbreaks often display multiple presentations of disease. For example, a 127-case Ugandan outbreak in 2006 produced 88% bubonic and 12% pneumonic cases (CDC 2009).

Clearly, though, diagnosis and case reporting are still a major problem in resource-poor countries, which have widely divergent diagnostic abilities and levels of treatment. This can lead to over-diagnosis that lowers the reported case fatality rate (Neerinckx et al. 2010). Late diagnosis and delayed treatment can also cause extreme differences in case fatality rates between the beginning and end of a single epidemic. So if the reported case fatality rate is cumulative, it will not distinguish between fatalities that occurred before and after antibiotic treatment began.

The incidence and case fatality rates reported to the WHO meeting in Antananarivo, Madagascar, in April of 2006 illustrate this problem (WHO 2008). At that meeting, the host country reported that plague cases between 2000 and 2005 were 94% bubonic with a fatality rate of 19%. The Democratic Republic of Congo reported a prevalent plague but could not offer reliable statistics for the years 2000 to 2005, because no records were kept between 2002 and 2003. Tanzania reported that about 90% of its cases were bubonic with an approximately 10% fatality rate. It also reported that deaths in family units were the result of secondary pneumonic plague caused by delayed treatment,[5] and that the human flea, *Pulex irritans,* was suspected as the vector in the absence of cat and dog fleas. Mongolia reported that 90% of its 160 cases between 1971 and 2000 were bubonic, with an astounding 40% developing secondary pneumonic plague due to lack of treatment. However, its officials also reported that only 4.2% of cases were primary pneumonic and reported a fatality rate of "up to 70%" due to lack of treatment and healthcare infrastructure. Neighboring China reported 630 cases between 1994 and 2004 with a case fatality rate of only 6.67%. China also reported that *Y. pestis* from southern foci (transmitted by the rat flea *X. cheopis*) caused bubonic plague with a very low fatality rate due largely to the relatively rapid provision of antibiotic treatment; yet *Y. pestis* from its northern foci was primarily transmitted to hunters who skinned animals, causing pneumonic and primary septicemic plague with a fatality rate over 50% due to the "remoteness" of the territory and delays in seeking and obtaining treatment. Little information on the Americas was offered at the meeting, but Peru did report an epidemic of 1,248 cases between 1992 and 1994. Peruvian representatives identified risk factors as "grain storage in the open air, which favors an abundance of rodents and fleas; promiscuity in housing; absence of rodent-proof devices, beds on the floor and infested with fleas; and the custom of raising guinea-pigs for their flesh" (WHO 2008: 20).

Plague reporting on routes of infection (or presentations) is similarly problematic. All individuals with fatal cases of plague develop a secondary septicemia before death. To put it simply, primary septicemic plague skips the initial inoculation phase that creates a bubo or manifests as pneumonia, and instead develops the systemic (body-wide) blood-borne infection immediately. The total rate of primary septicemic plague is therefore unknown, because it is usually only diagnosed by blood culture in the United States, where it represents approximately 30% of all cases (mostly contracted by handling or skinning animals) (Butler 2013). This suggests that primary septicemic plague is significantly under-diagnosed globally. It can be acquired while skinning or butchering animals via small cuts in the skin, giving *Y. pestis* direct access to the bloodstream. People handling

5 Secondary pneumonic plague is the development of plague pneumonia in a case of primary bubonic plague. Primary pneumonic plague outbreaks are begun by a case of secondary pneumonic plague in a human or animal index case.

plague victims or corpses could also be vulnerable to septicemic plague by extant wounds coming into contact with infected body fluids. In short, variations in modern standards of diagnosis and reporting mean that the data reported to WHO is suspect, serving as a further reminder that we need to be cautious when we use medieval data, too.

Although the vast majority of contemporary global cases appear to be bubonic, there have been a couple of recognizable pneumonic plague outbreaks in every recent decade. During this past winter of 2013–14, a pneumonic plague outbreak in Madagascar was widely reported in the news, but as of this writing it has not been formally reported to the scientific community. There was a pneumonic outbreak in Ecuador in 1998, and two nosocomial (hospital-acquired) pneumonic cases in Peru in 2010 (Schneider et al. 2014). Between 2000 and 2009, there were five natural pneumonic outbreaks affecting a dozen or more people: India (2002), Congo (2005 and 2006), Uganda (2006), and China (2009) (Joshi et al. 2009; Butler 2013; Bertherat et al. 2011; and Wang et al. 2010). The 2002 Indian outbreak in the Shimla district of Himachal Pradesh was caused by a strain distinct from the 1994 pneumonic epidemic in Surat (Kingston et al. 2009). The 2009 Chinese outbreak was chosen as a case study for a microbial forensic investigation (Yan et al. 2014) and was characterized as a 1.IN2 strain of *Yersinia pestis* (evolutionarily intermediate between the Second and Third Pandemic strain) and localized to Xinghai, in the Qinghai region of northwestern China.

The study of Yan and colleagues (2014) allows us to glimpse what future plague tracking and surveillance will look like when resources and databases mature. The unusually low genetic diversity of *Yersinia pestis* requires the comparison of whole genome sequences with reference to a global database of samples collected from animals and humans over the last century, in order to localize the source of the outbreak strain. This could be critically important for the success of a public health response. In the case of a biological attack, furthermore, the ability to trace the source of infection would also help the international community to identify the responsible state or terrorist organization (Koblentz and Tucker 2010). The seemingly random aspects of pneumonic plague transmission are typical of pathogens that spread by heterogeneous transmission (Lloyd-Smith et al. 2005). Like other respiratory "super-spreading" diseases, pneumonic plague is a high-impact, low probability event that can be explosive and catastrophic, as it was in Manchuria in 1910–11 (Summers 2012; Hinckley et al. 2012). With the variety of transmission methods, multiple vectors, and the potential for super-spreading events, existing plague foci are fertile grounds for initiating the next large epidemic, or even a pandemic, if the correct conditions emerge.

Uniting the Study of Past and Present, for the Future

Learning what we can from past epidemics is the best way to predict and prevent the next major epidemic. The careful analysis and contextualization of historical sources are therefore vitally important to our understanding of how plague functions as an epidemic pathogen. Combining historical data with a modern scientific knowledge also has the advantage of providing checks and balances to both humanistic and scientific study. It prevents researchers in all disciplines from stopping at the easy answers and being stymied by a mysterious aetiology.

Ancient and modern *Y. pestis* genetics suggest that current *Y. pestis* strains are good candidates for investigation by researchers in historic epidemiology. But while our understanding and use of aDNA data will continue and expand, it is still unlikely that a "smoking gun" will be found in the genome to explain its virulence or transmission patterns. Plague is created, amplified, and transported in man-made environments, whether it is transmitted by commensal rat fleas, human ectoparasites, or personal contact. The global distribution of plague reflects human movements more than any other host (Achtman 2012; Green, forthcoming). Plague epidemics have human fingerprints all over them, and that is why we need to know as much as we can about human interactions and global connectivity in the distant past: hence, this special issue of *The Medieval Globe.*

In the *Unnatural History of Emerging Infections* (2013), medical anthropologists Ronald Barrett and George Armelagos identify sustenance, settlement, and social order as primary drivers in the emergence of epidemic disease throughout human history. They reintroduce the metaphor of "seed and soil" (first used by physicians of the late nineteenth and early twentieth centuries, "who increasingly believed in Germ theory but continued to practice environmental medicine") to explain the relationship between microbes and the environment (Barrett and Armelegos 2013: 11). Whether or not genetically identical seeds (i.e., microbes) flourish is dependent upon the conditions of the soil (i.e., the environment). Understanding these conditions—of settlement, social order, nutrition—are historical issues that science alone cannot address. If the human components of epidemics are not understood (or are misunderstood), then our expensive preparations for the future will fail to mitigate not only the widespread return of diseases like plague, but also new emerging infectious diseases (Barrett 2006). The long history of plague gives us the rare opportunity to study a single disease over an unprecedented period of time.

Exploring the effects of nutrition on plague dynamics is a prime example of the need for interdisciplinary research. The expertise of historians is essential to the identification and analysis of sources that provide data on agricultural yields and practices of animal husbandry, food shortages and famine, trade networks and the diversification of foodstuffs, and all of the other activities that cultivate and sustain a food supply (e.g., Newfield 2012 and 2013). These efforts should dovetail with those of biologists working on the effects of nutrition on human immunology, *Y. pestis* itself, and rodent population dynamics (e.g., Crespo and Lawrenz 2014, in this issue; La Cava and Matarese 2004; Schaible and Stefan 2007). Biological anthropologists contribute, in turn, by analyzing bones for signs of malnutrition and disease, and tracing the sources and proportions of nutrients via isotopes (DeWitte 2014, in this issue). The work of climatologists provides a broader context for all of this historically informed research, by analyzing long- and short-term climate changes and their environmental and economic impact (e.g., Campbell 2010 and 2011). To understand the full complexity of plague, we need to pull together—rather than talk past each other.

A fine example of cross-disciplinary collaboration is that of anthropologist Sharon DeWitte and economic historian Philip Slavin (2013), who recently co-authored a study on the impact of the Great Famine (1315–17) and the food shortages resulting from the Great Bovine Epizootic (1319/20), which lasted until at least 1332. Their goal was to determine whether these catastrophic events had an impact on plague mortality, as reflected in London's East Smithfield cemetery, where victims of the Black Death were buried and where the full genome of *Y. pestis* was reconstructed in 2011. Slavin analyzed manorial accounts in order to document the depth and length of the famine and the subsequent food shortages resulting from the loss of cattle, while DeWitte assessed the ages and nutritional status of those individuals who lived through these privations only to die in the Black Death pandemic. Their failure to find a strong correlation between cohorts of people who survived the famine and food shortages, and increased susceptibility to the plague several decades later, is a good example of the checks and balances that the sciences and humanities can provide each other. The authors worked together to reach common conclusions, pose new questions, and suggest the next steps. Comparing bioarcheological evidence from one cemetery in the capital city of England to historical evidence from rural manorial accounts is a good start, but it does not settle the question of the influence of previous malnutrition on plague mortality, as they have noted. Many more collaborative studies of this kind are needed.

Settlement patterns, the conditions in which people live, and social stratification encompass another vast set of variables which must be understood from an historical perspective. As we saw in the case of Surat in 1994, socio-economic status can explain how plague moves through a large urban environment. What is the thread of social proximity that links together the earliest cases and therefore shapes the epidemic? Were some occupations at greater risk than others? What aspects of poverty might make people more vulnerable to plague? How are existing social, political, and religious tensions catalyzed by the stress of an epidemic disaster? How well does urban planning and the built environment correlate with plague incidence? What external factors (trade networks, new commodities, immigration) play a role in introducing or spreading disease? These are questions that historians and anthropologists are best suited to answer. Genetics and microbiology tell us little about these issues.

In turn, the methods and observations of modern epidemiology can illuminate the study of historic epidemics. The transmission of infection is now understood to be a continuum across hosts and environments (Lloyd-Smith et al. 2005). Heterogeneous transmission[6] is defined as "variability in the contribution of specific hosts or locations to the overall rates of pathogen spread" (Paull et al. 2012); extreme cases are better known by the more common term "super-spreading events" (SSE). *Yersinia pestis*, as we have observed, spreads by heterogeneous transmission, and the pneumonic form produces such super-spreading events (Lloyd-Smith et al. 2005). It is therefore possible that some historic outbreaks of bubonic plague were also super-spreading events fueled by disease hot spots.

Comparing plague to other insect-vectored zoonotic diseases provides further insight into transmission dynamics. Super-spreading events of Dengue fever, which like plague is transmitted by an insect vector that remains close to the place where it hatches, have been linked to sites where vector super-production intersects with human density (Padmanabha et al. 2012). In this study, vector super-production sites were as heterogeneous as would be expected of infection super-spreaders. Moreover, human density or traffic to these sites was as critical to disease transmission as vector production. Short distance or circular movements over the course of a day or week by humans has also been linked to increased risk of zoonotic disease transmission. For example, children at play or visiting friends can be exposed to more aspects or corners of a community than adults (Stoddard et al. 2009). A similar super-production of rodent fleas at sites of grain storage, which also draws in high human traffic, seems reasonable. It has often been remarked that outbreaks of plague

---

6 In contrast, homogenous transmission occurs when all hosts have an equal chance of becoming infected. See also Lambin et al. (2010) and Paull et al. (2012) for a discussion of some general principles of landscape epidemiology.

(past and present) disproportionally affect the poor more than the affluent (e.g., Wrightson 2011; Carmichael 1986), and it has been suggested that poverty-induced grain hoarding in crowded homes of poor construction create an environment where plague can flourish: this was the case in Surat (1994) as well as in Peru (1992–94) and in more recent outbreaks in Madagascar (Andrianaivoarimanana et al. 2013; WHO 2008). Testing such a hypothesis for historic epidemics requires good urban environmental histories of multiple locations and time periods, as proposed by Guy Geltner (2012) and Carole Rawcliffe (2013). We cannot rely on the traditional assumption that medieval cities were seething sites of filth and vermin; the historical reality is not only much more positive than these modern prejudices would credit, it is also more complex (Rawcliffe 2013).

So if there *were* historic plague hotspots in the medieval world, it will take much more research into the historical shaping of urban and rural environments in order to identify them: and this will require pulling together all available evidence, historical and scientific. So far, the eastern Mediterranean has been the most fruitful place to look for such sites, with the possible identification of an enzootic focus in the late antique Levant (Tsiamis 2010) and an environmental and documentary analysis of plague in Ottoman Egypt (Mikhail 2008). Indeed, Nükhet Varlık (2014, in this issue) argues convincingly for the Ottoman empire's central place in an historical understanding of plague. And importantly, Ann Carmichael (2014, in this issue) makes the first historical argument for a *European* plague focus. As part of an ongoing effort, the Environmental History Network for the Middle Ages is beginning to gather the environmental studies that are necessary to a contextualization of the plague and other medieval epidemics and epizootics.[7] Patterns of land use constitute another critical factor in creating an environment suitable for the establishment of plague. In modern Madagascar, for example, deforestation and bush fires (to clear land for agriculture) have been associated with plague outbreaks because they appear to disturb enzootic foci (Andrianaivoarimanana et al. 2013). Looking at plague incidence and severity in regions where the demographic effect of the Black Death substantially changed land use and agricultural methods could test these observations.

Related environmental change tends to occur after natural disasters like earthquakes and floods. An earthquake and monsoon flooding were both key catalysts for the 1994 outbreak in Surat (Barrett 2008). China has learned the importance of plague surveillance after earthquakes

7 ENforMA <http://www.medievaleh.org/> [accessed September 22, 2014].

around the Tibetan Plateau, where the plague is endemic and enzootic (and probably originated). The association between plague and earthquakes goes all the way back to the First Pandemic: Tsiamis and colleagues (2013) found an association between five earthquakes in the territories of the eastern Roman (Byzantine) empire and five plague outbreaks that occurred within a year of these respective events, in the era between 557 and 713. Extensive flooding was also associated with plague in Ottoman Egypt (Mikhail 2008), and the breakdown of infrastructures meant to regulate flooding and irrigation would have made matters worse (see Borsch 2014, in this issue). The first quantitative study of long- and short-distance transmission during the entire Third Pandemic in China showed that wet conditions facilitated spread of the plague: displacement of people and rodents by floods was proposed as a major factor in the increased velocity of transmission in South China (Xu et al. 2014). Indeed, a key feature in all of these natural disasters is that they displaced potential hosts (people, animals, rodents, insects) from their normal settings.

Environmental histories should accordingly make historical epidemiology more robust and comprehensive, because plague transmission is dependent upon the environment. It is necessary to approach the study of transmission from both the environmental context and the epidemiological result. Looking at one variable in isolation will not produce an accurate picture of transmission. If the epidemiological results do not match an expected plague pattern, then there is a missing piece to be found somewhere in the environment. For too long, plague researchers in both the sciences and the humanities were content to focus solely on the black rat and its flea, but we now know that over two hundred rodent species and their parasites carry and transmit *Yersinia pestis*; the black rat may be a common host but it is far from alone (Eisen and Gage 2011; Gage and Kosoy 2005). Moreover, fleas may be less abundant in the winter but some, such as *Oropysylla montana*, transmit *Yersinia pestis* effectively at temperatures as low as 6° C (42.8° F)—better, in fact, than at 23° C (73.4° F) (Williams et al. 2013). We must remember that *Yersinia pestis* evolved on the cold meadows of the Tibetan Plateau. It is not a tropical or near tropical disease.

Another environment that needs to be accounted for in studies of plague virulence is the landscape of the human body itself, and its co-infections and co-morbidities. What was the disease burden,[8] chronic

8 "Disease burden" is the total cost to a community of a type or category of disease. It can be measured in a variety of ways: mortality, birth rate and infant mortality, life expectancy, economic trends, declining productivity, etc. Each study should define its

and infectious, borne by the communities devastated by these epidemics? Expanding aDNA work to include other pathogens not only yields a better understanding of the disease burden of these communities but also looks for potential synergistic effects, or syndemics, between pathogens affecting the same populations (Barrett and Armelagos 2013). New methods are making the identification of all microbial contributions in an aDNA sample better and more efficient (Devault at al. 2014). Considering co-infection by other unrelated pathogens, such as malaria, is also important in estimating the overall health of the population and its response to plague. But again, because archeological remains always represent only a subsection of the population, this data must be balanced by study of surviving documentary sources. All of our evidence will always be a fraction of what once existed, so we must use all available sources to assess the overall health of earlier populations and their susceptibility to disease.

Identifying other pathogens, like typhus, can also tell us more about the parasite burden of these same populations (Tran et al. 2011a and 2011b). For example, it has recently been shown (experimentally) that lice can transmit the plague (Houhamdi et al. 2006; Drancourt, Houhamdi, and Raoult 2006; Tran et al. 2011a; Ayyadurai et al. 2010). During the Thirty Years' War (1618–48), there was a clear epidemiological transition between a dominant typhus phase yielding to a plague phase (Price-Smith 2009). Could the same species of louse that transmitted typhus during the first half of the war have been transmitting the plague in the second half, throughout the lands of Central and Eastern Europe—which were already devastated by violence, forced migration, destroyed crops, and the other catastrophic side-effects of war?

Conclusion

Interdisciplinary work is always a challenge, and it takes courage. It is daunting to confront another field with its own terminology and norms. But it is worth the effort. And happily, there are sources and people who can help to bridge the gap. In his *Evolutionary History: Uniting History and Biology to Understand Life on Earth* (2011), environmental historian Edmund Russell lays out a methodology for integrating biological information into historical studies and provides multiple examples of the difference that this makes. There are a variety of online forums for discussion, as well: these include the Medieval Medicine listserve (MEDMED-L)

---

criteria and methods for measuring disease burden, as appropriate for the community (and time period).

moderated by Monica Green, blogs (like my own *Contagions*) that also reach out to a general audience, and the above-mentioned Environmental History Network for the Middle Ages.[9] All are very welcoming to people from a variety of backgrounds, with diverse levels of expertise.

As I hope to have shown, all kinds of plague studies are relevant to understanding the modern experience of plague and are crucial to the development of strategies for handling future pandemic threats. There are multiple opportunities for interdisciplinary work and the formation of multidisciplinary partnerships that can lower the barriers between the sciences and the humanities. Linking historical studies to our current plague concerns is further proof of the important vital place of the humanities in our academic curricula and in the public sphere. Confirmation that the East Smithfield cemetery in London was founded and used only for the burial of Black Death victims would have been impossible without the analysis of surviving documents and artifacts. Archeology alone, even with data from carbon dating, will not be able to date graves accurately enough to distinguish between plague epidemics separated by a twenty-year hiatus. We cannot discern the epidemiology of historic plagues without knowledge of the historical environment and human ecology. Only when the sciences and the humanities work together can we really begin to understand the medieval phenomenon of "the Black Death" and put that knowledge to work in our own world.

9 I also recommend *Infectious Thoughts*, by microbiologist Siouxsie Wiles <http://sciblogs.co.nz/infectious-thoughts/>; *Powered by Osteons*, by bioarcheologist Kristina Killgrove <http://www.poweredbyosteons.org/>; and *Bones Don't Lie*, by anthropology graduate student Katy Meyers <http://www.bonesdontlie.com/> [all accessed September 22, 2014].

Bibliography

"40 al-Qaeda Terrorists Dead after Failed Experiment with Plague Weapon," *Homeland Security News Wire* (January 24, 2009) <http://www.homelandsecuritynewswire.com/40-al-qaeda-terrorists-dead-after-failed-experiment-plague-weapon> [accessed September 28, 2014]

Achtman, M. 2012. "Insights from Genomic Comparisons of Genetically Monomorphic Bacterial Pathogens," *Philosophical Transactions of the Royal Society B* 367: 860–67

Andrianaivoarimanana, V., K. Kreppel, N. Elissa, J.-M. Duplantier, et al. 2013. "Understanding the Persistence of Plague Foci in Madagascar," *PLoS Neglected Tropical Diseases* 7, no. 11: e2382

Arbaji, A., S. Kharabsheh, S. Al-Azab, M. Al-Kayed, et al. 2005. "A 12-case Outbreak of Pharyngeal Plague following the Consumption of Camel Meat, in North–Eastern Jordan," *Annals of Tropical Medicine & Parasitology* 99, no. 8: 789–93

Armstrong, M. 2012. "Rehearsing for the Plague: Citizens, Security, and Simulation," *Canadian Review of American Studies* 42: 105–20

Ayyadurai, S., F. Sebbane, D. Raoult, and M. Drancourt. 2010. "Body Lice, *Yersinia pestis Orientalis*, and Black Death," *Emerging Infectious Diseases* 16, no. 5: 892–93

Barrett, R.. 2006. "Dark Winter and the Spring of 1972: Deflecting the Social Lessons of Smallpox," *Medical Anthropology* 25, no. 2: 171–91

Barrett, R. 2008. "The 1994 Plague in Western India: Human Ecology and the Risks of Misattribution," in *Terrorism, War or Disease? Unraveling the Use of Biological Weapons*, ed. A. L. Clunan, P. R. Lavoy, and S. B. Martin, 49–71 (Stanford: Stanford University Press)

Barrett, R., and G. Armelagos. 2013. *An Unnatural History of Emerging Infections* (Oxford: Oxford University Press)

Bertherat, E., P. Thullier, J. C. Shako, K. England, et al. 2011. "Lessons Learned about Pneumonic Plague Diagnosis from Two Outbreaks, Democratic Republic of the Congo," *Emerging Infectious Diseases* 17: 778–84

Bin Saeed, A. A., N. A. Al-Hamdan, and R. E. Fontaine. 2005. "Plague from Eating Raw Camel Liver," *Emerging Infectious Diseases* 11, no. 9: 1456–57

Borsch, Stuart. 2014. "Plague Depopulation and Irrigation Decay in Medieval Egypt," *The Medieval Globe* 1: 125–156

Bowers, Kristy Wilson. 2013. *Plague and Public Health in Early Modern Seville* (Rochester: University of Rochester Press)

Butler, T. 2013. "Plague Gives Surprises in the First Decade of the 21st Century in the United States and Worldwide," *American Journal of Tropical Medicine and Hygiene* 89: 788–93

Cabanel, N., A. Leclercq, V. Chenal-Francisque, B. Annajar, et al. 2013. "Plague Outbreak in Libya, 2009, Unrelated to Plague in Algeria," *Emerging Infectious Diseases* 19, no. 2: 230–36

Campbell, Bruce M. S. 2010. "Nature as Historical Protagonist: Environment and Society in Pre-Industrial England," *Economic History Review* 63: 281–314

Campbell, Bruce M. S. 2011. "Panzootics, Pandemics and Climatic Anomalies in the Fourteenth Century," in *Beiträge zum Göttinger Umwelthistorischen Kolloquium 2010-2011*, ed. Bernd Herrmann, 177–215 (Göttingen: Universitätsverlag Göttingen)

Carmichael, Ann G. 1986. *Plague and the Poor in Renaissance Florence* (Cambridge: Cambridge University Press)

Carmichael, Ann G. 2014. "Plague Persistence in Western Europe: A Hypothesis," *The Medieval Globe* 1: 157–191

Centers for Disease Control and Prevention (CDC). 2009. "Bubonic and Pneumonic Plague – Uganda, 2006," *MMWR (Morbidity and Mortality Weekly Report* 58, no. 28: 778–81

Centers for Disease Control and Prevention. (n.d.). "Bioterrorism Agents/Diseases – by Category" <http://www.bt.cdc.gov/agent/agentlist-category.asp> [accessed February 3, 2014]

Christie, A. B., T. H. Chen, and Sanford S. Elberg. 1980. "Plague in Camels and Goats: Their Role in Human Epidemics," *Journal of Infectious Diseases* 141, no. 6: 724–26

Crespo, Fabian, and Matthew B. Lawrenz. 2014. "Heterogeneous Immunological Landscape and Medieval Plague: An Invitation to a New Dialogue between Historians and Immunologists," *The Medieval Globe* 1: 229–257

Cui, Y., C. Yu, Y. Yan, D. Li, et al. 2013. "Historical Variations in Mutation Rate in an Epidemic Pathogen, *Yersinia pestis*," *Proceedings of the National Academy of Science* 110, no. 2: 577–82

Devault, A. M., K. McLoughlin, C. Jaing, S. Gardner, et al. 2014. "Ancient Pathogen DNA in Achaeological Samples Detected with a Microbial Detection Array," *Scientific Reports* 4: <doi:10.1038/srep04245>

DeWitte, Sharon N. 2014. "The Anthropology of Plague: Insights from Bioarcheological Analyses of Epidemic Cemeteries," *The Medieval Globe* 1: 97–123

DeWitte, Sharon N., and P. Slavin. 2013. "Between Famine and Death: England on the Eve of the Black Death—Evidence from Paleoepidemiology and Manorial Accounts," *Journal of Interdisciplinary History* 44: 1–25

Drancourt, M., L. Houhamdi, and D. Raoult. 2006. "*Yersinia pestis* as a Telluric, Human Ectoparasite-Borne Organism," *Lancet Infectious Diseases* 6, no. 4: 234–41

Dutt, A. K., R. Akhtar, and M. McVeigh. 2006. "Surat Plague of 1994 Re-Examined," *Southeast Asian Journal of Tropical Medicine and Public Health* 37, no. 4: 755–60

Echenberg, Myron. 2007. *Plague Ports: The Global Urban Impact of Bubonic Plague, 1894–1901* (New York: New York University Press)

Eisen, R. J., and K. L. Gage. 2011. "Transmission of Flea-Borne Zoonotic Agents," *Annual Review of Entomology* 57: 61–82

Eisen, R. J., K. MacMillan, L. A. Atiku, J. T. Mpanga, et al. 2014. "Identification of Risk Factors for Plague in the West Nile Region of Uganda," *American Journal of Tropical Medicine and Hygiene* (March 31, 2014) <doi:10.4269/ajtmh.14-0035>

Esamaeili, S., K. Azadmanesh, S. R. Naddaf, M. Rajerison, et al. 2013. "Serologic Survey of Plague in Animals, Western Iran," *Emerging infectious Diseases* 19, no. 9: PMID:23968721.

Franco, C., and T. K. Sell. 2012. "Federal Agency Biodefense Funding, FY2012-FY2013," *Biosecurity and Bioterrorism: Biodefense Strategy, Practice, and Science* 10, no. 2: 162–81

Gage, K. L., D. T. Dennis, K. A. Orloski, P. Ettestad, et al. 2000. "Cases of Cat-Associated Human Plague in the Western U.S,. 1977–1998," *Clinical Infectious Diseases: An Official Publication of the Infectious Diseases Society of America* 30, no. 6: 893–900

Gage, K. L., and M. Y. Kosoy. 2005. "Natural Hhistory of the Plague: Perspectives from More than a Century of Research," *Annual Review of Entomology* 50: 505–28

Galimand, M., E. Carniel, and P. Courvalin. 2006. "Resistance of *Yersinia pestis* to Antimicrobial Agents," *Antimicrobial Agents Chemotherapy* 50, no. 10: 3233

Garrett, L. 2000. *Betrayal of Trust: The Collapse of Global Public Health* (New York: Hyperion)

Geltner, G. 2012. "Public Health and the Pre-Modern City: A Research Agenda," *History Compass* 10, no. 3: 231–45

Green, Monica H. 2014. "Taking 'Pandemic' Seriously: Making the Black Death Global," *The Medieval Globe* 1: 27–61

Green, Monica H. Forthcoming. "The Globalisations of Disease," in *From Colonisation to Globalisation: Species Movements in Human History*, ed. Michael Petraglia and Nicole Boivin (Cambridge: Cambridge University Press)

Hamblin, J. D. 2013. *Arming Mother Nature: The Birth of Catastrophic Environmentalism* (Oxford: Oxford University Press)

Harbeck, M., L. Seifert, S. Hänsch, D. M. Wagner, et al. 2013. "*Yersinia pestis* DNA from Skeletal Remains from the 6th Century AD Reveals Insights into Justinianic Plague," *PLoS Pathogens* 9, no. 5: e1003349

Hinckley, A. F., B. J. Biggerstaff, K. S. Griffith, and P. S. Mead. 2012. "Transmission Dynamics of Primary Pneumonic Plague in the U.S.A.," *Epidemiology and Infection* 140: 554–60

Holt, E., and S. Palazzo. 2013. "The Role of Rodents in the Disease Ecology of the Roman City," *Archaeological Review from Cambridge* 28, no. 2: 132–54

Horrox, Rosemary (ed. and trans.). 1994. *The Black Death* (Manchester: Manchester University Press)

Houhamdi, L., H. Lepidi, M. Drancourt, D. Raoult. 2006. "Experimental Model to Evaluate the Human Body Louse as a Vector of Plague," *Journal of Infectious Diseases* 194: 1589–96

Hufthammer, A. K., and L. Walløe. 2013. "Rats Cannot Have Been Intermediate Hosts for *Yersinia pestis* during Medieval Plague Epidemics in Northern Europe," *Journal of Archaeological Science* 40: 1752–59

Inglesby, T. V., R. Grossman, and T. O'Toole. 2001. "A Plague on Your City: Observations from TOPOFF," *Clinical Infectious Diseases: An Official Publication of the Infectious Diseases Society of America* 32: 436–45

Joshi, K., J. S.Thakur, R. Kumar, A. J. Singh, et al. 2009. "Epidemiological Features of Pneumonic Plague Outbreak in Himachal Pradesh, India," *Transactions of the Royal Society of Tropical Medicine and Hygiene* 103: 455–60

Kingston, J. J., U. Tuteja, M. Kapi, H. S. Murali, et al. 2009. "Genotyping of Indian *Yersinia pestis* Strains by MLVA and Repetitive DNA Sequence Based PCRs," *Antonie van Leeuwenhoek* 96: 303–12

Koblentz, G. D. 2010. "Biosecurity Reconsidered: Calibrating Biological Tthreats and Responses," *International Decurity* 34, no. 4: 96–132

Koblentz, G. D. 2012. "From Biodefence to Biosecurity: The Obama Administration's Strategy for Countering Biological Threats," *International Affairs* 88: 131–48

Koblentz, G. D., and J. B. Tucker. 2010. "Tracing an Attack: The Promise and Pitfalls of Microbial Forensics," *Survival* 52: 159–86

La Cava, A., and G. Matarese. 2004. "The Weight of Leptin in Immunity," *Nature Reviews Immunology* 4, no. 5: 371–79

Lake, Eli. 2009. "Al Qaeda Bungles Arms Experiment," *Washington Times* (January 19) <http://www.washingtontimes.com/news/2009/jan/19/al-qaeda-bungles-arms-experiment/#.UdWcKx5LLPg.gmail> [accessed October 12, 2013]

Lambin, E. F., A. Tran, S. O. Vanwambeke, C. Linard, et al. 2010. "Pathogenic Landscapes: Interactions between Land, People, Disease Vectors, and their Animal Hosts," *International Journal of Health Geographics* 9, no. 1: 54

Laudisoit, A., H. Leirs, R.H. Makundi, S. Van Dongen, et al. 2007. "Plague and the Human Flea, Tanzania," *Emerging Infectious Diseases* 13, no. 5: 687–93

Leslie, T., C. A. Whitehouse, C. Yingst, C. Baldwin, et al. 2010. "Outbreak of Gastroenteritis Caused by *Yersinia pestis* in Afghanistan," *Epidemiology and Infection* 139: 728–35

Lloyd-Smith, J. O., S. J. Schreiber, P. E. Kopp, and W. M. Getz. 2005. "Superspreading and the Effect of Individual Variation on Disease Emergence," *Nature* 438, no. 7066: 355–59

McKenna, M. 2013. "CDC Threat Report: 'We Will Soon Be in a Post-Antibiotic Era'," *Superbug* [*Wired* blog] (September 16) <http://www.wired.com/wired-science/2013/09/cdc-amr-rpt1/> [accessed September 22, 2014]

Mikhail, A. 2008. "The Nature of Plague in Late Eighteenth-Century Egypt," *Bulletin of the History of Medicine* 82, no. 2: 249–75

Neerinckx, Simon, E. Bertherat, and H. Leirs. 2010. "Human Plague Occurrences in Africa: An Overview from 1877 to 2008," *Transactions of the Royal Society of Tropical Medicine and Hygiene* 104, no. 2: 97–103

Newfield, T. 2012. "Epizootics and the Consumption of Diseased Meat in the Middle Ages," in *Religione e istituzioni religiose nell'economia europea, 1000–1800 / Religion and Religious Institutions in the European Economy, 1000–1800: atti della Quarantatreesima Settimana di Studi, 8–12 maggio 2011*, ed. Francesco Ammannati, 619–39 (Florence: Firenze University Press)

Newfield, T. 2013. "Early Medieval Epizootics and Landscapes of Disease: The Origins and Triggers of European Livestock Pestilences, 400–1000 CE," in *Landscapes and Societies in Medieval Europe East of the Elbe: Interactions between Environmental Settings and Cultural Transformations*, ed. S. Kleingartner, T. P. Newfield, S. Rossignol, and D. Wehner, 73–113 (Toronto: Pontifical Institute of Mediaeval Studies)

Oyston, P. C., and E. D. Williamson. 2013. "Prophylaxis and Therapy of Plague," *Expert Review of Anti-infective Therapy* 11, no. 8: 817–29

Padmanabha, H., D. Durham, F. Correa, M. Diuk-Wasser, et al. 2012. "The Interactive Roles of *Aedes aegypti* Super-Production and Human Density in Dengue Transmission," *PLoS Neglected Tropical Diseases* 6, no. 8: e1799

Pasternack, A. 2013. "Why the U.S. Is Building a High-Tech Bubonic Plague Lab in Kazakhstan," *Motherboard* (August 27) <http://motherboard.vice.com/blog/why-the-us-is-building-a-high-tech-plague-lab-in-kazakhstan> (repr. in *Popular Science* online [29 August 2013] <http://www.popsci.com/technology/article/2013-08/why-us-building-high-tech-bubonic-plague-lab-kazakhstan> [accessed October 23, 2014])

Paull, S. H., S. Song, K. M. McClure, L. C. Sackett, et al. 2012. "From Superspreaders to Disease Hotspots: Linking Transmission across Hosts and Space," *Frontiers in Ecology and the Environment* 10, no. 2: 75–82

Price-Smith, A. 2002. *The Health of Nations: Infectious Disease, Environmental Change and Effects on National Security and Development* (Cambridge, MA: MIT Press)

Price-Smith, A. 2009. *Contagion and Chaos: Disease, Ecology, and National Security in the Era of Globalization* (Cambridge, MA: MIT Press)

Rawcliffe, Carole. 2013. "'Less Mudslinging and More Facts": A New Look at an Old Debate about Public Health in Late Medieval English Towns," *Bulletin of the John Rylands Library* 89, no. 1: 203–21

Russell, Edmund. 2011. *Evolutionary History: Uniting History and Biology to Understand Life on Earth* (Cambridge: Cambridge University Press)

Schaible, U., and H. Stefan. 2007. "Malnutrition and Infection: Complex Mechanisms and Global Impacts," *PLoS Medicine* 4, no. 5: e115

Schneider, M. C., P. Najera, S. Aldighieri, D. I. Galan, et al. 2014. "Where Does Human Plague Still Persist in Latin America?," *PLoS Neglected Tropical Diseases* 8, no. 2: e2680

Sivaramakrishnan, K. 2011. "The Return of Epidemics and the Politics of Global-Local Health," *American Journal of Public Health* 101: 1032–41

Snowden, F. M. 2008. "Emerging and Reemerging Diseases: A Historical Perspective," *Immunological Reviews* 225: 9–26

Stein, R. A. 2011. "Super-Spreaders in Infectious Diseases," *International Journal of Infectious Diseases* 15, no. 8: e510–3

Stenseth, N. Chr., B. B. Atshabar, M. Begon, S. R. Belmain, et al. 2008. "Plague: Past, Present, and Future," *PLoS Medicine* 5, no. 1: e3

Stoddard, S. T., A. C. Morrison, G. M. Vazquez-Prokopec, V. Paz Soldan, et al. 2009. "The Role of Human Movement in the Transmission of Vector-Borne Pathogens," *PLoS Neglected Tropical Diseases* 3, no. 7: e481

Summers, W. C. 2012. *The Great Manchurian Plague of 1910–1911: The Geopolitics of an Epidemic Disease* (New Haven, CT: Yale University Press)

Tran, T.-N.-N., C. L. Forestier, M. Drancourt, D. Raoult, et al. 2011a. "Brief Communication: Co-Detection of *Bartonella quintana* and *Yersinia pestis* in an 11th–15th Century Burial Site in Bondy, France," *American Journal of Physical Anthropology* 145, no. 3: 489–94

Tran, T.-N.-N., M. Signoli, L. Fozzati, G. Aboudharam, et al. 2011b. "High Throughput, Multiplexed Pathogen Detection Authenticates Plague Waves in Medieval Venice, Italy," *PLoS ONE* 6, no. 3: e16735

Tsiamis, C. 2010. "Epidemic Waves during Justinian's Plague in the Byzantine Empire (6th–8th c. A.D.)," *Vesalius: Acta internationales historiae medicinae*, supp.: 12–18

Tsiamis, C., E. Poulakou-Rebelakou, and S. Marketos. 2013. "Earthquakes and Plague during Byzantine Times: Can Lessons from the Past Improve Epidemic Preparedness?," *Acta medico-historica adriatica* 11: 55–64

Urich, S. K, L. Chalcraft, M. E. Schriefer, B. M. Yockey, et al. 2012. "Lack of Antimicrobial Resistance in *Yersinia pestis* Isolates from 17 Countries in the Americas, Africa, and Asia," *Antimicrobial Agents and Chemotherapy* 56: 555–58

Varlık, Nükhet. 2014. "New Science and Old Sources: Why the Ottoman Experience of Plague Matters," *The Medieval Globe* 1: 193–227

Wagner, D. M., J. Klunk, M. Harbeck, A. Devault, et al. 2014. "*Yersinia pestis* and the Plague of Justinian, 541–543 AD: A Genomic Analysis," *Lancet Infectious Diseases* 14, no. 4: 319–26

Wang, H., Y. Cui, Z. Wang, X. Wang, et al. 2010. "A Dog-Associated Primary Pneumonic Plague in Qinghai Province, China," *Clinical Infectious Diseases* 52, no. 2: 185–90

Welch, T. J., W. F. Fricke, P. F. McDermott, D. G. White, et al. 2007. "Multiple Antimicrobial Resistance in Plague: An Emerging Public Health Risk," *PLoS ONE* 2, no. 3: e309

Wheelis, M. 2002. "Biological Warfare at the 1346 Siege of Caffa," *Emerging Infectious Diseases* 8, no. 9: PMID: 12194776

Williams, S. K., A. M. Schotthoefer, J. A. Montenieri, J. L. Holmes, et al. 2013. "Effects of Low-Temperature Flea Maintenance on the Transmission of *Yersinia pestis* by *Oropsylla montana*," *Vector Borne and Zoonotic Diseases* 13, no. 7: 468–78

World Health Organization (WHO). 2008. "WHO Interregional Meeting on Prevention and Control of Plague – Antananarivo, Madagascar, 7–11 April 2006," WHO/HSE/EPR/2008.3 <http://www.who.int/csr/resources/publications/WHO_HSE_EPR_2008_3/en/index.html> [accessed September 22, 2014]

Wrightson, K. 2011. *Ralph Tailor's Summer: A Scrivener, His City, and the Plague* (New Haven, CT: Yale University Press)

Xu, Lei, L. Chr. Stige, K. L. Kausrud, T. Ben Ari, et al. 2014. "Wet Climate and Transportation Routes Accelerate Spread of Human Plague," *Proceedings of the Royal Society B: Biological Sciences* 281, no. 1780: 20133159

Yan, Y., H. Wang, D. Li, X. Yang, et al. 2014. "Two-Step Source Tracing Strategy of *Yersinia pestis* and its Historical Epidemiology in a Specific Region," *PLoS ONE* 9, no. 1: e85374

Michelle Ziegler (zieglerm@slu.edu) is a biologist with interests in the history of infectious disease and in science communication. She is particularly interested in the ways that science and history can inform each other, toward a greater understanding of plague. Her blog *Contagions* <http://contagions.wordpress.com> focuses on the intersection of science and history, and is intended to be a bridge between them, explaining scientific studies for people without a science background and exploring the historical contexts of infectious diseases under investigation today. She received an MS in Biological Science from Southern Illinois University at Edwardsville and an MS in Biosecurity and Disaster Preparedness from Saint Louis University. She is currently on the staff of the DNA Diagnostics Laboratory in the Department of Pathology at Saint Louis University.

Abstract This essay summarizes what we know about the spread of *Yersinia pestis* today, assesses the potential risks of tomorrow, and suggests avenues for future collaboration among scientists and humanists. Plague is both a re-emerging infectious disease and a developed biological weapon, and it can be found in enzootic foci on every inhabited continent except Australia. Studies of the Black Death and successive epidemics can help us to prepare for and mitigate future outbreaks (and other pandemics) because analysis of medieval plagues provides a crucial context for modern scientific discoveries and theories. These studies prevent us from stopping at easy answers, and they force us to acknowledge that there is still much that we do not understand.

Keywords Black Death, epidemiology, biosecurity, global history, public health, re-emerging infectious diseases.

EPILOGUE: A HYPOTHESIS ON THE EAST ASIAN BEGINNINGS OF THE *YERSINIA PESTIS* POLYTOMY

ROBERT HYMES

FOR THE HISTORIAN of premodern Eurasia, the 2013 study of historical variations in *Yersinia pestis* mutation rates by Yujun Cui and others signals a new departure in the cumulative study of the genetics of the bacillus over the preceding fifteen years. Whereas previous studies had been moving to define *Y. pestis*'s place of origin and dissemination only in a broad chronological framework of up to 20,000 years (Achtman et al. 2004; Morelli et al. 2010), Cui and colleagues' work makes a historical claim of much greater precision: that the evolution of *Y. pestis* since its divergence from its most recent common ancestor may have occurred within the past three to four thousand years, and more importantly that a polytomy (simultaneous or nearly simultaneous genetic divergence of multiple lineage branches) or "Big Bang" that yielded most of the current strains of *Y. pestis*, as well as the 1348 Black Death strain, took place between 1142 and 1339 (Cui et al. 2013: 580, table 1; their time interval has a confidence level of 95%). Their further finding, that the bacillus originated in or near the Qinghai-Tibet Plateau, offers historians both a period and place to look for human events that could produce a punctuated genetic divergence. I will offer as a hypothesis that the "Big Bang" can be placed in space and time in historical sources, too: that the polytomy first manifests itself historically in the long destruction, by the Mongols under Cinggis-Qan (Genghis Khan), of the Xia state of the Mi or "Tangut" people in the early 1200s, and continues with the movement of the Mongols into north China, south China, and much of Eurasia. The new genetic evidence, I argue, merits revisiting the documentary evidence of epidemics in thirteenth- and fourteenth-century Central Asia and China, epidemics that earlier authors had proposed as possible *Y. pestis* outbreaks. No piece of evidence I offer argues unambiguously for plague: in particular, the Chinese sources have little to say about clinical symptoms and nothing to say about rodents. The case I propose rests rather on how bits of evidence fit together and, as a starting point, on their fit with the Cui team's findings on the Big Bang's timing and the region of plague's origin; and I point forward to the need for new research on China and Inner Asia.

Table 7. States of "China," 976–1644

<table>
<tr><th>Northwest (Gansu corridor)</th><th>North China</th><th>South China</th></tr>
<tr><td rowspan="2">Xia (Tangut)
1038–1227</td><td colspan="2">Song (Chinese) 976–1127
except for sixteen prefectures in far north under Liao (Khitan)</td></tr>
<tr><td>Jin (Jurchen)
1126–1234</td><td rowspan="2">Song (Chinese)
1127–1279</td></tr>
<tr><td colspan="2">Yuan (Mongol) 1227/1234–1279</td></tr>
<tr><td colspan="3">Yuan (Mongol) 1279–1368</td></tr>
<tr><td colspan="3">Ming (Chinese) 1368–1644</td></tr>
</table>

In 1205, the Mongols under Cinggis-Qan's leadership began a series of incursions south into the state of Xia, founded almost two centuries before by the people whom some of their neighbors called (and historians usually call) Tangut.[1] The Mongols attacked Xia cities in separate campaigns in 1205, 1206, 1209, 1217, and 1224. In 1225 Cinggis planned a final conquest, and in 1226–27 a pincer attack by two large armies, from the west and from the north, attacked and captured almost every Xia city until the capital, Zhongxing Fu, fell after a six-month siege. (For these campaigns, see Wu 1982: 122–38.)

What may make this destruction of a now obscure state important for the history of plague is that the territory of Xia, lying in the corridor between highlands encompassed today by the Chinese province of Gansu, directly adjoined the Qinghai-Tibet Plateau pointed to by Cui and colleagues: Xia lay just north and northeast of the Qilian mountains that mark the Plateau's northern edge.[2] The western pincer of the 1226 assault traced a west-east line very close to the Qilian, thus to the Plateau. Today, Gansu lies within the range of the Himalayan marmot (*Marmota himalayana*) that lives on the plateau just to the south and in which plague today is more or less stably resident, and is home to many other species of rodent that might carry or serve as intermediary transmitters of the dis-

1 They called themselves "Mi" or "Mi-nia." The name for the state more commonly applied by modern historians, *Xi Xia* or its translation "Western Xia," was an informal name used by Song scholars. "Great Xia" (*Da Xia*), or simply *Xia*, was its formal Chinese name. See Dunnell 1996: xiii–xiv.

2 The more recent article of Yan et al. (2014) points much more specifically to "a small region east of Qinghai Lake" as the possible origin point of *Y. pestis*. This area of Qinghai happens to be the closest part of the province to the territory of the Xia state in the early thirteenth century.

ease as well. A two-year campaign on separate routes by two large armies surely damaged the natural as well as human economy of the region, and long encampments using carried provisions and producing heaps of refuse will attract rodent scavengers. When armies moved on, such rodents and their fleas may have hitched rides in stores and feedbags. My hypothesis requires that Gansu, in the thirteenth century, lay within the bacillus's homeland posited by geneticists, and that of the rodents that carry it today (questions for future research); and my proposal is that the Mongols unwittingly carried rodent plague hosts and their fleas eastwards into Jin and Song China as passengers in their stores.[3] The Chinese sources begin recording new deadly epidemics exactly in the years of the Mongols' spasmodic and then systematic Xia conquest.

William McNeill argued forty years ago that the Black Death that struck Central and Western Europe and the Mediterranean in the fourteenth century began in East Asia, riding with the Mongols (McNeill 1976: 132–75). Michael Dols showed that many Middle Eastern plague accounts at the time assumed an eastern origin (Dols 1977: 38–43; for another view see Norris 1977; and see Dols's reply in Dols 1978 and Norris's further rejoinder in Norris 1978; cf. also Sussmann 2011). In 1995, Cao Shuji, using Chinese primary sources directly, built a similar argument—though placing the plague's geographic origin in Mongolia itself rather than positing the Mongol passage through Yunnan in the 1250s as crucial, as McNeill does in one version of his hypothesis. (Cao 1995; McNeill 1976: 143, but see also 145).[4] I owe many primary source passages I cite here to Cao's work, which has been a crucial foundation for my own, though our arguments differ in important ways.

Despite McNeill and Cao, historians of China remain skeptical about an East Asian origin of plague or indeed about any plague in China as early as the Song, Jin, or Yuan dynasties.[5] The path-breaking volume on the Song-Yuan-Ming "transition" was noncommittal on the question (Smith and von Glahn 2003: 8–9); Timothy Brook's recent general history of Yuan and Ming China is skeptical (2010: 64–66). In a more recent and thorough examination, Paul Buell (2012) has vigorously rejected the idea. Among

3 For known long-distance travel by plague-bearing rodents and/or fleas in bags of grain etc., see Benedictow 2010: 150–93.

4 On Cao's much more comprehensive 2006 treatment in collaboration with Li Yushang, see the afternote to this essay.

5 From outside the China field, see also the skeptical account in Sussman 2011, which however takes very little account of even the genetic work already known at that time.

his arguments are: that early Ming (1393) population figures that seem to show huge losses since the end of the Song dynasty (1279) cannot be taken "at face value"—true, on simple methodological grounds; that the records McNeill used as evidence for epidemics (and those used in Twitchett 1979, an inquiry into possible plague in China in the seventh through ninth centuries) are unevenly distributed across China, often vague, and faulty in other respects—true, and I attempt to improve to some degree on McNeill's sources here; that Mongol movement (and movement of trade) from east to west in the fourteenth century was by no means as easy as some have imagined, thanks to the division of their empire into often competing domains; and that plague could not travel via the Indian ocean, as distance would burn out any shipborne outbreak. I return to each of these points (except the problem of McNeill's sources) at least briefly below, but I plan to consider all of Buell's arguments at length elsewhere, as there is not room to treat them fairly here. Taken together, they still seem to me to leave room for an argument for plague drawing on evidence that Buell did not consider or have available. In particular, he seems unaware of Cao Shuji's work on Song-Yuan epidemics, though he cites Cao's later article on plague in the Ming and Qing (Buell 2012: 139).

Buell's assertion that "there was no demonstrable mass outbreak [of] plague in China" (2012: 129) bids to close the question prematurely: Is it "demonstrable" now? No—but this is what we want to find out. And till very recently, the same assertion would have held true for Europe, as important authors found it far from demonstrable that the Black Death itself was plague. That controversy is largely resolved after the multi-threaded genetics work of this millennium, culminating (for my purposes here) in the Cui team's work.[6] Monica Green (2014b, in this issue) suggests that the polytomy Cui et al. identify may have been "caused by the organism moving into new climatic environments and new hosts." If we look for historical opportunities for such movement, the fact that these dates span the first explosive expansion of the Mongols is hard to miss.

This is the background against which to consider the materials on thirteenth-century epidemics in China that Cao Shuji compiled in 1995, along with two sources he does not cite (see points 2, 4, and 5 below). I treat these in chronological order. Note that items 1–3 emerge from exactly the period of the Mongols' long conquest of Xia.

---

6 On the arguments against plague and the swing of the pendulum the other way in the last decade or so, see Little 2011 and Bolton 2013. The major challenges were mounted in Twigg 1984; Scott and Duncan 2001; and Cohn 2002. On the genetics work, see Green 2014b, in this issue; Bolton 2013; and Little 2011.

1. In 1211, the chief minister of the Jin state that governed the northern half of what is now China, then facing a Mongol incursion of its own, advised his ruler to submit to Cinggis to avoid costly direct conflict; and added, apparently as reassurance that Mongol dominance could not last: "I have heard that the men and horses of the Tartars [i.e., Mongols], not appropriate to the water and land [in which they find themselves], are experiencing pestilence" (*Yuanchao mishi* 1228/2005: 173; see also Cleaves 1982: 184; Cao 1995: 186). Note his clear opinion that the Mongols had not always suffered "pestilence" but had acquired it while in new country.
2. The physician Li Gao, in his account of the 1232 Kaifeng epidemic that appears in item 4 below, reported major epidemics in Dongping, Taiyuan, Fengxiang, and other cities of the Jin empire in the years between 1213 and 1222. Cao (1995: 187) notes the Kaifeng epidemic, citing Tuotuo et al. (1345b/2004, 1: 309a), but not the others, and does not cite Li Gao.
3. In 1226, the Yuan-period Chinese scholar Tao Zongyi (1316–?) tells us that the Khitan advisor Yelü Chucai (1190–1244) joined in the conquest of two cities in Chinggis Qan's Xia campaign. "The commanders competed to seize boys, girls, jades, and silks; [Yelü] alone took only several volumes of documents and two camel-loads of rhubarb. Later there was epidemic in the army, and only those who received rhubarb were curable: nearly ten thousand men were saved" ([1366]/1959: chap. 2; quoted in Cao 1995: 189, with no reference). Here, both the association of epidemic in the Mongol army with the invasion of Xia and the strange mention of rhubarb as a medicine to treat it are important. On rhubarb see item 8 below.
4. The Jin dynasty doctor Li Gao, founder of the "internal damage" school of Chinese medicine, claimed to have witnessed the Mongols' 1232 siege of the Jin's southern capital Daliang (modern Kaifeng, Henan):

   At the time of the change of eras, in the *renchen* year [1232], the capital was at maximum readiness by the last ten days of the third month [April 24 to May 4].[7] In all it had been half a month since the enemy's arrival, and after the siege was lifted,[8] not one or two out of ten thousand of the

7 According to the official Jin history, the siege began on April 28 (Tuotuo et al. 1345b/2004, 1: 309a).

8 The siege was lifted on May 8 according to the official history (Tuotuo et al. 1345b/2004, 1: 310a).

> people of the capital did not become sick, and the sick who died followed another without end. At each of the capital's twelve gates, [the dead] sent out each day were two thousand at most and no less than one thousand at fewest, and this was so for almost three months. Could all these million people have contracted wind-cold external damage? Needless to say, people in the besieged city had been harmed by irregular eating and drinking and by excess toil. From two or three months of hunger in the morning and gorging at night, rising and resting irregularly, and suffering cold and heat through displacement, their stomach *qi* had long been exhausted. Suddenly to eat their fill to great excess injures people, and if furthermore their [medical] treatment is inappropriate, they are certain to die. It was not only in Daliang that things were this way. Further back, during the Zhenyou and Xingding eras [1213–22], [cities] like Dongping, like Taiyuan, or like Fengxiang were all the same in the illness and death they suffered after their sieges were lifted.[9]

"Wind-cold external damage" here refers to the "cold damage" school of Chinese medical theory and therapeutic practice, which had gained dominance in the preceding two centuries precisely for its perceived value against epidemics; its therapeutic methods had naturally been tried against this one. Li Gao recounts several treatments he saw other doctors apply in accordance with the theory, noting that they elicited changes in presentation that mimicked real cold damage, though the patients all died. He thus writes an entire book to distinguish "external" cold damage from the "internal damage" he finds in the 1232 events—damage caused, as we see in his account, by poor or erratic nutrition and by "excess toil" in the siege. What is important for my argument is that he clearly perceives the phenomena he is confronting as new to medicine, requiring new methods. Further, he sees the same process at work in a number of cities of north China—he lists three, but signals with his recurrent "like . . ." that these are three of a larger number—starting about twenty years before. The three are major cities scattered widely across the north China plain:

9 *Neiwaishang bianhuo lun, bian yinzeng, yangzheng*, in Li Gao (1247/1993: 8–9). The Jin official history's account (Tuotuo et al. 1345b/2004, 1: 309a–311a) is independent of Li's, mentioning dates he does not and setting deaths at 900,000 instead of a million. Li Gao's account has finer-grained numbers: his "million" estimates what by his own details would lie somewhere between 600,000 and 1.2 million. I thank my student Stephen Boyanton for calling my attention to this passage. My translation has started from his but diverges on some points. I thank him also for several productive conversations on the question of plague and for other source help cited below. He is exploring the larger significance of Li Gao's shift from "cold damage" to "inner damage" in work of his own. See Boyanton 2014 and forthcoming.

even taken by themselves, let alone if typical of a larger number as he suggests, they and Kaifeng would represent mass death in north China spread across two decades. In Kaifeng itself, mortality seems to have been at least 40%, as its population when it finally surrendered to the Mongols the next year was about 1.4 million[10] (Song et al. 1370/1976, 11: 3459]; Cao 1995: 187). Most important, Li Gao places the moment of outbreak in all four cities not during a process of siege but *at the lifting* of a siege (each a step in the twenty-year Mongol conquest of north China and the Jin state), thus at a point of contact by Mongol troops either with city populations or with Jin troops who then relieved the cities.[11] These two points—the perception of the epidemics as something new, and their association with contact with the Mongols—are critical, and will recur.

5. In 1235, the Mongol court debated the failure of already-conquered regions to submit fully to their rule. Some urged that Muslims from Central Asia ("the western regions") be used to subdue China, and northern Chinese to subdue Central Asia. Yelü Chucai opposed this, arguing that "the water and land are of different appropriateness (*yiyi*); epidemics will arise" (Song et al. 1370/1976, 11: 3460; not cited in Cao 1995). Again, epidemic is blamed (now from experience, perhaps) on movement of peoples into lands not "appropriate" to them.
6. In 1241, when the Mongols attacked Shouchun, in Song territory just south of the Huai River, they faced long summer rain. Li Zhen, a scion of the Western Xia royal house who had gone over to Yuan, told his commander: "If we camp the army below the walls, in the summer rain an epidemic will arise, and we will fail . . . I ask that you retreat

10 I say "at least forty per cent" because of probable increase over time in the denominator. The population of Kaifeng in 1232, at the time when the Mongols began their siege, was presumably greatly swelled by refugees from the surrounding countryside, probably to a considerable distance. A million people out of the resulting population, Li tells us, died in the epidemic. But in the year between this epidemic and the Mongols' final taking of the city, its population would presumably have been increased again by new refugees fleeing the Mongols' second arrival. Thus one cannot treat the 1.4 million remaining in the city at its final fall as the number left over after the epidemic a year before; that number may have been considerably smaller.

11 In Kaifeng, the official Jin history makes clear that the siege was lifted (temporarily) after the Jin sent a delegation out of the city to negotiate with the Mongols (Tuotuo et al. 1345b/2004, 1: 310a). For the other three cities, the siege appears to have been lifted after battle with the Mongols by Jin troops sent to relieve them, who would then have entered the cities themselves (Tuotuo et al. 1345b/2004, 1: 253, 258, 263, 265, 270, 272, 278, 284–85, 292, 306–07). Direct contact with Mongol troops outside the city was thus common to all four cases.

several *li* [a few kilometers], and I will go myself to invite them [to yield]." The plan worked, but of interest here is the connection that Li, who had served in the Kaifeng attack in 1232, saw between sieges and epidemics (Song et al. 1370/1976, 10: 3051; Cao 1995: 187, cites Li Zhen for his death in the 1259 campaign below, but does not cite Li's testimony on sieges).

7. Several potential references to plague center on the Mongol invasion of Sichuan in 1258–59. The official Yuan history records that, in 1258, the general Shi Yuanze "followed Xianzong [Möngke] to attack the Song, entering via western Shu [Sichuan]. In the summer of *jiwei* [1259] he camped at Mt. Diaoyu in Hezhou; there was a great epidemic in his army" (Song et al. 1370/1976, 12: 3660; Cao 1995: 187). The same year, Xianzong ordered another officer "to prepare medicated leaven [yeastcake] to treat the epidemic in the army" (Song et al. 1370/1976, 11: 3279; Cao 1995: 187). Elsewhere we read that, at this time, a Song general "was newly occupying [the Sichuanese city of] Chengdu, and his troops and horses could not tolerate the water and land and grew sick and died in great numbers" (Song et al. 1370/1976, 10: 3145; Cao 1995: 187).[12] Here it is Song troops who suffer from being in places unfit for them; but this makes sense in the text's terms, as Sichuan for most Song people was far from home.[13] Song accounts record the sudden death of the Song general

12 It might be asked whether this particular outbreak should be disqualified as plague because it affected horses. That would be premature, I think, though the question is worth asking. Horses do not commonly contract plague in the usual way, because fleas do not infest them. But Alexandre Yersin, after whom *Y. pestis* is named, did succeed in infecting horses (the usual host for serum manufacture at the time) in order to produce a therapeutic serum against plague. Yersin "was able to obtain a certain degree of immunity in a horse by injecting small quantities of the plague bacillus subcutaneously, and afterwards, *as this produced suppuration*, by making intravenous injections of the plague bacillus, these injections being repeated from time to time as *the temperature went down, the glandular enlargements and joint tenderness disappeared*, and the animal came to its normal condition" (emphasis mine). That is, Yersin produced *suppuration*, *fever*, and *glandular enlargements* in a horse even with carefully graduated small quantities of the bacillus: see "Plague" in *The British Medical Journal* (6 February 1897: 357). This was by direct injection, of course, and it does not necessarily follow that horses can contract plague in other ways; but the possibility that they could become sick by ingestion of the bacillus in contaminated food at least deserves further investigation.

13 The text has earlier referred to large-scale *nueli* among Niulin's own troops, a term that in modern discourse means "malaria," and in the testimony of the Persian historian Rashid-al-din the epidemics of this campaign are called variously

Wang Deng: "He had agreed [with the Mongols] on a day for battle, and the night before was arranging army affairs when he suddenly collapsed, emitting blood from all five viscera."[14] Within moments he died (Tuotuo et al. 1345a/1977, 35: 12385; Cao 1995: 188 notes that Wang Deng's troops had already been suffering epidemic disease, but offers no citation).

8. In 1273, as the Song state fell, a certain Liu Fu joined the loyalist minister Chen Yizhong for a last-ditch campaign against the Yuan, but died on reaching Luofu in Guangdong.

> Before this, Chen dreamed someone told him: 'This year a Heaven-sent disaster will spread, and nearly half the people will die; those who take rhubarb will live'. Afterward a great epidemic arose, and those who took [rhubarb] indeed did not die. When Liu was sick, [Chen] had him take it, but he could not be saved. (Tuotuo et al. 1345a/1977, 35: 12249; Cao 1995: 188)

This is the second mention of rhubarb as a treatment for these epidemics we have seen. It may be that this was simply a regional folk remedy of which Yelü Chucai gained knowledge in the conquest of Xia and which he brought with him from Gansu, and that knowledge of it had spread to the Song side by the 1270s. Rhubarb is a commonplace item in Chinese traditional pharmacology, but almost always as one element in a compound: to use rhubarb alone is quite unusual. In the great imperially sponsored Song compendium of prescriptions, the *Prescriptions by Imperial Grace of the Taiping Era* of 992, I have found just seven listings for rhubarb alone out of the many thousands of prescriptions the work collects. Only one of these appears in a section directly concerned with epidemic diseases, in this instance called literally "seasonal ethers" (*shi qi*). There rhubarb is the sole component of a prescription specifically for "pea sores in epidemics."[15]

"dysentery" and "cholera" (Boyle 1971: 228, 248). Cao Shuji quotes the latter passage in Chinese, and his term is *huolan*, the word for cholera in modern Chinese; but as he points out, none of these terms can necessarily be taken as equivalent to any modern biomedical disease entity, and the diarrhea suggested by Rashid al-din's "dysentery" and "cholera" as well as the high fever suggested by the Yuan history's *nueli* are consistent with plague (Cao 1995: 187).

14 "Blood from the five viscera" in this context probably means that Wang Deng bled from all bodily orifices.

15 Wang 992/1958: 428; the description of "pea sores" appears on p. 427; another description in connection with "cold damage" disorders (also epidemics) appears on p. 285. Interestingly, three other prescriptions in the compendium that specify rhubarb

"Pea sores" (*wandou chuang*) are described as raised sores, white or red, that are shaped like a pea (or "emerge like a pea") and that are probably meant to be understood as pea-sized. Given their size, I think there is virtually no chance that the "pea sores" described here are buboes, and I would certainly not argue for plague as something widely enough known in China in 992 to make its way into an imperial compendium. If, however, one imagines that an official faced with an epidemic in 1226 or 1273 might consult this rather old but still quite authoritative volume, then the only entry for epidemic he would have found that specified rhubarb alone as a treatment was *one intended specifically for an epidemic involving raised sores*. To put it differently, if an official consulted this compendium about an epidemic and came away with rhubarb as a sole treatment, he must have been looking for help with a disease that involved raised sores. He would have been generalizing somewhat from a prescription originally meant for an epidemic involving a different *kind* of raised sores; but surely this would be a rational procedure in the face of a new disease. Again, we cannot know that the rhubarb treatment came from consulting this work, as opposed to from local knowledge in 1226 Gansu and/or 1273 south China, or from sheer improvisation; but it is possible that the mentions of rhubarb in items 3 and 8 may carry, for us, a tantalizing though indirect hint that the epidemics of this period involved raised sores.

Cao Shuji judges the episodes he cites to be plague based on several factors: their mortality levels, clearest for 1232 Kaifeng (and the others that Li Gao likens to it, which Cao does not cite); their timing, as he goes on to trace epidemic records in the Yuan official history through the fourteenth century, a series that he appears to see as leading up to the spread of plague to Europe; and their association, in two sources, with rhubarb—to which I return below. My own reason for urging that we take these scattered records as possible evidence of plague is also timing, but from a different angle: that the encounters with epidemic by Yuan armies, and then by those they invade, begin just when Mongol troops pass in force, and with great destruction, through a region that abuts the Qinghai-Tibet Plateau and where plague is now endemic in marmots and other mamma-

---

as the sole treatment also involve raised sores: these are a prescription against "fluid-filled vesicles" on the face (p. 1213); one against "vermilion toxin sores," i.e., large raised swellings on the skin (p. 2990); and one against "pox-like rash" in children: the section that includes this one mentions "cold damage" in its introductory matter, so we must take it as intended for a context of epidemic as well, though specific to children. The remaining three rhubarb-only prescriptions, none for epidemic contexts, are for two kinds of jaundice and for delirious speech in fever (pp. 480, 1685, and 1686).

lian hosts. But one must also note (with Cao) the extraordinary mortality reported by the Jin history for Kaifeng, and by Li Gao for Kaifeng and three other cities: 40% or more is a level attested in Eurasia, to my knowledge, for no pre-nineteenth-century infectious disease but plague.

The history of medicine, some time ago, moved away from "retrospective diagnosis" toward attending to the constructions that historical actors themselves placed on the phenomena of illness or health they experienced and recognized. This approach has illuminated much, though as a sole lens it may also obscure. The present volume, of course, is precisely focused on redefining "retrospective diagnosis" by incorporating the diagnostic capabilities of a new type of microbiological analysis. Yet one would still hope to know just what construction(s) contemporary actors placed on the thirteenth-century epidemics in China. Since all our sources (except perhaps Li Gao's eyewitness account) lie at a considerable temporal distance from events,[16] and (as works of official history) are the products of the state and of literati elites, it is very unlikely that they even come close to exhausting the constructions that contemporaries placed on these illnesses; we can only ask what *our sources* "construct." But that is still worth asking. First, they see simply *epidemic*: *yi* or *wen*. For Chinese medicine at the time it was arguably "epidemicity" itself, and not specific symptoms, that most dictated classification: "cold damage" theory had arisen to treat epidemics as a single category. More importantly, our sources—brief mentions in chronicle-style accounts or in the biographies of officials or military officers taking part in campaigns or in debates over policy *versus* the enemy—are the kinds least likely to be specific about symptoms. Second, very importantly, they see something *new*: for Li Gao this required a remaking of the medicine of his time because it was an epidemic that *resisted usual epidemic treatment*; for others, it needed explanation, significantly, in the movement of people into spaces not customary for them. Third, they see something connected to *the lifting of siege*, thus to contact with the besieging Mongols. And fourth, in two cases (nos. 3 and 8), they see something treatable with rhubarb, which as I have suggested above may convey indirectly our only hint about symptoms.

---

16 One diary of the Kaifeng siege has survived, as far as I know, written by Liu Qi (1203–50) and included in his miscellany *Guiqian zhi*. Surprisingly, his more or less month-by-month and sometimes day-by-day record jumps from the fourth month of 1232 straight to the seventh month, simply skipping the entire period that our other sources tell us encompassed the epidemic. It seems to me very likely that he had left the city during that period. I am grateful to Stephen West for letting me know of Liu Qi's diary.

I would argue that, rhubarb aside, these are just the terms in which a Chinese-literate audience might well construct bubonic plague that they recognized as coincident with Mongol armies moving through their states and sacking their cities. They had no exact terms for it because, as they saw, it was new, and older exact terms were (according to Li Gao) failing. Most striking were its mortality (which should strike us too) and its speed, but perhaps these simply made it a particularly dangerous *yi*. Finally, as Cao suggests, the epidemics presented themselves to all involved as concomitants of war and dynastic change, thus as just one of the forms of death and destruction prominent across China (Cao 1995: 190). If Chinese records do not proclaim a "Black Death" as European records do, this does not tell us that demographically damaging plague was absent: the Chinese could construct such damage in other terms.

But is there, in any case, evidence of the demographic damage one would expect from plague? Were there large population losses in the Song-Yuan or Yuan-Ming transitions? Buell says no, but other serious scholars have thought so. In their book on Chinese population history, not (in Buell's words) "taking at face value" official Ming totals but critically mining local sources as well, Zhao Wenlin and Xie Shujun place the combined population of Song and Jin (ruling south and north respectively) in 1210 at just over 108 million; the total population under Yuan (ruling both north and south) at a bit more than 75 million in 1292 and about 87 million in 1351; and the total under Ming (also ruling both north and south) in 1381 at about 67 million (Zhao and Xie 1984: 310, 333, and 364). Significantly, the population losses have different distributions: massive loss in the north from Song to Yuan, large loss in the south from Yuan to Ming. It is interesting to compare this distribution to Cao Shuji's material. After his discursive treatment of thirteenth-century outbreaks, Cao simply lists epidemics from the Yuan official history for 1297 through 1362 (Cao 1995: 190–01). These impressively number thirty-one for the sixty-five years and cover many prefectures and all regions, but offer little detail,[17] most simply noting "great epidemic" for each place, with few numbers or percentages of dead. If we add Cao's earlier cases to his post-1297 list, six cases of recorded epidemic emerge between 1211 and 1292 in the north, only two in the south (the 1259 Sichuan campaign and the 1273 Guangdong case), matching the higher northern population loss that Chao and Hsieh find across just those decades. At the other end the match is less

17 Cao does not provide citations for this list, but the relevant passages I have been able to trace are in Song (1370/1976, 2: 413, 416, and 559; 3: 603, 620, 625, 740, 764, 784, 800, 820, 912, 914, 918, 944; and 4: 1080 and 1111).

clear: between 1351 and 1381 (without Ming data for 1369 on), we find eight epidemics recorded in the north to five in the south. The difficulty here is that by the 1350s China was in chaos, with civil war in the south, so that the Yuan court in the far north was in a poor position to record southern epidemics. Nor should we expect plague, if it was there, to do all the demographic work in a region constantly at war. We may never sort out the relative weight of war and disease here; yet no evidence we have excludes a role for plague in southern population loss.

Gaps in this picture cry out for research. As epidemic records after the Yuan conquest are (even) less circumstantial than those of the Sung-Yuan transition, Cao Shuji (1995) simply assumes that many of the epidemics in his post-1297 list are plague because he believes he has shown that earlier ones are. This is hardly sufficient and badly needs to be reinforced by further evidence. Some obstacles that seemed serious to earlier plague researchers, however, no longer seem so. No particular speed of local spread is too fast, any longer, to represent plague, as the potentially quite slow "blocked flea" mechanism of older theories is, we now know, not the only one available mode: newer research on early-phase transmission by "unblocked" ground-squirrel fleas, prairie-dog fleas, and even rat fleas has settled that problem and made rapid person-to-person spread via fleas plausible.[18] Thus, for plague to ravage a city the size of Kaifeng (swollen, as we have seen, to something perhaps near 2.4 million by refugees from the countryside) and to kill nearly a million within fifty days presents no serious epidemiological problem as far as speed is concerned. All this also means that we do not need to find reports of mass rat death in our sources to find plague plausible: even if the sources were likely to attend to such things, neither rat epizootics nor rats themselves are necessary to spread plague.[19] The apparent patchy character of plague in China (if many of these epidemics are plague)—now here, then silent for a while, then over there—need not be a problem either, as we now know that plague can be carried great distances even without rodents sick enough to die quickly: in food or feed contaminated by rodent or flea feces, or by fleas themselves

18 Eisen et al. 2006; Eisen et al. 2007; Wilder et al. 2008; for a general review of this point, see Gage 2012: 86–91. Note that the ground-squirrel and prairie-dog fleas investigated are of the same genus, *Oropsylla*, as the marmot flea.

19 Katherine Royer shows brilliantly the process by which an awareness of a variety of mechanisms for plague transmission among early twentieth-century scientific plague researchers was transmuted into a collective and very long-lasting conviction that rats, the rat flea, and mass rat death were essential features of plague (Royer 2014).

(cf. especially Benedictow 2010: 150–93). I argue that it may also travel in (transported) rodents from populations with a history of coping with the disease: Gansu rodents—like those that I am suggesting hitched rides with the Mongols—having lived for a very long time in a region where the plague bacillus had long been present too, may offer this possibility.[20] Finally, where other populations of potential host rodents are available, the bacillus may settle down in a new (or old) reservoir for a considerable time without new epizootic or epidemic activity. Many such reservoirs, or more accurately regional assemblages of reservoirs, are known in the world today.

This is a central point. We know that the reservoirs of plague-bearing rodents in contemporary North America, for instance, are the result of movements of people, rodents, and fleas from Asia in the late nineteenth and early twentieth centuries during the Indian and Chinese plague outbreaks that stimulated the first scientific work on plague and *Y. pestis*. It is reasonable to assume (in fact it is the direct implication of Cui and colleagues' work), and we should investigate the likelihood, that some of the other reservoirs known to exist in China and Eurasia were created by similar processes of movement in much earlier periods.[21] Ann Carmichael (2014, in this issue) proposes that the formation of such reservoirs in the Alpine marmot population can account for the periodic recurrence of plague in Europe after 1348 without necessarily new imports of rats,

---

20 Wang et al. (2009) have shown the reservoir status of Himalayan marmots in Sichuan. Zhang et al. (2012) demonstrate actual plague tolerance and thus reservoir capacity in Central Asian great gerbils. Eisen and Gage (2009: 2) are skeptical of the idea of "truly independent epizootic and enzootic cycles" that they note "has dominated the literature." Yet there seems no doubt that plague is resident long-term in certain rodent reservoirs, Himalayan marmots (as in the Wang et al. 2009 above) and California ground squirrels among them, and Eisen and colleagues' explanation by difference of "rates of transmission and numbers of hosts infected," though replacing a dichotomy with a possible continuum, may offer an explanation for the phenomenon more than deny it. The question would then be what factors can affect these transmission rates and numbers of infected.

21 Cao Shuji (1995: 186) appears to assume that the Mongolian reservoir predates the Mongol conquests, and McNeill (1976: 145) appears to make the same assumption for both Mongolia and Yunnan. Yet Julia Riehm and her team (2012) argue from genetic data that the Second Pandemic strain did not come to Mongolia before about six hundred years ago, and my hypothesis here implies that the Mongols brought plague from Gansu both to Yunnan in their incursion in the 1250s and back to Mongolia at some later date. Cf. also Varlık (2014, in this issue), dealing with a late Ottoman context: "It may be erroneous to assume that the active foci of the eighteenth and nineteenth centuries also existed before that time."

fleas, or bacilli from port cities or by major trade routes. Part of the burden of my hypothesis is that at least some of the existing rodent reservoirs in China and the rest of Eurasia were established by the movements of Mongol armies and are thus historical, human (not merely biological or zoological) artifacts with specific moments of origin that new research, both genetic and historical, may establish. Significantly, the work of Julia Riehm and colleagues shows that Mongolia itself seems to have become a reservoir for post-polytomy strains only after the Mongol conquests in the south.[22] Are local rodent populations too, or their attendant flea populations, historical human imports in some cases? On the human side we need archeological work combined with genetic ancient-DNA analysis to determine whether *Y. pestis* can be found in thirteenth- and fourteenth-century Chinese and Central Asian bones or teeth as it has been found in Black Death victims in Europe. The hypothesis I offer here may not be finally confirmable except by such evidence.

I offer no specific solution for how the plague gets from East (or Inner or Central) Asia to the specific Mongols at Caffa in 1346 (if that story stands), but if the Mongol expansions of the previous century or more did indeed establish new rodent reservoirs for plague in other parts of Eurasia, there may be no reason to assume an immediate Chinese origin for the events of 1347 and after in the Mediterranean basin and Western Europe; and in this respect Buell could be right. Alternatively, and I think more probably, his point about the Mongol empire's division could explain plague's presence in China and Central Asia for more than a century (1211–1340s?) before it goes west to the Golden Horde, to produce the Caffa incident. But we should also consider the possibilities of a second route. In the south there are major epidemics in 1331, 1333, 1344, and 1345, suggesting continuous presence by that time; and merchant ships sailing to the Indian Ocean, which since mid-Song had carried an extensive Chinese trade with both south Asia and the Middle East, departed from the south (Sen 2006; Chaffee 2006; Clark 1991; So 2000). Especially interesting in this connection are the epidemics recorded for 1333 and 1344. In 1333, the prefectures affected included Songjiang, Jiaxing, and Hangzhou. The three lie in a northeast-to-southwest arc along the southeast China coast in what is now Zhejiang; more importantly, the major Shanghai and Ganpu ports where the emperor Khubilai had established official Offices of Maritime Affairs to tax but also encourage trade with the south seas lay within Songjiang and Hangzhou respectively: here, then, were major epidemics in 1333

22 Riehm et al. 2012; see n. 21 above.

at or near two of the four officially sponsored ports through which most Yuan trade with the Indian Ocean passed. The most important of those four ports, however, was Quanzhou in Fujian.[23] The epidemics in 1344 were concentrated in Fujian and affected Fuzhou, Yanping, Shaowu, and Tingzhou prefectures. Quanzhou is not specifically listed, but both Fuzhou and Yanping bordered it directly, while Shaowu and Tingzhou were mountain prefectures joined by overland trade and downriver traffic to the prefecture in which Quanzhou port lay. Goods infested with rodents, fleas, or their feces could have found their way from any of these epidemic prefectures to the Quanzhou port and onto South Sea trading ships. The considerations on distant transmission that I have already touched on seem to me to leave it possible that plague moved from China to, for example, the Persian Gulf by sea and thus contributed, if not to the European Black Death (it may be difficult to posit plague's passage north from the Gulf to the Golden Horde's territories), perhaps to its Middle Eastern equivalent.[24] There is also the problem of siege conditions, and why plague would seem so strongly associated with them in China. This may go back to the identity of the rodent: if (for instance) marmots, or other rodents from the plague foci in Gansu and the Qinghai-Tibet Plateau, are unlike rats in being able to live for extended times as stable carrier-populations for the bacillus, then perhaps it is siege that turns stable carriers into unstable ones. If so—and this is speculation apart from my main hypothesis—perhaps nutrition is key. Perhaps in sieges the rodents brought from far away, like humans, begin to starve, or switch to new foods, and this changes their relation to the bacilli that some of them carry. We still know too little about how enzootic turns to epidemic; and a key element that my hypothesis glosses over for now is the identity of the plague-carrying rodents I am proposing came with the Mongols from the territory of Xia. Marmots seem to be the main, though not necessarily the only, carriers of plague in that region today; but does *Marmota himalayana* descend low enough from the

23 For Khubilai's decree establishing Quanzhou, Shanghai, Ganpu, and Qingjiang as sites of Offices of Maritime Affairs, see Song et al. 1370/1976, 94: 2401.

24 On the practicality of sea-borne transmission, cf. Benedictow (2010: 185–87); on the possibility of Indian Ocean transport of plague, though not necessarily from China, see Green (2014b, in this issue). See also her introduction, in which she suggests that the genetic evidence may support the notion of two sources for plague in Anatolia and North Africa (Green 2014a, in this issue). This possibility is strengthened and extended to Europe by the work of Stephanie Haensch's team (Haensch et al. 2010), showing that distinct strains seeming to belong to separate points on the polytomy later identified by Cui's team are both present in European Black Death victims. This may support the possibility of separate transmissions both overland and by sea.

mountain slopes of the region to have had significant enough encounters with the Mongols and their encampments? Are marmots capable of entering something like a commensal relation with human beings, at least for long enough to be transported into other regions of China in their store-wagons and feedbags?[25] If not, could other rodents in the Gansu corridor have played this role? Studies of the distribution of plague among rodents in the larger region have concentrated more on Qinghai than on Gansu,[26] so new work may be needed there. And ultimately we need to know about Gansu rodents in the thirteenth century more than now, which argues a need for bio-archeological work in the old territory of Xia.

As a final point for further research there is the question of rhubarb. We have seen it used twice against the epidemics I have traced here, and I have traced how those mentions might constitute a hint as to symptoms. But the story of rhubarb and plague in China may not end there. Cao Shuji cites the traditional Chinese physician Li Jianshi who, in 1935, claimed success in treating bubonic plague with very high rhubarb doses (Cao 1995: 189; I have not so far been able to obtain Li's book). Biomedically trained physicians in China are currently undertaking research on *why* rhubarb is effective against *Y. pestis*, apparently having already concluded that it is (Bai et al. 2008). We need not take our Song-Yuan sources' word when they tell us that everybody who took rhubarb survived in order to believe that some ameliorative effect may have been at work. Where did Li Jianshi and current researches get the idea of trying rhubarb against plague in

25 Voluntary stowing-away need not be the only plausible means for marmots to move with the Mongol armies into China. The *Secret History of the Mongols*, Marco Polo, and contemporary Chinese observers all report that the Mongols, in their native territory, hunted marmots for food (Cleaves 1982: 29; Smith 1984: 223; Buell and Anderson 2000: 45). It is likely that they made use of the pelts as well. John Masson Smith (1984: 227) has considered the possibility that marmots were an important food for Mongol armies on the move, and concluded that they "must have been a supplementary rather than a basic component of Mongol rations." But a supplementary role would suffice for the purpose of my hypothesis if it should motivate Mongol troops in Xia territory to capture local marmots and transport them for future use, either as food or as furs. If Mongols were already eating or clothing themselves in marmot in Xia territory, a plague epidemic in their army might have begun there; but as this epidemic was likely also either to burn itself out or destroy the army outright on the spot, it is probably easier to account for the pattern of siege-related epidemics in China if we suppose that marmots carrying the plague bacillus, but not yet sick and transmissive, were transported alive to China and transmitted the disease to humans later under siege conditions.

26 See for instance Yang et al. 2014. I am grateful to Monica Green for making me aware of this article.

the first place? Did a belief in its effectiveness descend historically from Yelü Chucai and others in the thirteenth century? from the *Prescriptions by Imperial Grace* of 992? from local knowledge in Gansu? Does rhubarb actually inhibit *Y. pestis*, and if so, how?[27] There is historical, medical-historical, and perhaps even medical investigation to be undertaken here.

I am proposing, in sum, that we may need to place the "beginnings of the Black Death" more than a century earlier than we have been accustomed to place them. My suggestion that the expanding Mongols were the

27 Here I might risk an even more speculative expansion on my speculative suggestion above, about nutrition in rodents. Oddly enough, the Qinghai-Tibet-Gansu region that is the original home of plague is a natural botanical home of undomesticated rhubarb as well (Wang et al. 2010; Foust 1992). Marmots—again, the most frequent rodent carrier of plague in that region—are reported by contemporary travelers to eat large quantities of rhubarb leaves (Anon. 2013: 2). Awareness of a connection between marmots and rhubarb in this region is much older, however: the first European hunters of rhubarb for medical purposes noted how commonly marmot burrows were to be found surrounded and shaded by rhubarb plants, and argued that marmots were enabling the growth of rhubarb by aerating the soil with their burrowing activities: see Burke (1767: 84–85, quoting John Bell's memoirs of his travels, in this instance with regard to Mongolian marmots and rhubarb). Rhubarb leaves are toxic to humans because of their high oxalic acid content; the content of the stems and roots, though lower, is significant as well. (Traditional Chinese medicine always used the root, dried; it should be noted however that drying vegetables typically doubles the proportion of oxalic acid; cf. Paul et al. 2012: 313, especially table I.) Oxalic acid compounds (oxalates) have been used by *Y. pestis* researchers to breed non-virulent strains *in vitro* (Higuchi and Smith 1961) or to detect virulent strains by their inhibited reproduction on oxalate-rich agar (Bhaduri, Chaney-Pope, and Smith 2011). This works, it seems, because oxalic acid binds calcium, which the bacillus needs for its virulence plasmid: batches raised in calcium-poor conditions develop either without the plasmid or with drastically reduced reproductive rates. Rhubarb is not the only plant food high in oxalic acid: two more are oats and buckwheat, which a horse-borne army might carry with it in grain bags, just the way rats and fleas hitched train rides during the Indian and Chinese plagues of the last century (Benedictow 2010: 160–61). Alongside rhubarb we have seen "medicinal leaven" or yeastcake as a treatment for the disease in our sources (no. 7, above); and after the 1232 siege and epidemic the Jin government, needing money to repair the city wall, put a special tax on tea-leaf sellers—along with coffin-makers, clergy, and physicians—because all these had "arrogated great profit to themselves since the epidemic began" (Tuotuo et al. 1345b/2004, 1: 311a). Coffin-makers for the dead, doctors for the sick, clergy for prayers and funerals, of course; but tea-leaf sellers? Tea-leaves, it turns out, are extremely high in oxalic acid, and so are many yeasts. Does *in vitro* modulation of *Yersinia pestis* virulence or reproduction via oxalates work to some extent *in vivo* too? Had Central Asian marmots benefited from this for millennia, and did some Mongols, Jurchen, and Chinese benefit from it, though of course theorizing its benefit in quite other ways, in a thirteenth century crisis?

agents of plague's spread is hardly new, but my hypothesis places the critical moment neither in the Mongols' emergence from their native steppe, in itself, nor in their passage through Yunnan into Sichuan fifty years later, but in their repeated assaults on and eventual highly destructive conquest of a state that sat cheek-by-jowl with what the new genetic evidence is telling us was probably the first home of plague. It has been crucial for the framing of the hypothesis that the genetic evidence points not only to a region but to a well-defined period. Most people in the world today have never heard of the state of Xia, or of the Mi (Tangut) people who founded it and successfully defied or coexisted with powerful neighboring Chinese and then Jurchen states for almost two hundred years. But if the hypothesis I articulate here is correct, the Mongols' choice to make Xia their first conquest outside of Mongolia has had enormous consequences for the history of the medieval and modern worlds.

Afternote

When Monica Green kindly invited me to contribute to the present issue, I had been away from the direct study of plague in Song-Yuan China for many years and had not followed all new developments. Thus, it was only when this article had reached its final stages that I was able to acquire Cao Shuji's more recent book on the history of plague in China and its association with war, coauthored with Li Yushang (Cao and Li 2006). I have been able to undertake only a quick review of the historical sections so far, and have not yet tracked down all the source passages that Cao and Li cite. On the Mongol-associated epidemics I discuss here, their evidence is essentially the same as in Cao's 1995 article (Cao and Li 2006: 79–99). More potentially problematic is their position, new for Cao, on certain epidemics of the early Jin (1139–48), which they also believe to be plague (Cao and Li 2006: 60–65).

Space does not allow a thorough examination of their evidence, but on my examination so far I find it very hard to agree that the *datou wen*, literally the "big-head epidemic" that their sources describe for the early Jin epidemics, is plague. Among the sources they cite, only retrospective accounts of Yuan or even Ming date mention sores of any kind (by which time, on my hypothesis, plague was known from recent experience in north China and later in south China, and retrospection could conceivably have conflated two different epidemic-associated diseases); and all their sources seem to describe a condition of general swelling of the throat-and-neck and often of the face, which they further describe as regularly involving "the throat closing" and an inability to open the eyes, a "filling" of the eyes and ears obstructing sight and hearing, and a "head like an ox." I have not encountered any accounts elsewhere of blindness, deafness, inability to open the eyes, throat-closing, or generalized swelling of the neck-and-face area as standard symptoms of plague. A Ming source (cited by Cao and Li 2006: 57–67 but especially 60–65) that associates "big-head epidemic" with the popular disease names "frog epidemic" and "cormorant epidemic" similarly seems to point to a generalized swelling of the throat-and-neck, since a frog puffs out its whole throat and a cormorant famously expands its throat when it swallows a large food item. Neither seems a likely simile for a discrete bubo on the neck.

I am currently undertaking deeper research into the medical sources Cao and Li cite on these issues, as well as other medical sources of the same period, and will publish my findings on them separately elsewhere. The scholarly discourse on plague among non-Chinese scholars has yet to take any notice, as far as I know, of this book. Nor has work in that discourse (that I am aware of, other than my own) paid proper attention to Cao's 1995 article and his first heroic assembly of sources there. Such notice is well overdue.

Bibliography

Achtman, Mark, Giovanna Morelli, Peixuan Zhu, Thierry Wirth, et al. 2004. "Microevolution and History of the Plague Bacillus, *Yersinia pestis*," *Proceedings of the National Academy of Sciences* 101, no. 51: 17837–42

Anonymous. 2013. "How to Party in Mongolia, Bhutan, and Burma," *Panoramic Journeys* (blog) <www.panoramicjourneys.com/wp/index.php/how-to-party-in-mongolia-bhutan-and-burma> (dated April 11, 2013) [accessed October 4, 2014]

Bai, Q., Y. Jia, X. Da, H. Xiao, et al. 2008. "[Study of Rhubarb Anti-*Yersinia pestis* Based on DNA Microarray]," *Zhonghua liuxing bingxue zazhi* [*Chinese Journal of Epidemiology*] 27, no. 6: 602–05

Benedictow, Ole. 2010. *What Disease was Plague? On the Controversy over the Microbiological Identity of Plague Epidemics of the Past* (Leiden: Brill)

Bhaduri, S., K. Chaney-Pope, and J. L. Smith. 2011. "A Procedure for Monitoring the Presence of the Virulence Plasmid (pYV) in *Yersinia pestis* under Culture Conditions," *Foodborne Pathogens and Disease* 8, no. 3: 459–63

Bolton, Paul. 2013. "Looking for *Yersinia pestis*: Scientists, Historians, and the Black Death," in *Society in an Age of Plague*, ed. Linda Clark and Carole Rawcliffe, 15–37 (Woodbridge: Boydell)

Boyanton, Stephen. 2014. "The Ambiguity of Epidemics: Epidemic Febrile Illness and the Creation of Internal Damage as a Medical Specialty" (paper presented at the annual meeting of the Association for Asian Studies in Philadelphia, 29 March 2014)

Boyanton, Stephen. Forthcoming. "The *Treatise on Cold Damage* and the Formation of Literati Medicine: Social, Epidemiological, and Medical Change in China, 1000-1400" (doctoral dissertation, Columbia University)

Boyle, J. A. 1971. *The Successors of Genghis Khan: Translated from the Persian of Rashīd al-Dīn* (New York: Columbia University Press)

Brook, Timothy. 2010. *The Troubled Empire: China in the Yuan and Ming Dynasties* (Cambridge, MA: Belknap at Harvard)

Buell, Paul D. 2012. "Qubilai and the Rats," *Sudhoffs Archiv* 96, no. 2: 127–44

Buell, Paul D., and Eugene Anderson, 2000. *A Soup for the Qan: Introduction, Translation, Commentary, and Chinese Text* (London: Kegan Paul)

Burke, Edmund. 1767. "Some Curious Particulars relative to the Growth of Rhubarb; How an Animal Called the Marmot Contributes to its Propagation, and How the Natives Dry the Root," *Annual Register of World Events* 10: 84–85

Cao Shuji曹树基. 1995. "Dili huanjing yu Song-Yuan shidai de chuanranbing 地理环境与宋元时代的传染病," *Lishi yu dili* 历史与地理 12: 183–92

Cao Shuji 曹树基 and Li Yushang 李玉尚. 2006. *Shuyi: Zhanzheng yu heping — Zhongguo de huanjing yu shehui bianqian, 1230–1960 nian* 鼠疫:战争与和平:中国的环境与社会变迁 (1230–1960 年) (Ji'nan: Zhongguo huabao chubanshe)

Carmichael, Ann G. 2014. "Plague Persistence in Western Europe: A Hypothesis," *The Medieval Globe* 1: 157–191

Chaffee, John. 2006. "Diasporic Identities in the Historical Development of the Maritime Muslim Communities of Song-Yuan China," *Journal of the Economic and Social History of the Orient* 49, no. 4: 395–420

Chen Boyi 陳博翼. 2008. "Review of Cao Shuji and Li Yushang, *Shuyi: Zhanzheng yu heping — Zhonnguo de huanjing yu shehui bianqian, 1230–1960 nian* 鼠疫：戰爭與和平—中國的環境與社會變遷 (1230–1960年)," in *Lishi renleixue xuekan* 歷史人類學刊 6, no. 2: 286–89

Clark, Hugh. 1991. *Community, Trade, and Networks: Southern Fujian Province from the Third to the Thirteenth Century* (Cambridge: Cambridge University Press)

Cleaves, Francis Woodman (ed. and trans.) 1982. *The Secret History of the Mongols: For the First time Done into English out of the Original Tongue and Provided with an Exegetical Commentary, vol. 1* (Cambridge, MA: Harvard University Press)

Cohn, Samuel K. Jr. 2002. *The Black Death Transformed: Disease and Culture in Early Renaissance Europe* (London: Arnold)

Cui, Y., C. Yu, Y. Yan, D. Li, et al. 2013. "Historical Variations in Mutation Rate in an Epidemic Pathogen, *Yersinia pestis*," *Proceedings of the National Academy of Science* 110, no. 2: 577–82

Dols, Michael. 1977. *The Black Death in the Middle East* (Princeton: Princeton University Press)

Dols, Michael. 1978. "Geographical Origin of the Black Death: Comment," *Bulletin of the History of Medicine* 52, no. 1: 112–13

Dunnell, Ruth. 1996. *The Great State of White and High* (Honolulu: University of Hawaii Press)

Eisen, R., S. W. Bearden, A. P.Wilder, J. A. Montenieri, et al. 2006. "Early-Phase Transmission of *Yersinia pestis* by Unblocked Fleas as a Mechanism Explaining

Rapidly Spreading Plague Epizootics," *Proceedings of the National Academy of Sciences* 103: 15380–85

Eisen, R., and K. L. Gage, 2009. "Adaptive Strategies of *Yersinia pestis* to Persist during Inter-Epizootic and Epizootic Periods," *Veterinary Research* 40, no. 2: 1

Eisen, R., A. P. Wilder, S. W. Bearden, J. A. Montenieri, et al. 2007. "Early-Phase Transmission of *Yersinia pestis* by Unblocked *Xenopsylla cheopis* (Siphonoptera Pulicidae) is as Efficient as Transmission by Blocked Fleas," *Journal of Medical Entomology* 44, no. 4: 678–82

Foust, Clifford M. 1992. *Rhubarb: The Wondrous Drug* (Princeton: Princeton University Press)

Green, Monica H. 2014a. "Editor's Introduction to *Pandemic Disease in the Medieval World*," *The Medieval Globe* 1: 9–26

Green, Monica H. 2014b. "Taking 'Pandemic' Seriously: Making the Black Death Global," *The Medieval Globe* 1: 27–61

Haensch, S., R. Bianucci, M. Signoli, M. Rajerison, et al. 2010. "Distinct Clones of *Yersinia pestis* Caused the Black Death," *PLoS Pathogens* 6, no. 10: e1001134

Higuchi, K., and J. Smith. 1961. "Studies on the Nutrition and Physiology of *Pasteurella Pestis* VI.A: Differential Planting Medium for the Estimation of the Mutation Rate to Avirulence," *Journal of Bacteriology* 81, no. 4: 605–08

Li Gao 李杲. 1247/1992. *Nei wai shang bian huo lun*, in *Dongyuan yiji* 东垣医集, ed. Ding Guangdi 丁光迪 and Wang Kui 王魁 (Beijing: Renmin Weisheng Chubanshe)

Little, Lester K. 2011. "Plague Historians in Lab Coats," *Past and Present* 213: 267–90

McNeill, William H. 1976. *Plagues and Peoples* (New York: Anchor)

Morelli, G., Y. Song, C. J. Mazzoni, M. Eppinger, et al. 2010. "*Yersinia pestis* Genome Sequencing Identifies Patterns of Global Phylogenetic Diversity," *Nature Genetics* 42, no. 12: 1140–45

Norris, John. 1977. "East or West? The Geographic Origin of the Black Death," *Bulletin of the History of Medicine* 51: 1–24

Norris, John. 1978. "Response" [to Dols 1978], *Bulletin of the History of Medicine* 52: 114–20

Paul, V., S. Verma, S. Paul, and A. Paul. 2012. "Effect of Cooking and Processing Methods on Oxalate Content of Green Leafy Vegetables and Pulses," *Asian Journal of Food and Agro-Industry* 5, no. 4: 311–14

Riehm, J. M., G. Vergnaud, D. Kiefer, T. Damdindorj, et al. 2012. "*Yersinia pestis* Lineages in Mongolia," *PLoS ONE* 7, no. 2: e30624

Royer, Katherine. 2014. "The Blind Men and the Elephant: Imperial Medicine, Medieval Historians, and the Role of Rats in the Historiography of Plague," in *Medicine and Colonialism: Historical Perspectives in India and South Africa*, ed. Poonam Bala, 99–110 (London: Pickering & Chatto)

Scott, Susan, and C. J. Duncan. 2001. *Biology of Plagues: Evidence from Historical Populations* (Cambridge: Cambridge University Press)

Sen, Tansen. 2006. "The Formation of Chinese Maritime Networks to Southern Asia, 1200–1450," *Journal of the Economic and Social History of the Orient* 49, no. 4: 421–53

Smith, John Masson, 1984. "Mongol Campaign Rations: Milk, Marmots, and Blood?," *Journal of Turkish Studies* 8: 223–28

Smith, Paul Jakov, and Richard von Glahn. 2003. *The Song-Yuan-Ming Transition in Chinese History* (Cambridge, MA: Harvard University Asia Center)

So, Billy K. L. 2000. *Prosperity, Region, and Institutions in Maritime China: The South Fukien Pattern, 946–1368* (Cambridge, MA: Harvard University Asia Center)

Song Lian 宋濂 et al. 1370/1976. *Yuan shi* 元史, 15 vols. (Beijing: Zhonghua shuju)

Sussman, George. 2011. "Was the Black Death in India and China?," *Bulletin of the History of Medicine* 85: 319–55

Tao Zongyi 陶宗儀. [1366]/1959. *Chuogeng lu* 輟耕錄 (Beijing: Zhonghua shuju)

Tuotuo 脫脫 et al. 1345a/1977. 1977. *Song shi* 宋史, 40 vols. (Beijing: Zhonghua shuju)

Tuotuo 脫脫 et al. 1345b/2004. *Jin shi* 金史, ed. Ershisi shi quan yi 二十四史全譯, 3 vols. (Shanghai: Shiji chubanjituan – Hanyu da cidian chubanshe)

Twigg, Graham. 1984. *The Black Death: A Biological Reappraisal* (London: Schocken)

Twitchett, Denis. 1979. "Population and Pestilence in T'ang China," in *Studia Sino-Mongolica: Festschrift für Herbert Franke*, ed. Wolfgang Bauer, 35–68 (Wiesbaden: Steiner)

Varlık, Nükhet. 2014. "New Science and Old Sources: Why the Ottoman Experience of Plague Matters," *The Medieval Globe* 1: 193–227

Wang Huaiyin 王懷隱 et al. 992/1958. *Taiping shenghui fang* 太平聖惠方 (Beijing: Renmin weisheng chubanshe)

Wang, L. M., Z. D. Luo, Q. Yue, Y. J. Duan, et al., 2009. "[Study on the Natural Foci of *Marmota himalayana* Plague in Sichuan Province]," *Zhonghua liuxing bingxue zazhi* [*Chinese Journal of Epidemiology*] 30, no. 6: 601–05

Wilder, A. P., R. J. Eisen, S. W. Bearden, J. A. Montenieri, et al. 2008. "Transmission Efficiency of Two Flea Species (*Oropsylla tuberculata cynomuris* and *Oropsylla hirsuta*) Involved in Plague Transmission Epizootics among Prairie Dogs," *EcoHealth* 5: 205–12

Wu Tianchi 吴天墀. 1983. *Xi Xia shi gao* 西夏史稿 (Chengdu: Sichuan renmin chubanshe)

Wang, X., X. Hou, Y. Zhang, and Y. Li. 2010. "Distribution Pattern of Genuine Species of Rhubarb as Traditional Chinese Medicine," *Journal of Medical Plant Research* 4: 1865–76

Yan, Y., H. Wang, D. Li, X. Yang, et al. 2014. "Two-Step Source Tracing Strategy of *Yersinia pestis* and its Historical Epidemiology in a Specific Region," *PLoS ONE* 9, no. 1: e85374

Yang, Y., M. Wang, X. Zhao, Z. Zhao, et al.. 2014. "[Analysis on the Results of Etiology and Serology of Plague in Qinghai Province from 2001 to 2010]," *Zhonghua yufang yixue zazhi* [*Chinese Journal of Preventative Medicine*] 48, no. 2: 124–27

Yuanchao mishi 元朝秘史. [1240?]/2005. Ed. Bao Sitao 鲍思陶 (Ji'nan: Qilu shushe)

Zhang, Y., X. Dai, X.Wang, A. Maituohuti, et al. 2012. "Dynamics of *Yersinia pestis* and its Antibody Response in Great Gerbils (*Rhombomys opimus*) by Subcutaneous Infection," *PLoS One* 7, no. 10: e46820

Zhao Wenlin 赵文林 and Xie Shujun 谢淑君. 1988. *Zhongguo renkou shi* 中国人口史 (Beijing: Renmin chubanshe)

Robert Hymes (hymes@columbia.edu) is H. W. Carpentier Professor of Chinese History at Columbia University. He received his BA from Columbia College (1972), and his MA (1976) and PhD (1979) from the University of Pennsylvania. Much of his work so far has focused on the social and cultural history of middle period and early modern China, drawing questions and sometimes data from cultural anthropology as well as history, and using the methods of the local historian to study elite culture, family and kinship, medicine, religion, and gender. His publications include *Statesmen and Gentlemen: The Elite of Fu-chou, Chiang-hsi, in Northern and Southern Sung* (Cambridge, 1987); *Ordering the World: Approaches to State and Society in Sung Dynasty China* (Berkeley, 1993, co-edited with Conrad Schirokauer); and *Way and Byway: Taoism, Local Religion, and Models of Divinity in Sung and Modern China* (Berkeley, 2002). Both *Statesmen and Gentlemen* and *Way and Byway* won the Joseph Levenson Prize of the Association for Asian Studies for the best book on pre-1900 China in their years of publication. He is now working on two (he hopes) book-sized projects simultaneously: one on the notion of "belief" (*xin*) in the mentalités of middle-period China, and one on the origins of the Black Death in Central and East Asia, of which the present article is a preliminary product.

Abstract The work of Cui et al. (2013)—in both dating the polytomy that produced most existing strains of *Yersinia pestis* and locating its original home to the Qinghai-Tibet Plateau—offers a genetically derived specific historical proposition for historians of East and Central Asia to investigate from their own sources. The present article offers the hypothesis that the polytomy manifests itself in the Mongol invasion of the Xia state in the Gansu corridor in the early thirteenth century and continues in the Mongols' expansion into China and other parts of Eurasia. The hypothesis relies to a considerable extent on work of Cao Shuji (1995), but argues for a different means and direction for the spread of plague than either Cao or William McNeill have previously posited.

Keywords Plague, Mongols, China, Black Death, Song Dynasty, Yuan Dynasty, Jin Dynasty, Xia, Gansu, rhubarb, oxalic acid.

FEATURED SOURCE

DIAGNOSIS OF A "PLAGUE" IMAGE: A DIGITAL CAUTIONARY TALE

MONICA H. GREEN, KATHLEEN WALKER-MEIKLE, and WOLFGANG P. MÜLLER

A PARTICULAR OBJECTIVE of this special issue of *The Medieval Globe*, "Pandemic Disease in the Medieval World: Rethinking the Black Death," is to interrogate how scientific and humanistic approaches to plague's histories can enrich and expand one another. Science, we have argued, has developed methods to reconstruct the deep histories of pathogenic organisms in addition to studying them as they exist in the present-day world. At the same time, the humanistic disciplines retain their power to reconstruct human activities that may have contributed to *Yersinia pestis*'s amplification throughout the world and to describe and explain how humans responded to that threat. All disciplines involved in the analysis of the past have rigorous standards of what constitutes evidence and what kinds of interpretations are valid. Multidisciplinary work demands due respect for those traditions.

This short essay offers a lesson in caution. It is a story of error, but also an opportunity to be reminded of the care needed to properly contextualize all our evidence—to be reminded, as L. P. Hartley famously said, that "the past is a foreign country: they do things differently there." To negotiate this country successfully, we need to learn its language.

The image on the following page (**Plate 3**) has been reproduced in the past decade in a variety of popular media: *Wikipedia*, pamphlets for sale at tourist sites, the cover of an encyclopedia devoted to the Black Death, an exhibit on the Black Death at the Museum of London in 2012, a *NOVA* documentary, and an essay in one of the world's leading science journals. It even appeared in one of our own publications, inserted by an editor without con-

Our thanks to Lucy Freeman Sandler for her wise counsel on the correct "reading" of the *Omne bonum* images; to Peter Murray Jones, for help transcribing the manuscript; and to the members of the 2012 National Endowment for the Humanities Summer Seminar, "Health and Disease in the Middle Ages," for help spotting popular uses of the "plague" image. Monica H. Green's contribution to this study was written, in part, during a leave supported by the Institute for Advanced Study, Princeton, and funded by the National Endowment for the Humanities and the Willis F. Doney Membership Endowment. Any views, findings, conclusions or recommendations expressed in this essay do not necessarily represent those of the National Endowment for the Humanities.

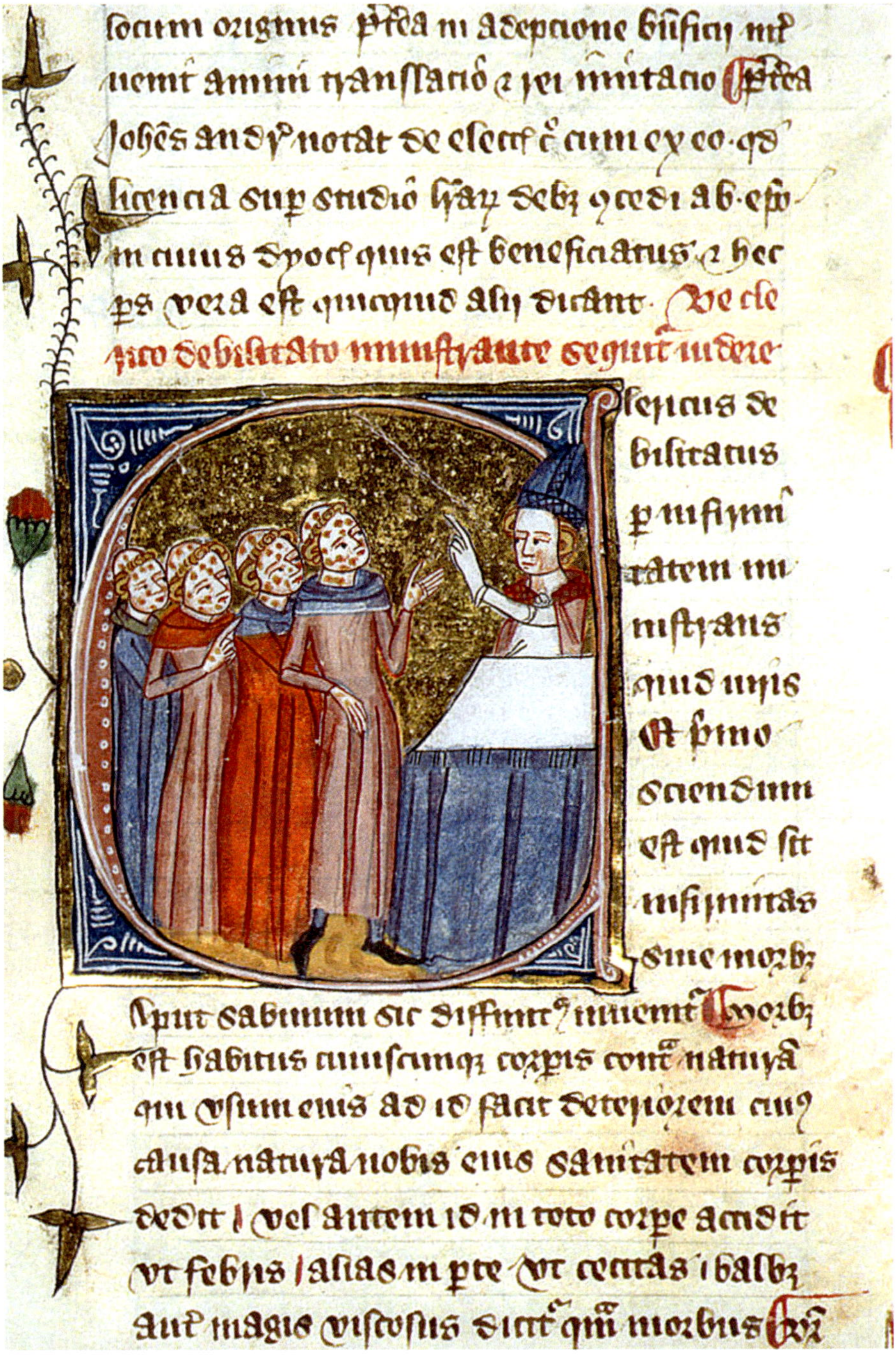

Plate 3. James le Palmer, *Omne bonum*. London, British Library, MS Royal 6 E VI, vol. 2, fol. 301rb (detail). *Reproduced in accordance with the British Library's guidelines for the reproduction of images in the public domain.*

sultation (Green 2011). It is accompanied by captions such as "monks, disfigured by the plague, being blessed by a priest" or "Plague victims blessed by priest."[1] Perhaps its most significant use was in Callaway 2011, which was an interpretive essay in *Nature* accompanying the announcement of the complete sequencing of the *Yersinia pestis* genome retrieved from the mid-fourteenth-century London Black Death Cemetery, the first pathogen fully sequenced from historic remains (Bos et al. 2011). There, it bore the caption "Historical descriptions of the Black Death have helped link *Yersinia pestis* with the disease." One could say it has become the iconic representation of the Black Death. Available for download on the British Library's website since at least 2007, it is ubiquitous, and people have accepted it as a representation of "plague" because they have been told that it is.

There is certainly reason to connect the image to the Black Death, at least on chronological grounds. The medieval manuscript from which it comes has been securely dated to a couple of decades after the arrival of plague in England late in 1348. Moreover, the fact that all the "victims" are represented with similar lesions would suggest, from our biomedical perspective, that this is indeed an infectious disease.

But connecting it specifically with plague is wrong. The modern captions attached to the image offer several misreadings. First, medieval iconographic conventions indicate that the "priest" is not a priest but a bishop, shown with the distinctive bishop's mitre. Second, his hand gesture tells us that he is not "blessing" the individuals in front of him but giving them instruction on the performance of their duties. The "plague victims" are all tonsured, indicating their clerical status, a fact one caption reflected by identifying them as "monks." But clerics of various statuses were tonsured, so "monks" is too precise.

So how should the image be "read?" It is an illuminated initial in a manuscript (specifically, the letter "C"), meaning that we know precisely the context for which it was made. The image (which measures 7.2 cm × 7.6 cm in the original manuscript) illustrates a passage in a two-volume encyclopedia of knowledge called *Omne bonum*, "All That Is Good," an unfinished opus by a London clerk, James le Palmer (b. before 1327, d. 1375), who was employed in the royal Court of the Exchequer (Sandler 1996).[2]

1 The quotations come, respectively, from the British Library's *Images Online* page (first accessed May 3, 2011) and the *Wikipedia* entry for "The Black Death" (first accessed February 12, 2007; most recently accessed April 24, 2014, where the reference to the "priest" is now gone). On the British Library site, see below.

2 London, British Library, MSS Royal 6 E VI (letters A–D) and 6 E VII (E–Z), together comprising almost 1100 folios, more than 1350 entries, with more than 750 historiated initials. All the images in the two manuscripts can be consulted free of charge at the

The topic of the chapter which it illustrates (transcribed and translated below) asks whether clerics should lose their benefices on account of (chronic) infirmity or sickness. The general answer (which varies depending on the cleric's rank) is that if the debility is *leprosy* clerics below the rank of bishop should be removed from office, but a bishop should be given an assistant who receives part of the prelate's income.

If we look back at the image now—with a full understanding of its accompanying text—we see it anew. We notice, first, that the "victims" are standing, not lying prostrate as we would expect were they afflicted with a quickly lethal disease like plague. We see no buboes so characteristic of the bubonic form of that disease. While that is not a decisive indicator (after all, neither the quickly lethal pneumonic nor the septicemic plague would necessarily have produced visible buboes), the prominent, widely dispersed spots on these "victims" are a telling trait. Petechiae and ecchymoses (skin hemorrhages of varying sizes) are known to be an occasional complication in severe cases of plague (Carniel 2008, 118–19). However, that is not what spotted skin meant in medieval iconographic traditions. Depicting skin as spotted was the traditional way of representing leprosy in medieval European painted art (Boeckl 2011). Indeed, this conventional iconography is found elsewhere in this same manuscript, used to depict the Emperor Constantine (d. 330 CE), who is alleged to have been cured of his leprosy when he converted to Christianity (MS Royal 6 E VI, vol. 1, fol. 394r). In other words, a correct "diagnosis" of the depicted condition—"correct" in terms of medieval Europe's own categories of analysis (an *emic* approach; see Green 2014, in this issue)—is that this image shows victims of leprosy, not plague.

At what point, then, did this image become a depiction of "plague"? Medical historians have long referenced the *Omne bonum*'s useful images of anatomy, bathing, circumcision, dentistry, and surgery (MacKinney 1965; Jones 1984 and 1998); but none associated its illustrations with either leprosy or plague. In 1996, art historian Lucy Freeman Sandler's masterful two-volume study of Le Palmer's work correctly identified this image as a reference to leprosy (Sandler 1996, 2: 110).[3]

That correct association with leprosy seems to have broken down, however, in two stages. In 2007, the British Library's online *Catalogue of Illuminated Manuscripts*, though drawing broadly on Sandler's work, described the image on fol. 301rb of the *Omne bonum* without any diag-

British Library's *Catalogue of Illuminated Manuscripts* site: <http://www.bl.uk/catalogues/illuminatedmanuscripts/welcome.htm> [accessed April 24, 2014].

3 On le Palmer's medical interests, which "fall into the category of the endemic rather than the epidemic," see Sandler 1996, 1:120-21.

nostic specificity: "Detail of a historiated initial "C"(lericus) of a bishop blessing four clerics with faces covered with spots."[4] That diagnostic void in interpreting the "spots" was then filled in the British Library's *Images Online* webpage (where high quality images are sold for a fee), when a photo of the historiated initial, posted around the same time, was newly interpreted with the caption "Plague victims blessed by priest."[5] The caption is still there, at the time of this writing.

Thus, the widespread error in "reading" the *Omne bonum* image as if it depicted plague is not an example of the dangers of retrospective diagnosis: the taking of modern diagnostic categories and projecting them into the past (an *etic* approach; see Green 2014, in this issue). Sandler had in fact "diagnosed" it correctly as "leprosy," a "reading" of the image supported by both the surrounding text and medieval iconographic traditions. The confusion surrounding the *Omne bonum* image had its genesis rather in mundane, very modern phenomena: the mislabeling of the image in the act of separating it from its textual home in the British Library's *Images Online* database, and then the willingness of users of that database to accept the label rather than attempt to recontextualize the image in its original manuscript or historical context. Moved to an online venue, stripped of its textual surroundings, the image acquired a free-association connection to plague. And from there it went (if you'll pardon the phrase) viral. Had proper rules of analysis been applied when labeling the image, no error would have been generated. But given the nature of the Internet, it will now have an extended life under that mistaken rubric.

This error is instructive in reminding us how important context is to the evaluation of the often meager evidence that survives from the medieval past, whether that be fragments of microbial DNA or chance references to illness in chronicles. In the case of the *Omne bonum*, which gathered together all sorts of information that contemporary clerics might need, leprosy—a disease prevalent throughout Europe since the early Middle Ages and a topic of concern in canon law since the twelfth century—was the more pressing concern, as its slowly debilitating effects impinged on clergy members' ability to perform their tasks. The issue took on new urgency in fourteenth-century England, since a few decades before the *Omne bonum* was assembled the abbot of St. Albans and noted astronomer Richard Wallingford (d. 1336) had had a contentious period of rule,

4 British Library, *Illuminated Manuscripts Online*, <http://www.bl.uk/catalogues/illuminatedmanuscripts/ILLUMIN.ASP?Size=mid&IllID=40313> [accessed April 24, 2014].

5 British Library, *Images Online*, <imagesonline.bl.uk/> [accessed April 24, 2014], image #062047.

marked in part by claims that his leprosy disqualified him from office. Both the pope and the king became involved in the controversy. Notably, Richard Wallingford is depicted with spots on his face in the two known likenesses of him.[6]

The error in "diagnosis" that prompted this investigation is also instructive in raising the question: "Should we expect visual depiction of a catastrophe of such scope as the Black Death?" James le Palmer, who died in 1375, must certainly have witnessed plague strike England in 1348–50, when he was a young adult, and again in 1361–63, when he had already started work on the *Omne bonum*. But *what images* did he *himself* have of that experience? We cannot know. The crowded cemetery he depicts in the *Omne bonum* (fol. 267v) may have had no more personal resonance for him than the images of (to take other examples from the letter "C") *coruscacio* (lightning), *corvus* (raven), or *crocus* (the flower crocus). In contrast, the Belgian chronicler and abbot Gilles le Muisit (d. 1353), who was himself nearly blind at the time of the Black Death (Chareyron 1996), paid an artist handsomely to include illustrations in his *Chronicle* (d'Haenens 1969). These included three images that rightly remain emblematic of the social disruptions of the Black Death: a depiction of the burning of a community of Jews, a procession of flagellants, and a mass burial.[7] Gilles's project was, to be sure, unusual as an illustrated monastic chronicle (Vanderputten 2005), and it would not be until the fifteenth century that most of the images we associate with the experience of plague and a macabre outlook on life take hold in Western European culture (Boeckl 2000 and Gertsman 2010).

No images that seem to depict plague are known from the late medieval Islamic world, and none have yet been noted in Chinese sources.[8] In neither case does that absence of visual evidence constitute evidence of absence of the disease. But it may reflect differing understandings of art or death or the functions of symbolism (Jones 2007). And that is the "foreign country" whose languages we must continually attempt to learn.

---

6 North 2004; cf. Rawcliffe 2006: 253–54 and 266–67. The likenesses are London, British Library, MS Cotton Nero D.vii, fol. 20r; and MS Cotton Claudius E.iv, pt 1, fol. 201r. On medieval leprosy generally, see Rawcliffe 2006 and Demaitre 2007. On the rich canon law tradition of discourse about leprosy among the clergy, see Fowler 1972. On bioarcheological and genetics work on the form of leprosy caused by *Mycobacterium leprae*, see Mendum et al. 2014.

7 Brussels, Bibliothèque royale de Belgique, MS 13076–77 (1349–52), fol. 12v, Jews being burned alive on a bonfire; fol. 16v, procession of Flagellants; and fol. 24v, plague (mass burial) in Tournai in 1349.

8 We thank Stuart Borsch, Justin Stearns, and Emilie Savage-Smith for their counsel on this matter.

APPENDIX 1

TEXT OF *OMNE BONUM*, "DE CLERICO DEBILITATO MINISTRANTE SEQUITUR VIDERE"

THE FOLLOWING PORTION of *Omne bonum* was transcribed from the manuscript London, British Library, Royal 6 E. VI, vol. 2, fols. 301rb–302ra. Its author, James le Palmer, originally pieced this passage together from two sets of sources.

Lines 2–63 (lines 2–64 of the English translation in Appendix 2, below) constitute an extensive excerpt from Hostiensis (d. 1271), *Summa aurea* X 3.6, a text which survives in numerous late medieval manuscripts, incunabula, and early modern printed editions (including Basle: apud Thomam Guarinum, 1573, cols. 702–03, digitally available through the website of the Bayerische Staatsbibliothek in Munich, Germany). Lines 64–109 (in the English translation: lines 65–112) are a miscellany of notes derived from the *Glossae ordinariae* on the *Liber extra* (lines 64–82; English: 65–83) and the *Decretum Gratiani* (lines 105–109; English: 107–112), plus an extensive quotation (lines 83–96; English: 84–98) from a statute of Pope Boniface VIII, inserted under the same title (*De clerico debilitato*) in his *Liber sextus* VI 3.5.1 (compiled 1298), along with portions of its *Glossa ordinaria* by Johannes Monachus (lines 97–104; English: 99–106). The Ordinary Glosses can be consulted in any edition of the *Corpus iuris canonici* published before the 1620s.

The spelling of the text follows the Latin original, except for consonantal 'u' and 'i', which have been regularized to 'v' and 'j'; both the capitalization of words and the punctuation have been modernized. Textual emendations are shown in pointed brackets (<...>). The shortened legal references (in round brackets) are given in full in Appendix 2.

[fol. 301rb] *Clericus debilitatus ministrans.*

Clericus debilitatus per infirmitatem ministrans, quid juris? Et primo sciendum est quid sit infirmitas sive morbus. Aput Sabinum sic diffinitus invenitur: Morbus est habitus cuiuscunque corporis contra naturam qui usum eius ad id facit deteriorem cuius causa natura nobis eius sanitatem corporis dedit. Vel autem id in toto corpore accidit ut febris, alias in parte ut cecitas. Balbus autem magis viscosus dicitur quam morbus.[1] Videtur autem morbus sonticus id est dampnosus scilicet recidivus qui incidit in hominem postquam sanatus est. Sontes enim nocentes dicuntur.

An propter infirmitatem sive morbum amittat clericus beneficium suum distingue utrum sit prelatus. Et is etiam propter lepram non **[fol. 301va]** removetur, sed datur ei coadjutor cui porcio competens reddituum episcopatus assignatur. Sic intelligas e<odem> titulo, De rectoribus (X 3.6.3). An sit sacerdos parochialis vel minister inferior et talis propter lepram removetur, e<odem> titulo, Tua nos (X 3.6.4). Alia distinctio loquitur utrum morbus provenerit[2] a natura: et sic loquitur capitulum, De rectoribus (X 3.6.3); aut divino judicio, et sic loquitur capitulum, Tua nos (X 3.6.4). Cuius cognicionem, determinationem et discrescionem physicis[3] relinquo. Et potest esse divino judicio quia cognovit mulierem inmediate post leprosum[4], vii q. ii c. Nuper (C.7 q.2 c.2). Hec tamen solutio reprobatur vii q. i <Cum> percussio (C.7 q.1 c.2). Vincentius dixit quod quamdiu potest quis in collegio remanere non removetur. Sed ex quo non potest removetur, sicut judex mutatur si non posset judicio operam dare.

Et si queras quid fiet si servire non potest, respondeo: si est prelatus dabitur ei coadjutor ut in dicto capitulo, De rectoribus (X 3.6.3). Si vero fuerit inferior sive simplex dabitur ei vicarius secundum Goffredum qui exponit illam decretalem, Tua (X 3.6.4) sicut Laurentius scilicet quod ibi removetur scilicet non a titulo, sed ab executione officii sue administracionis. Thomas[5] notavit idem excepto morbo lepre, propter quem removetur indistincte quicunque ipsum incurrerit sive sit prelatus sive alius. Et hoc conprobatur in antiqua compilacione, De concessione prebende et ecclesie non vacantis, capitulo Ex transmissa (2 Comp. 3.7.1); que hodie tamquam iniquitatem continens remota est secundum Goffredum. Bazianus distinctit utrum morbus esset curabilis et sic loquitur capitulum, De rectoribus (X 3.6.3), vel incurabilis et sic loquitur Tua (X 3.6.4). Prior intellectus magis placet et ipsum magis approbo, eodem titulo, Ex parte (X 3.6.5).

---

1 A marginal entry to the right of this line reads: *Nota hic plene et ex alia parte folii quando clericus amittit beneficium suum propter morbum et quando non videas* (Note here in detail and also check on the next page of the folium when a cleric loses his benefice because of disease and when he does not).

2 MS: *prevenerit*. The likely formal source of *Omne bonum*, the *Summa aurea* of Hostiensis, has *provenerit*.

3 MS: *prohibitis*; Hostiensis: *physicis*.

4 Cf. the commentary in Appendix 2 below, note 2.

5 MS: *Thomas*; Hostiensis correctly has: *T<ancredus>*.

Sed que est ratio quod speciale sit in episcopis quod propter lepram non removeantur, inferiores vero removentur? Hoc est quod difficulter removetur episcopus, ut extra, De translatione, capitulo Quanto (X 1.7.3). Quamvis enim metropolitanus et episcopi possint cognoscere de crimine super quo accusatur episcopus non tamen possunt episcopum deponere sine legitima proprietate, iii q. vi Quamvis (C.3 q.6 c.7) et capitulo Dudum (ibid., c.9). Timendum enim est, ne concussis columpnis corruat edificium. Sed minores ex levioribus causis removentur. Sed propter alias infirmitates quam propter lepram non sunt clerici privandi beneficiis suis, sed pocius dandus est coadjutor etiam si paraliticus sit is de quo agitur, ne terreantur volentes Deo militare, ut e<odem> titulo, Percuscio (X 3.6.1), quia non est addenda afflicto afflictio ut ibidem. Idem est si factus sit impotens non ex culpa sua, e<odem> titulo, capitulo ii (X 3.6.2). Secus si culpa sua, ut notatur infra ubi agitur de corpore viciato. Alii distingunt inter morbum perpetuum et temporalem, sed reprobatur e<odem> titulo, capitulo penultimo et ultimo (X 3.6.5-6).[6]

Unum tamen non omitto quod si clericus leviter pateretur vel haberet veterem **[fol. 301vb]** quartanam que merito sperni posset et esset intentus circa negocia propria, nichil percipiet nisi serviret. Supradicta vero non de ficta infirmitate sed vera et gravi intelliguntur, <ff.>, De re judicata, <l.> Quesitum[7], et si clericus infirmus potest officium suum exercere, nisi vexetur a demonio vel epilentico morbo et caderet assidue vel emissione vocis confuse et jactacione spume, vii q. ultima (C.7 q.2) per totum. Si vero raro caderet cum annua expectacione posset celebrare, xxxiii di. Communiter (D.33 c.3), ita tamen quod habeat vicini solaminis adjutorem, vii q. i Illud (C.7 q.1 c.15).

Item abbates facti inutiles penitus removentur, e<odem> titulo, Tua nos (X 3.6.4), secundum glossam et secundum Innocentium.

Quid si ecclesia non potest sufficere utrique, scilicet leproso et substituto? Dic quod ille qui servit habebit redditus et leproso providebit episcopus, ut in dicto capitulo, De rectoribus (X 3.6.3), secundum glossam.

Et coadjutor datus egrotanti habet generalem et liberalem administrationem et invito dandus est coadjutor, vii q. i Scripsit (C.7 q.1 c.1), secundum glossam.

An presbiter qui amisit digitos cum medietate palme poterit missam celebrare? Dic quod non quia nec secure propter debilitatem, nec sine

6 A finger pointer appears here in the left margin of the ms.

7 MS: *extra, de re iudicata, c. Omnium*, is a garbled, non-existent allegation, probably reflecting a lack of familiarity with Roman legal references. The text here properly cites the passage from Justinian's *Digesta* as given by Hostiensis.

scandalo propter[8] deformitatem, sed ceteris officiis sacerdotalibus fungi potest, e<odem> titulo, Presbiterum (X 3.6.2).

Item nec potest infirmus ex certa sciencia vel ex affectata ignorantia sumere cibum sive potum ad debilitandum corpus suum quia faceret contra caritatem quia debet corpus suum diligere ut in eo deserviat Deo, extra, De homicidio, capitulo Tua nos (X 5.12.19).

An archidiacono percusso morbo paralitico sit dandus coadjutor? Dic quod sic. Et idem est dicendum si amiserit officium oculorum, extra, e<odem> titulo, capitulo ultimo (X 3.6.6), secundum glossam.

Item episcopus senio aut infirmitate gravatus ut suum officium nequeat exercere potest auctoritate apostolica duos coadjutores secum assumere ad dictum officium exeguendum et si episcopus factus fuerit demens et coadjutorem habere noluerit, tunc eius capitulum vel due partes auctoritate apostolica debent assumere unum vel duos curatores sive coadjutores ad dictum officium exeguendum. Sed si episcopus senio vel incurabili morbo gravatus noluerit habere coadjutorem tunc nichil innovabit capitulum, sed capitulum intimabit pape statum et conditionem episcopi et ecclesie et facti circumstancias et tunc fiet quod per papam fuerit ordinatum et coadjutores isti habebunt sumptus moderatos de proventibus episcoporum in quorum auxilium assumuntur. Sed bona prelatorum non alienabunt et reddituri sunt rationem episcopo si postea fuerit sane mentis eidem seu successori episcopi, extra, e<odem> titulo, capitulo Pastoralis, libro sexto (VI 3.5.1).

Nec isti coadjutores possunt conferre beneficia vacancia quia in generali commissione non continetur beneficiorum collacio, e<odem> capitulo (VI 3.5.1), secundum Johannem **[fol. 302ra]** Monachum et Guidonem.

Item nec per metropolitanum est dandus coadjutor, sed per sedem apostolicam vel auctoritate eiusdem, ut in dicto capitulo, Pastoralis (VI 3.5.1), nec mirum quia solum potest metropolitanus in sua provincia sibi decreta quod a jure reperitur concessum vel ex prisca consuetudine introductum, ut in dicto capitulo (X 3.5.1) secundum Johannem Monachum.

An sacerdos leprosus posset licite missam celebrare? Dic quod populo non debet celebrare propter scandalum. Si autem velit celebrare privatim non est prohibendus dum tamen non sit nimis debilis vel deformis. Et dicit Hugo quod cessabit a ministerio suo quoad sanos, sed leprosis poterit cantare et ministrare divina, xlix di. Hinc etenim[9] (D.49 c.1).

---

8 At this point, the word *debilitatem* is first added and then deleted by the scribe.

9 MS: *Sed hec entenim*; corrected after Hostiensis.

APPENDIX 2

OMNE BONUM, "ON MINISTRATION BY A DISABLED CLERIC"

THE ENGLISH TRANSLATION of this passage contains numerous references to the textbooks of late medieval jurisprudence which, in accordance with current scholarly convention, have been abbreviated as follows:

2 Comp. 0.00.00	*Compilatio secunda*, book 0, title 00, chapter 00, ed. Emil Friedberg, *Quinque compilationes antiquae necnon Collectio canonum Lipsiensis* (Leipzig: Tauchnitz, 1882).
C.00 q.00 c.00	*Decretum Gratiani*, part II: Causa 00, quaestio 00, capitulum 00, ed. Emil Friedberg, *Corpus iuris canonici* 1 (Leipzig: Tauchnitz, 1879).
D.00 c.00	*Decretum Gratiani*, part I: Distinctio 00, chapter 00, ed. Friedberg, *Corpus iuris canonici* 1 (Leipzig: Tauchnitz, 1879).
Dig. 00.00.00	*Digesta Iustiniani*, book 00, title, 00, lex 00, ed. Paul Krüger and Theodor Mommsen, in: *Corpus iuris civilis*, 1: *Institutiones, Digesta* (Berlin: Weidmann, 1895).
VI 0.00.00	*Liber sextus decretalium*, book 0, title 00, chapter 00, ed. Friedberg, *Corpus iuris canonici* 2 (Leipzig: Tauchnitz, 1881).
X 0.00.00	*Decretales Gregorii IX* (*Liber extra*), book 0, title 00, chapter 00, ed. Friedberg, *Corpus iuris canonici* 2 (Leipzig: Tauchnitz, 1881).

For further information on the legal references and most of the juristic authors quoted (indirectly) in the subsequent section of *Omne bonum*, see Brundage 1995: 190–232.

On Ministration by a Disabled Cleric

What is the law regarding ministration by a cleric who is disabled by illness? First, it has to be known what an illness or disease is. This definition is found in Sabinus[1]: A disease is an unnatural condition of a body which weakens its use for the purpose that Nature assigned when it gave health to our bodies. This happens either to the whole body, as with a fever; or to one part as with blindness. Stuttering, however, is more of an impairment than a disease. A disease appears to be *sonticus*, that is harmful and causing a relapse, when it inflicts a person after she or he has recovered. For *sontes* means "harmful ones."

[The next question is] whether on account of infirmity or disease a clerk should lose his benefice. It depends on whether he is a prelate. Then he is not removed even because of leprosy, but he is given a coadjutor to whom a suitable portion of the bishopric's revenue is assigned. This is how you should understand X 3.6.3. Or he is a parish priest or lesser minister and someone like that is removed because of leprosy, as in X 3.6.4. Another distinction asks whether the disease happens naturally, and this is discussed in X 3.6.3, or [whether it happens] by divine judgment, as is said in X 3.6.3. The recognition, assessment, and differential diagnosis of this I leave to the physicians; and it may be by divine judgment, because he had sex with a woman immediately after (she has had sex with) a leper[2], C.7 q.2 c.2. This solution, however, is rejected in C.7 q.1 c.2. Vincentius[3] said that as long as someone is able to stay in his clerical community, he is not removed. But if he is unable to remain, he is removed, just as a judge is changed if he is not able to render judgment.

And if you ask what will be done if he is not able to serve, the answer is that if he is a prelate, a coadjutor will be given to him as explained in X 3.6.3. But if he is of a lower order or a simple priest, a vicar will be

1 The ensuing definition of illness (lines 4–8) is attributed to Sabinus, an ancient Roman lawyer, in Dig. 21.1.1.7.

2 This passage is problematic in its extreme brevity. Nevertheless, our rendering accords with certain medical understandings about the transmission of leprosy. For example, a *quaestio* from the "Prose Salernitan Questions" ([*c.* 1200]/1979: 9) reads: "Queritur si leprosus accedit ad mulierem mulier non leditur, qui vero post illum prius ad eam accedit quare leprosus efficitur?" (It is asked: Why if a leper has relations with a woman, the woman is not harmed, but if another man comes to her later, the latter man is affected?) The answer explains that the "corruption" of the leper remains in the woman's womb, which is then sucked out by the penis of the next man with whom she has sex.

3 Vincentius Hispanus (d. 1248); cf. Brundage, *Medieval Canon Law* 228.

given to him according to Goffredus[4] who explains this decretal, X 3.6.4, just as Laurentius[5] does, that is to say, that he is removed there not from the entitlement to his office but from the execution of the office under his administration. Thomas[6] has noted the same except for the disease of leprosy, because of which everyone who incurs it is removed without distinction, be he a prelate or another, and this is proved in the ancient compilation, 2 Comp. 3.7.1, according to Goffredus.

Bazianus[7] distinguished whether the disease was curable, as in X 3.6.3, or incurable, as in X 3.6.4. The prior interpretation is more convincing and I rather approve of it, X 3.6.5. But what is the reason for the special treatment of bishops in that they are not removed from office on account of leprosy, whereas those in lower orders are removed? This is because it is difficult to remove a bishop as in X 1.7.3. For although a metropolitan and [his] bishops are able to investigate a crime of which a bishop is accused, they cannot depose a bishop without legitimate due process, C.3 q.6 c.7 and c.9. Because it is to be feared that by smashing the columns the whole edifice [of the Church] will collapse. But those in minor orders are removed for lighter reasons. But clerics must not be removed from their benefices for other diseases than leprosy. Rather, a coadjutor must be given even if he who is concerned is paralyzed lest those wishing to be God's soldiers be scared away, as in X 3.6.1, because an affliction must not be added to those afflicted, as is explained there.

Likewise, if he happens to become debilitated through no fault of his own, as in X 3.6.2. It is different if the fault is his, as is noted below[8] where the defective body is considered. Others distinguish between a chronic disease and one that comes and goes, but this is rejected in X 3.6.5-6.

One topic I do not omit is what to do if a cleric suffers lightly or has an inveterate fever that recurs every fourth day and can simply be ignored, and who is willing to do his work? He will receive nothing unless he

---

4 Goffredus de Trano (d. 1245); cf. Brundage, *Medieval Canon Law* 211–12.

5 Laurentius Hispanus (fl. 1215); Brundage, *Medieval Canon Law* 216.

6 "Thomas [Aquinas]" is a misreading in *Omne bonum* for "T(ancredus)" in the *Summa aurea* (ed. Basle, 1573), col. 702. It was uncommon for canonistic commentators like Hostiensis to cite theologians. On Tancred (fl. 1220), see Brundage, *Medieval Canon Law* 227-228.

7 Bazianus (fl. 1180–90) was a canonist not to be confused with the contemporary Roman lawyer, Johannes Bassianus; cf. Donahue 2003.

8 MS: *infra, ubi agitur de corpora viciato*; Hostiensis, *Summa aurea* (ed. Basle, 1573), col. 703, reads: *supra, de corpore viciato* (above, on the defective body), a legal reference to X 2.20.

serves. What is said above, though, needs to be understood in the case not of an imagined illness, but a real and serious one, as in Dig. 42.1.60. And if the sick cleric is able to perform his duties, unless he is vexed by a demon or the falling sickness and falls frequently or with confused speech and foaming at the mouth, as in C.7 q.2 throughout. But if he rarely falls, he can celebrate Mass if he has no incident for a year[9], D.33 c.3, but in such a way that he has a coadjutor ready to help out, C.7 q.1 c.15.

Likewise abbots who have become useless are removed entirely, as in X 3.6.4, according to the Ordinary Gloss and Innocent[10].

What if a church is not able to support both a leprous cleric and his substitute? Say that he who serves will keep the revenue and the bishop will provide for the leper as in X 3.6.3, according to the Ordinary Gloss. And the coadjutor given to the sick man has general and free administration, and the coadjutor is given even against the sick man's will, C.7 q.1, according to the Ordinary Gloss.

[If asked] whether a priest who is missing his fingers with half of his palm is able to celebrate Mass, say that he cannot because he cannot do it safely due to the debility nor without scandal due to the deformity, but he can serve in the other priestly functions, as in X 3.6.2.

Similarly, a sick person cannot take food or drink to weaken his body either out of certain knowledge or feigned ignorance, for he would do so against charity because he ought to take good care of his body so he may serve God in it, X 5.12.19.

[It is asked] whether an archdeacon struck by a paralytic disease must be given a coadjutor? Say that he must be, and the same must be said if he loses the use of his eyes, X 3.6.6, according to the Ordinary Gloss.

Likewise an aging bishop, or one aggrieved by illness so that he cannot perform his duties, can by apostolic authority assume two coadjutors to help him perform his office, and if the bishop has become demented and does not wish to have a coadjutor, then his chapter or two thirds of it must assume by apostolic authority one or two curators or coadjutors in order to perform the said office.

But what if a bishop who is senile or burdened with an incurable disease does not want to have a coadjutor? Then the chapter will not undertake anything, but the chapter will inform the pope about the state

9 MS: *cum annua expectatione*; cf. the alleged D. 33 c.3: *quousque unius anni spatio* [...] *inveniantur ab incursu demonum liberati* (provided they are found to be free of demonic possession for a year).

10 Pope Innocent IV (Sinibaldo dei Fieschi, d. 1254), a famous canonist; Brundage, *Medieval Canon Law* 225–26.

and condition of the bishop and the actual circumstances of the church. And then that will be done which is mandated by the pope, and these coadjutors will have their moderate expenses covered by the bishops' income in whose aid they are assumed. But they will not alienate the prelates' goods and must render account to the bishop if afterward he returns to his sound mind or to the successor of the bishop, VI 3.5.1.

Nor are these coadjutors able to confer vacant benefices because in their general commission the collation of benefices is not contained, as in VI 3.5.1 according to Johannes Monachus[11] and Guido.[12]

Likewise the coadjutor must not be given by the metropolitan, but by the Apostolic See or through its authority, as in VI 3.5.1. And this is not surprising because the metropolitan can only do in his assigned province what is found permitted by law or introduced by ancient custom, as in VI 3.5.1, according to Johannes Monachus.

[It is asked] whether a leprous priest is licitly able to celebrate the Mass? Say that he must not celebrate before his flock on account of scandal. But if he wishes to celebrate it privately he must not be prohibited, at least as long as he is not too disabled or deformed. And Hugo[13] says that he should cease his ministry among the healthy, but he may sing and minister the divine office to lepers, D.49 c.1.

11 Johannes Monachus, author of the Ordinary Gloss (of 1302) on the *Liber sextus*; see Brundage, *Medieval Canon Law* 218.

12 Guido de Baysio (fl. 1300), who composed another gloss apparatus on the Liber sextus; Brundage, *Medieval Canon Law* 212–13.

13 Huguccio (fl. 1188–90); Brundage, *Medieval Canon Law* 214.

Bibliography

Boeckl, C. M. 2000. *Images of Plague and Pestilence: Iconography and Iconology* (Kirksville, MO: Truman State University Press)

Boeckl, C. M. 2011. *Images of Leprosy: Disease, Religion, and Politics in European Art* (Kirksville, MO: Truman State University Press)

Bos, K. I., V. J. Schuenemann, G. B. Golding, H. A. Burbano, et al. 2011. "A Draft Genome of *Yersinia pestis* from Victims of the Black Death," *Nature* 478, no. 7370: 506–10

Brundage, James. 1995. *Medieval Canon Law* (London: Longman)

Byrne, Joseph P. 2012. *Encyclopedia of the Black Death* (New York: ABC-CLIO)

Callaway, Ewen. 2011. "The Black Death Decoded," *Nature* 478: 444–46

Carniel, Elisabeth. 2008. "Plague Today," *Medical History Supplements* 27: 115–22

Chareyron, Nicole. 1996. "Chirurgien et patient au Moyen Âge : l'opération de la cataracte de Gilles le Muisit en 1351," *Revue belge de philologie et d'histoire* 74: 295–308

Demaitre, Luke. 2007. *Leprosy in Premodern Medicine: A Malady of the Whole Body* (Baltimore: Johns Hopkins University Press)

Donahue, Charles, Jr. 2003. "Bassianus, That Is to Say, Bazianus? Bazianus and Johannes Bazianus on Marriage," *Rivista internazionale di diritto commune* 14: 41–82

Fowler, Linda. 1972. "Innocent Uselessness in Civilian and Canonist Thought," *Zeitschrift der Savigny-Stiftung für Rechtsgeschichte: Kanonistische Abteilung* 58: 107–65

Gertsman, Elina. 2010. *The Dance of Death in the Middle Ages: Image, Text, Performance* (Turnhout: Brepols)

Green, Monica H. 2011. "'History of Medicine' or 'History of Health'?," *Past and Future* 9: 7–9

Green, Monica H. 2014. "Taking 'Pandemic' Seriously: Making the Black Death Global," *The Medieval Globe* 1: 27–61

Haenens, Albert d'. 1969. "Pierart dou Tielt, enlumineur des oeuvres de Gilles Li Muisis: note sur son activité à Tournai vers 1350," *Scriptorium* 23: 88–93 and plates 23–30

Jones, Peter Murray. 1984. *Medieval Medical Miniatures* (London: British Library)

Jones, Peter Murray. 1998. *Medieval Medicine in Illuminated Manuscripts*, rev. ed. (London: British Library by arrangement with Centro Tibaldi)

Jones, Peter Murray. 2006. "Word and Image in Medieval Medicine," in *Visualizing Medieval Medicine and Natural History, 1200–1550*, ed. Jean A. Givens, Karen M. Reeds, and Alain MacKinney (Berkeley: University of California Press)

Mendum, T. A., V. J. Schuenemann, S. Roffey, G. M. Taylor, et al. 2014. "*Mycobacterium leprae* Genomes from a British Medieval Leprosy Hospital: Towards Understanding an Ancient Epidemic," *BMC Genomics* 15: 270 [8 unnumbered pages]

North, J. D. 2004. "Wallingford, Richard (c. 1292–1336)," *Oxford Dictionary of National Biography*, online ed. (Oxford: Oxford University Press) [accessed May 14, 2014]

The Prose Salernitan Questions: Edited from a Bodleian Manuscript (Auct. F.3.10). [c. 1200]/1979. Ed. Brian Lawn (London: Oxford University Press for the British Academy)

Rawcliffe, Carole. 2006. *Leprosy in Medieval England* (Woodbridge: Boydell)
Sandler, Lucy Freeman. 1996. *Omne bonum: A Fourteenth-Century Encyclopedia of Universal Knowledge*, 2 vols (London: Harvey Miller)
Vanderputten, Steven. 2005. "Une iconographie de l'historiographie monastique: Réalité ou fiction?," in *Medieval Narrative Sources: A Gateway into the Medieval Mind*, ed. Jean Goossens, Ludo Milis, Werner Verbeke, 251–70 (Leuven: Leuven Uni versity Press)

Monica H. Green (Monica.Green@asu.edu) is a historian of medieval European medicine and global health. In 2009 and 2012, she ran a National Endowment for the Humanities Summer Seminar in London on "Health and Disease in the Middle Ages," which had as its central goal the exploration of ways that the scientific and humanistic disciplines could engage in productive dialogue about the history of disease and health-seeking behaviors. During this same period, she has also argued for the development of a new field, "Global History of Health," which explores the evolution of the major pathogens that have afflicted the human species since its origin up to the present day, and the ways that human cultural changes have facilitated or hindered those pathogens' trajectories. In addition to many works on the cultural history of medieval medicine, she is the author of "The Value of Historical Perspective," in *The Ashgate Research Companion to the Globalization of Health*, ed. Ted Schrecker (Aldershot: Ashgate, 2012), pp. 17–37; and "The Globalisations of Disease," which will be published in 2015.

Kathleen Walker-Meikle (kathleen.walker-meikle@york.ac.uk) is currently a research assistant on the Tradamus project (Saint Louis University) and is co-authoring, with Monica Green, a digital edition of the *Antidotarium magnum*: a large and influential late eleventh-century pharmaceutical text. Her own research focuses on the role of animals in medical texts and the interaction between natural history and medicine in the Middle Ages. She is currently completing a study on learned medical treatment of animal bites in the Middle Ages, a project funded by the Wellcome Trust. Other recent work examines animal substances in experimental literature. She holds a PhD from University College London.

Wolfgang P. Müller (wmueller@fordham.edu) is Professor of History at Fordham University in New York City. His main research area is the legal history of Western Europe and especially medieval jurisprudence, which through its insistence on forensic fact-finding was instrumental in fostering demand for medical professionals and science at the time. His most recent monograph, *The Criminalization of Abortion in the West: Its Origins in Medieval Law* (2012), includes a chapter on "Abortion Experts and Expertise"; writing it sparked an abiding appreciation for inquiries into the history of medicine.

Abstract This brief study examines the genesis of the "misdiagnosis" of a fourteenth-century image that has become a frequently used representation of the Black Death on the Internet and in popular publications. The image in fact depicts another common disease in medieval Europe, leprosy, but was misinterpreted as "plague" because of a labeling error. The error was then magnified because of digital dissemination. This mistake is a reminder that interpretation of cultural products continues to demand the skills and expertise of humanists. Included is a full transcription and translation of the text which the image was originally meant to illustrate: James le Palmer, *Omne bonum*, cap. "De clerico debilitato ministrante sequitur videre" (On Ministration by a Disabled Cleric), London, British Library, Royal 6 E. VI, vol. 2, fols. 301rb–302ra.

Keywords *Omne bonum*; James le Palmer; Gilles le Muisit; art history; plague imagery; leprosy; canon law; Black Death, disability history.

INDEX